Caring for Mental Health in the Future

Scenario Committee on Mental Health and Mental Health Care

Chairman: prof. Ph.A. Idenburg
Mental Health Research Team
Principal Researchers: Dr. E. Ketting
R.V. Bijl
Netherlands Institute of Mental Health

Caring for Mental Health in the Future

Future Scenarios on Mental Health and Mental Health Care in the Netherlands 1990-2010

Scenario report commissioned by the Steering Committee on Future Health Scenarios

1992
Springer-Science+Business Media, B.V.

Distributors

Steering Committee
on Future Health Scenarios
P.O. Box 5406
2280 HK Rijswijk
The Netherlands
Telephone (31-70) 3407205

Translation by Jonathan Phillips from the Dutch original: 'Zorgen voor geestelijke gezondheidszorg in de toekomst'.

ISBN 978-0-7923-1565-0 ISBN 978-94-011-2638-0 (eBook)
DOI 10.1007/978-94-011-2638-0

Contents

Preface

This study of mental health issues breaks new ground. The task set by the Steering Committee on Future Health Scenarios was twofold, encompassing issues relating both to mental health and to mental health care. Discussions of mental health normally narrow down immediately to a focus on its care; this study, in contrast, seeks to deal with mental health as a theme in its own right alongside that of mental health care.

This task led to the establishment of a broadly based committee whose members possessed a wide range of knowledge and experience in the field. The study was carried out by an equally expert team from the Netherlands Institute of Mental Health.

In the course of the study over a hundred people with wide-ranging expertise took part in consultative panels. No-one among these committee members, researchers and panel participants would claim to be familiar with the entire field of mental health and its care.

The enormous scale and diversity of the field set their stamp on the whole project. First of all the widely varying backgrounds of those involved meant that, for the sake of mutual understanding, it was vital to adopt the clearest possible use of language from the scenario committee's first meeting onwards. Then attention focused on four strategically selected themes within the overall field of mental health. While the results of the four thematic studies produced material which was interesting in its own right, the purpose of the exercise was to contribute to the development of policy in respect of the whole field of research.

Looking back down the long road which led from the initial development of ideas to the completion of the final report it is clear that a great debt of gratitude is owed to the many people involved. It is owed in the first place to the research team of the Netherlands Institute of Mental Health, who responded in creative fashion to the study's ever changing requirements and showed cheerfulness and perseverance in coping with every new bump and bend on the way.

The members of the committee, all of them volunteers who had to tear themselves away from busy jobs, showed admirable dedication and considerable good humour in dealing with the many concepts (and concepts of concepts) involved. In the course of several weekend conferences they succeeded in achieving a substantive exchange of ideas which has left its mark on the end product.

The four panels were the main source of expert knowledge and ideas in the four areas covered. Every one of their members devoted many hours to extensive questionnaires, while their participation in group discussion again demonstrated the value of the Delphi process used.

The report contains a large volume of information, ideas and suggestions of relevance to policy-making. This is gratifying. At the same time there is an essential imbalance in the nature of the suggestions made in the different fields, reflecting the nature of the future expectations on which these suggestions are made.

The expectations set out in the report cover many different areas. A distinction may be made between those that are specific and concrete and those that are more general or abstract. Among the more concrete, for example, is the expectation that the number of elderly demented patients needing care will rise by 74% over the next twenty years. The number of patients can be estimated with a high degree of probability, as can the duration of their illness. Given the desire to maintain current levels of care, the measures needed and their cost can be determined with reasonable accuracy.

Of a more general nature are the expectations that the balance of youth care will shift from the justice/welfare services to the medical services and that a widening social divide will open up with major qualitative implications for children and adolescents. While large numbers of young people are involved here, we cannot begin to estimate how many: the research data available are too scanty. In the causal sphere the factors mentioned include inadequate opportunities and insufficient emphasis in school on personal and social education and parents' uncertainties as to the best ways of bringing up children; in the sphere of possible solutions importance is attached to policy on the spread of incomes and employment - broad recommendations, not easily implemented. However, we must not lose sight of the broader and more general trends through an overconcentration on more specific issues to which concrete policy responses are possible.

In the light of the examples given - albeit, it must be said, extreme ones - there can be no doubt that the report is a disturbing one from the viewpoint of those who must make policy. It is clear that in terms of personal suffering and its duration and long-term cost, the problems of children and adolescents are at least as serious as those arising in connection with dementia, but because the latter are visible, demonstrable and concrete they are likely to receive considerably greater attention from politicians and policy-makers.

In the course of the study researchers and committee members were made aware almost daily of the widespread public interest in mental health issues. Almost no day goes by without an issue or dispute in this field reaching the front pages of the newspapers, bearing witness to the political nature of the problems concerned. The public at large seems to assume that something can and should be done: action is demanded on sexual child abuse, suicide, the maltreatment of the elderly, shortcomings in the treatments available to the mentally ill and so on. This brings out one of the core themes of this study, namely the extent to which social choices and developments influence both how problems are defined and what responses they elicit in the field of mental health. The recognition that many mental health problems are culturally determined implies that they need to be not only controlled and treated but above all interpreted. Even more than in other areas of health and health care, a scenario study concerned with mental health thus confronts society with a responsibility which many would rather ignore. Those who are prepared to face that responsibility will recognize the far-reaching, and twofold, significance of this study for the development of policies which look to the future. On the one hand many of its recommendations can serve directly as starting points for policy-making; on the other it ventilates issues which will no doubt play a part in determining the course of public policy in general, and health policy in particular, over the coming decades.

The committee members and researchers involved in the report's production hope that it will be read in this way.

Ph.A. Idenburg, Chair Scenario Committee
February 1990

Summary

This scenario project on the future of mental health and mental health care was carried out by the Scenario Committee on Mental Health and Mental Health Care and the Netherlands Institute of Mental Health at the request of the Steering Committee on Future Health Scenarios.

The question on which the project focused was this: *'What developments are possible over the next two decades in the area of mental health and the associated need for care, what are their implications, and to what extent can they be influenced?'*

The project was thus concerned both with mental health problems occurring in the population and with specialized care services. The two topics do not by any means fully coincide, in that only a small proportion of mental health problems, about 10-20%, receive specialized treatment. For the purposes of this study the need for care was operationalized as the utilization of care services.

The investigation involved on the one hand a review of the literature and data analysis and on the other intensive consultations with panels of experts. The panels were formed around four themes, namely dementia, schizophrenia, occupational incapacity due to mental disorders and emotional and behavioural problems in children and adolescents. Weighty reasons underlay this choice: the themes represent major categories of mental ill-health, giving rise to service utilization on a large scale and to correspondingly high costs, and their widely differing nature reflects the great diversity of mental health problems.

The notion of mental health at community level has changed over the last fifty years. In the period following the Second World War the stress was on the creation of social conditions and on changes in education and upbringing which were considered to promote mental health; later on the term came to refer simply to the aggregate of mental health problems in the population and to the care provided. The concept thus shifted from one focusing on social action to one which was neutrally descriptive.

Diagnosable psychiatric problems are very common - international statistics indicate that between one in four and one in six people are affected - and as a result among other things of the aging of the population and of a range of adverse social and cultural trends we must expect their prevalence to rise further. Current best estimates indicate that in the Netherlands around 250 people in every thousand are affected by mental health problems in any one year; of these, around 140 come to the attention of the primary-care services and 43 receive specialist care, seven of them as hospital or nursing-home inpatients.

The number of people receiving specialist mental health care at any one time is rising; the following table summarizes current trends and the prospects for the future if present policies are maintained.

	1980	1990	2000
Numbers receiving treatment at 1 January	186,000	274,000	405,000
Numbers receiving treatment per 1000 population	13.2	18.4	25.8
Cost of mental health care in millions of guilders (adjusted for inflation)	4,000	5,000	6,100

It should be stressed that this growth in the utilization of services cannot be explained simply by a growth in the number of people with problems. Two other developments are also highly relevant, namely the shift from intramural hospital care to extramural ambulatory care and the shortening duration of admissions, leading to an increase in the numbers reentering treatment; the number of patients presenting for treatment is thus rising more quickly than the number of people receiving it at any one time.

The study focused on four specific themes. In each case a background ('baseline') analysis was compiled, assembling the latest scientific data on the numbers of people affected by the condition concerned, its causes, possible treatments and cures and trends in the utilization of services.

Those developments which the experts making up the panels felt to be most likely are brought together in *reference scenarios* for the next twenty years; other possible trends, less likely but no less important, are covered in two *alternative exploratory scenarios* for each theme; and objectives for the year 2010 which, though bold, are viewed by the experts as attainable are set out in *target-setting scenarios*.

There are thus two distinct categories: the exploratory scenarios (including the reference scenarios) look ahead from the present to the future and indicate possible developments; the target-setting scenarios are normative, in the sense that they look back towards the present from a desired future situation and indicate the measures and interventions needed to achieve that situation.

An initial indication of costs and benefits is given for each scenario.

The vast scope of the topic and the great diversity of care provision for children and adolescents with emotional and behavioural problems hampered the construction of scenarios for this theme; the conclusions formulated are thus more general and speculative in nature.

Dementia

The reference scenario envisages an increase in the number of elderly demented patients - reflecting the increasing numbers of old people in the population, the growing life expectancy of dementia sufferers and the earlier diagnosis of the condition - from 100,000 at present to 150,000 in 2010, over 60% of whom will be over 80 years old. Little or no progress is expected in the prevention or cure of dementia. Nursing-home capacity will lag behind the rise in demand for places, despite a rapid expansion of extramural services and home support by professional carers. Less care will be available from patients' families and friends.

The two alternative exploratory scenarios envisage on the one hand a radical expansion of the professionals' role in the care of demented patients and their families and on the other a strengthening of informal care.

The target-setting scenario details the measures needed in the areas of diagnosis, prevention, training, treatment and care if the objective of ensuring that *the quality of dementia-related care provided at all stages of the condition is considerably higher in 2010 than under the reference scenario* is to be achieved over the next twenty years.

Annual expenditure directly attributable to the care of the demented elderly, corrected for inflation, rises in twenty years by over 1,100 million guilders under the reference scenario; under the target-setting scenario the increase is cut by 300 million.

Schizophrenia

Here the reference scenario envisages that the number of people who can be said to have schizophrenia will remain roughly constant at around the 70,000 mark; chronicity will be prevented slighly more often and patients' average level of functioning will improve, as will the treatments available. More informal care will be provided by families and there will be an increase in partial hospitalization, usually day treatment, sheltered-living provision and extramural care. Even so, most schizophrenia care will remain concentrated in the psychiatric hospitals.

The two alternative exploratory scenarios envisage on the one hand a trend towards the social marginalization of schizophrenics and on the other growing tolerance to sufferers and improvements in their quality of life.

The target-setting scenario outlines the broad conditions and specific measures needed over the next twenty years to achieve the objective of ensuring that *by 2010 the quality of life of those vulnerable to schizophrenia will be considerably better than under the reference scenario (unchanged policy)*.

While annual expenditure directly attributable to the care of schizophrenics rises at roughly the same rate under all four scenarios, the psychiatric hospitals' share is 78% under the reference scenario and only 54% under the target-setting scenario.

Occupational incapacity due to mental disorders

The reference scenario envisages an increase in mental health problems in the labour force, due among other things to more demanding working conditions, and a rise from 185,000 at present to 320,000 in 2010 in the number of people receiving disability benefit in connection with such problems. Women and migrants will be particularly at risk. While the assessment agencies will become more alert to mental health problems at work, no significant progress will be made towards greater competence, uniformity and objectivity in the determination of the limitations on work skills resulting from such problems. Help for those incapacitated by mental disorders will be provided mainly by general practitioners, with the specialist mental health services playing a much smaller role. The likelihood of re-employment will remain small.

The two exploratory scenarios envisage on the one hand an intensification of preventive activities by employers and on the other a trend towards passive attitudes on the part of industry and government.

The target-setting scenario describes the measures needed over the next twenty years to achieve the threefold objective of:

- a structural decline in mental health problems in the workforce as compared with 1990;
- a fall in the number of disability-benefit claimants with a 'mental disorder' diagnosis to 2% of the workforce (a decline in terms of

individuals from 185,000 in 1990 to 145,000 in 2010);
- the gradual creation of a situation in which 90% of claimants (i.e. over 20,000 people every year) can return to some appropriate form of employment within two years of becoming entitled to benefit.

Under the target-setting scenario the annual cost of benefit payments to those incapacitated by mental disorders is almost five billion guilders, less than half the sum envisaged under the reference scenario. Investment in health care, company health services and rehabilitation programmes is recouped in the form of billion-guilder savings in benefit expenditure.

Emotional and behavioural problems in children and adolescents
Here expectations are gloomy. Around 200,000 under-18s are currently affected by emotional and behavioural problems and the number is thought likely to grow as developments tending to prevent such problems (such as many children's growing capacity to deal with problems thanks to information and support at school) are offset by more adverse trends. The relative deterioration in the social position of some low-status groups, notably ethnic minorities, is seen as a major factor in the worsening situation; another is the continuing erosion of the family. In addition the demands placed on children and adolescents are likely to become heavier and the expectations entertained regarding their functioning higher, producing a widening gap between what children can achieve and what adults regard as desirable or normal and hence a growing risk of problems.

Growing numbers of children and adolescents are expected to need care of one form or another. The existing division between the justice/welfare system and the health services is likely to widen.

Two objectives were emphasized by the experts, who also made many suggestions as to the measures needed for their achievement: the prevalence of emotional and behavioural problems in children and adolescents should be considerably reduced and the integration into society of youngsters with problems should be improved.

Finally the study's principal findings are placed in a broader historical and sociological perspective, in which framework they are interpreted and, where possible, generalized to the whole field of mental health and its care.

Various developments point to mental health problems being recognized more and earlier and to a growing tendency to seek professional help. This trend is related in part to the growing availability of such help and in part to people's decreasing willingness to endure mental health problems. The latter, it is argued, reflects the fact that such problems are increasingly, and increasingly automatically, seen as a form of illness.

The resulting demand for services forces policy-makers to seek ways of distinguishing those more severe problems which require professional care from those, less serious, for which such care is not strictly necessary. Science has not so far proved very helpful in this connection, being inclined to expand rather than limit the area of problems requiring professional intervention.

The growing demand for professional care reflects not so much medical as social and cultural factors. Two trends appear relevant in this connection: first, in many areas of life the boundaries of what is considered normal and acceptable are being drawn ever more narrowly and, second, the individual is increasingly required independently to develop his or her own identity. At the individual level these trends can easily manifest themselves as mental health problems.

The fact that the growth of mental health problems for which treatment is desirable is associated with social and cultural changes does not make them any the less real or serious. It does imply, however, that care provision needs to be supplemented with a more socio-cultural focus on mental health problems.

The report ends by outlining three options for future policy. The first involves meeting the growing need for professional help to only a limited extent; this, it is expected, would tend to open up a division in society between those who are still able to cope with the psychological demands of contemporary society and those who can no longer do so. The second option is to expand professional services at a rapid rate - by 2% a year - in order to keep pace with the growing need for care. The third option focuses on prevention and on relevant aspects of other policy areas, the argument being that, given the background of mental health problems, the most desirable approach is a broad social and cultural one. Such a policy cannot be formulated or implemented immediately, because our knowledge in this area is deficient and because the necessary social awareness does not yet exist. The first step must therefore be to focus on and develop the concept of community mental health.

1 Introduction

This project on possible future developments in the area of mental health and its care was implemented as part of the forecasting exercise which the State Secretary of Welfare, Health and Cultural Affairs instituted in 1983 with the aim of enhancing the ability of health policy to anticipate future trends.

In 1986 the Steering Committee on Future Health Scenarios (*Stuurgroep Toekomstscenario's Gezondheidszorg*, STG) asked the Netherlands Institute of Mental Health (*Nederlands centrum Geestelijke volksgezondheid*, NcGv) to study the feasibility of a scenario project in the area of mental health and its care. The results of this study led the STG to commission such a project in mid 1987. A scenario committee under the leadership of Professor Ph.A. Idenburg was appointed at the beginning of 1988 by the STG chairman, Professor J. van Londen; the NcGv was given the job of carrying out the necessary research.

Close and fruitful cooperation was established between the NcGv research team and the scenario committee, the latter determining the broad outlines of the project and the former gathering and analysing the relevant information. In addition individual scenario-committee members gave practical suggestions and advice, in the light of their own areas of expertise, to the research team. This final report is thus the joint product of the scenario committee and the research team.

The scenario committee and the research team were given the task of exploring future developments in the area of mental health and its care. This field differs sharply from others which have been covered by forecasting exercises (such as cardiovascular disease, cancer or even the aging of the population) in that it does not focus on one condition with various causes or one causative factor with various implications for health and health care: instead it relates to an entire field of care, extending over various levels and specialties. While much of the care needed in connection with mental health problems is provided by the primary sector, in particular family doctors, it was decided to do no more than touch on such care in this study (mainly because a scenario project was also under development for primary care). The proportions of care provided at the various levels are covered in chapter 3 on the basis of the Goldberg and Huxley model.

Mental health at the level of the community is a concept with several dimensions, not only covering the aggregate of mental problems or conditions in the population but also referring to certain characteristics of society. In elaborating our task and designing this study this duality of mental health and its care was borne in mind at all times.

A major feature of the field is the 'high elasticity of demand': in contrast with most other health problems, in mental health the linkage between the incidence of certain problems or conditions among the population and the need for or utilization of professional services is a rather loose one. While epidemiological studies regularly find some 15-25% of the population to be suffering mental problems of varying degrees of severity, only around 2-4% of people in the Netherlands present for specialized psychiatric care (the percentage depends among other things on the time period studied). The situation in other western countries is similar. This fact is of crucial importance, since it implies both that the demand for professional services cannot be used as an indicator of the general mental health situation and that the latter cannot tell us what services need to be provided. In other words, mental health and its care cannot simply be incorporated into some form of mathematical model: to an important extent they move independently of one another and each depends in some degree on a variety of factors. Between the two there is a multiplicity of factors - among them the extent of social support and integration, practitioners' referral habits, how problems are defined, interpreted and dealt with - which in all probability are more important than the prevalence of mental problems as determinants of the need for services. Whether or not professional care is sought depends not just on the nature of mental problems but also on the individuals concerned, the situation in which they find themselves and the involvement, professional or otherwise, of third parties. This study therefore devotes considerable attention to such intervening factors.

The dual perspective - mental health and mental health care - guides and permeates the study. Chapter 2 sets out the questions which arise from it, the analytical model developed to answer them and the research strategy adopted. It also amplifies the considerations which led to the focus on four specific themes.

Chapters 3 and 4 cover the whole field of mental health and its care. Chapter 3 focuses on two questions. The first concerns the nature of mental health problems and its implications for public policy, while the second is epidemiological: what problems affect what categories of the population, and to what degree?

Chapter 4 is concerned with quantitative aspects of mental health care, looking at the relative importance of the various sectors and types and the shifts taking place between them. As well as outlining recent developments chapter 4 looks forward over the next decade, basing its forecasts on the hypothetical assumption that the same trends and developments will continue unchanged.

Chapters 5-8 form the core of the study. Dealing with separate themes as they do, each chapter constitutes in some measure a study in its own right, albeit the procedure followed and structure used are the same in each case. Each chapter opens with a socalled baseline analysis of its theme, comprising a systematic overview of the scale of the problem, its backgrounds and causes, the scope for intervention and the utilization of services. Areference scenario is then presented outlining the most likely developments over the next twenty years, together with two alternative exploratory scenarios deemed to be less likely; both these types of scenario take the present as the starting point for their exploration of possible future developments. Finally, a target-setting scenario, looking back to the present from a desired future situation, seeks to determine what measures are needed to achieve that desired situation. Each chapter ends with an exploration of the various scenarios' cost implications.

Chapter 5 looks in the manner just outlined at the subject of dementia and chapter 6 at that of schizophrenia. Chapter 7 is concerned with occupational incapacity due to mental disorders, while chapter 8 focuses on emotional and behavioural problems in children and adolescents.

Finally, chapter 9 brings the various results together, seeking to interpret them and set them in a broader social context. It also formulates a number of central conclusions and policy options of relevance not only to the Ministry of Welfare, Health and Cultural Affairs but also to other ministries, local government and social organizations.

As noted earlier, the report as a whole is the collective product of the scenario committee and the research team, who bear joint responsibility for it. The preparation of the report involved the following division of functions within the research team: R.V Bijl, who was a member of the team from the start, prepared the texts of chapters 2, 3 (from section 3.3 onwards), 5 and 7. M.A. Jansen, who joined the project at a later stage, drew up the draft texts of chapter 6 and, jointly with J.D. Kroon, chapter 8. Chapters 1, 4 and 9 were prepared by Dr E. Ketting, who also undertook the general coordination of the study. C. Jacobs made a major contribution to the collection and processing of data for chapter 4. Professor P. Schnabel, while not a member of the research team, drew up the basic text of chapter 3 (sections 3.1 and 3.2) and the first section of chapter 4. Finally, R.F. Koenders, who was on placement with the research team for the first half of the project, gave general assistance.

2 Design and implementation of the study

2.1 *Introduction*

In November 1986 the Steering Committee on Future Health Scenarios (STG) asked the Netherlands Institute of Mental Health (NcGv) to make a preliminary study of the scope for a forecasting exercise using scenario methods in the area of mental health and its care. This feasibility study was carried out in the period from December 1986 to May 1987; the main activities were the charting and demarcation of the potential research field and familiarization with the methodology of futures research. The results of this work are set out in the Report on the Preliminary Study for the Scenario Project in Mental Health and Mental Health Care (Bijl & Ketting 1987).

The main study began in August 1987. Since the report on the preliminary study did not include a blueprint for the activities to be undertaken and principles and strategic choices had yet to be finalized on certain points, the first six months of cooperation between the scenario committee and the research team were mainly taken up with determining the theoretical principles of the study and making a number of fundamental choices.

On a limited number of points this led to some discrepancy between the proposals emerging from the preliminary study and what was eventually done. The four themes investigated were not specifically mentioned in the preliminary study, for example, while the strongly functional, client-centred, approach to mental health care advocated at the preliminary stage proved very difficult to maintain in a future-oriented study and is therefore a less prominent feature of the final results.

2.2 *Problem definition*

The main problems and difficulties in the area of mental health and its care which already face us or are expected to arise in future are concerned chiefly with the relationship between the prevalence of mental health problems and the consequent need for services on the one hand and on the other the match or mismatch between the demand for and supply of services and ways of influencing it. It is this observation that underlies the question on which the scenario project focuses:

'What developments are possible over the next two decades in the area of mental health and the associated need for care, what are their implications, and to what extent can they be influenced?'

The general issue was refined into three more specific questions which guided the subsequent design of the study:

a. Are any quantitative or qualitative changes in mental morbidity likely in the medium-to-long term (to the year 2010)?
b. What prospect is there for socially acceptable health-promotion measures and what effect might they have on mental morbidity?
c. What care options exist for non-avoidable mental health problems?

From this formulation it follows that there are two dependent variables for study, namely mental morbidity in the Dutch population and the need for care resulting from the mental health problems concerned. Determinants can be distinguished for both variables which influence the extent of both morbidity and the need for care. It is important to note that while mental morbidity is a dependent variable for the purposes of this study it is also one of the determinants (albeit far from the only one) of the need for care.

Since 'need for care' is a very vague and ambiguous concept (Bijl & Mastboom 1986), it has been operationalized in this study in the empirically measurable form of the 'utilization of services'. We return to this issue in section 2.5.

2.3 *Principles and fundamental choices*

The kind of research carried out as part of this project inevitably runs the risk of vagueness and ambiguity and consequently of producing irrelevant results. To minimize that risk the following fundamental principles and choices were formulated with a view to providing direction throughout the project.

1. *Beneficiary groups*: the results of the study were intended to be of use to the government, the health care institutions, patients'/clients' organizations and other groups in society concerned in any way with mental health and its care in the Netherlands.

2. *Goals*: the project had a twofold purpose, on the one hand to initiate and stimulate *thinking and debate* among the various beneficiary groups on the future of mental health and its care, and on the other to identify options for influencing developments and concrete *strategies* for achieving the various groups' aims and to indicate their consequences and side-effects. It should be emphasized that the purpose of the study was not to *predict* future developments in the area of mental health and its care.

3. *Mental health problems*: these are of many kinds and degrees of severity. Our society seeks where possible either to prevent such problems arising or to treat or otherwise palliate them with a view to rendering them bearable from the viewpoint of the individuals immediately concerned and/or those around them. Since mental health problems are part of human existence and indeed can sometimes have a positive impact on individuals' personal development, the aim is not, and cannot be, their complete elimination. We return to this point in chapter 3.

In this study 'mental health problem' means any problem or disorder leading to a concrete demand for care; whether such a problem or disorder is best classified symptomatologically under a psychiatric, psychosocial or some other heading is of secondary importance in this connection. Where particular disorders or conditions have clear care structures of their own (notably epilepsy and mental retardation) they are not regarded as mental health problems for the purposes of this study. Section 2.4 describes the specific themes that were studied in some detail.

4. *Mental health care*: these are primarily taken to encompass all those persons and institutions customarily regarded by society as providing such services (the institutional approach), with distinctions being made between intramural, semi-mural or intermediate and extramural (ambulatory) services. This perspective recurs in chapter 4. Wherever possible, however, five 'functions of care' of a substantive nature are distinguished within this formal threefold structure, namely treatment, nursing care, general care, residence and occupational functions. The interactions with other sectors in the health care system and elsewhere made it necessary and desirable that the scenario study should not remain limited to mental health services in a narrow sense but should also extend to adjacent sectors (notably primary care and family and home care).

5. The *principal elements of the study* were as follows:

Baseline analysis: a description and interpretation of the current situation in the particular area of mental health and its care and of the developments and relevant factors (determinants) which have produced that situation. Four of these background analyses were carried out, reflecting the four themes that were examined in detail.

A scenario model: an analytical model bringing out the links between the two dependent variables ('mental morbidity' and 'utilization of care') and the determinants emerging as most relevant from the baseline analyses. The scenario model is intended to show in simple fashion what variables and links can be varied and can provide a starting point for the future scenarios to be elaborated at a later stage. The scenario model used is discussed in detail in section 2.5.

Future analysis: the design of a number of scenarios, partly on the basis of views obtained from experts using the Delphi process (see section 2.6). A choice is possible from scenarios of various types. Of great importance here is the distinction between developments which are autonomous (i.e. cannot be altered to any significant extent by deliberate interventions), such as demographic changes, and those which can be influenced by measures or interventions in the area of mental health and its care.

It was decided to compile both *exploratory* and *target-setting* scenarios. The exploratory scenarios take the present as their starting point and consider possible or conceivable developments and their implications for the future; the target-setting scenarios, in contrast, start by formulating a desired future situation and go on to determine what measures and strategies are possible, desirable or necessary to achieve it. Section 2.7 describes the method whereby the scenarios were compiled.

Effect analysis: the consequences of the various scenarios needed to be investigated. Important focuses of attention here included the flows of patients into the various mental health institutions and sectors and the consequences for adjacent sectors (such as primary care) and the analysis of costs and benefits in financial and wherever possible also non-financial terms (e.g. possible health gains from each scenario).

6. *Empirical basis*: the baseline analyses are the foundation of the project. In order to ensure adequate reliability and validity these baseline analyses ought only to cover themes and topics on which empirical data are available, but in looking to the future it was both inevitable and desirable that use be made of data of varying degrees of 'hardness', ranging from future trends with a firm empirical basis to 'informed guesswork' by experts.

2.4 *Selection of four themes: dementia, schizophrenia, emotional and behavioural problems in children and adolescents, occupational incapacity due to mental disorders*

To ensure that worthwhile and relevant research could be carried out within the project's time and budget constraints it was necessary to select a limited number of topics for detailed analysis within the broad field of mental health, mental health problems and mental health care.

The research team and the scenario committee based their final choice on the following *considerations*:

- The choice of themes should reflect the diversity of the mental health field in terms both of the range of problems encountered and the kinds of response made.
- The themes chosen should represent a large proportion of the overall field of mental health and its care. To maximize the study's social and political relevance the choice should be such as to ensure that the research results (scenarios) for each theme could wherever possible serve as examples for more general future developments in the field of mental health and its care in the Netherlands.
- The third consideration was a very pragmatic one, namely that adequate research data should be available: scenarios for the future cannot be built on inadequate empirical foundations.

The nature both of the problems, diseases and circumstances covered by the 'mental health problems' label and of the efforts and activities aimed at preventing, alleviating or resolving them varies widely in many respects.

The main criterion adopted by the research team and scenario committee for the purpose of choosing four themes to bring out that diversity concerned *'the extent to which a mental health problem or the care associated with it is socially and culturally determined'*. This criterion reflects the fact that there is a continuum of mental health problems, ranging from those which in relation to their causes, treatment and care are not predominantly socio-culturally determined (to the point perhaps of being entirely biologically determined) at the one extreme to those which are primarily determined or defined by social and cultural factors at the other.

There are many other dimensions to the diversity of the research field, and we return to this topic in chapter 3. Other dimensions of diversity reflected in the final choice of themes were these:

- The *causes* of problems may be psychological, organic or socio-cultural in nature and often combine all three; the *scope for prevention* are therefore also very varied.

- The *severity* of symptoms varies within a single condition as well as from one condition to another, depending on the stage reached. Severity has many aspects, both qualitative and quantitative, in part flowing directly from the mental health problem itself and in part associated with the responses and attitudes, positive or negative, of carers and family. The following oppositions can help illuminate the notion of severity:

chronic	*versus*	transient
incurable	*versus*	curable
great personal suffering	*versus*	little personal suffering
requiring intensive care	*versus*	requiring extensive care
causing considerable nuisance	*versus*	causing little nuisance
socially incapacitating	*versus*	not socially incapacitating
common	*versus*	relatively rare

- The *manifestations* of mental health problems are very diverse, even within the same diagnostic category, with both the duration and the course of conditions varying widely.
- The need for, necessity of and options for *treatment or other care* vary widely from one problem to another, and indeed the treatment of the same condition can range in terms of duration and nature from short-term drug-based outpatient care to long-term intramural psychotherapy.
- *Community concern*, i.e. the extent to which society (public opinion) feels concern on moral, financial or other grounds at the occurence of particular problems within particular social groups or about the functioning of particular services. Such concern varies widely and fluctuates over time.

These various considerations - the need to reflect the diversity of the mental health field, the representativeness of the conditions studied and the availability of sufficient data - led to the choice of the four themes.

The first two are concrete problem categories obviously involving illness, namely:

- *Dementia.* Major considerations here were the growing incidence of dementia as the numbers of old people increase and more people survive into advanced old age, the heavy demands on care provision and the high level of community concern.
- *Schizophrenia.* Here the major considerations were the condition's

fairly constant prevalence and generally chronic course, the long-term hospitalization which it often necessitates, the large proportion of intramural care currently devoted to schizophrenic patients and the limited level of community concern.

The third theme is one with clear links with mental health problems, predominantly set in a socio-cultural context:

- *Occupational incapacity due to mental disorders.* Relevant considerations here were the heavy demands notably on primary and extramural services, the enormous social cost in terms of loss of output and benefit payments, growing community concern (not least on account of the huge financial cost) and the fact that the problem can be influenced by policy actions.

The fourth theme concerns a social group with mental health problems of a generally socio-cultural nature:

- *Emotional and behavioural problems in children and adolescents.* The considerations leading to this choice were the fact that such problems have proved more common than was until recently supposed and could continue to grow and that their potential long-term effects are serious, the very fragmented use made of treatment and care facilities, the high level of community concern and the possibility that the situation is susceptible to policy action.

Between them these four themes cover a very large and important part of the overall field of mental health in the Netherlands and of the services available to people with mental health problems. Even so, their choice excluded a wide range of problems and their treatment or care, among them personality disorders, addictions, organic disorders other than dementia, phobias, anxiety, depression, dissociative disorders and physiological dysfunction due to mental conditions (affecting eating, sleeping or the sexual function). However, we can assume that the three largest problem categories not specifically covered in this study (anxiety, depression and addiction) are strongly represented under the heading of occupational incapacity due to mental disorders.

2.5 *The scenario model*

The scenario project needed a model which could bring out the links between the two dependent variables and their determinants in relatively simple fashion and could be fleshed out as concretely as possible. A complex model was rejected for two reasons. First, there is a strong tendency to try to design a structure capable of bringing out 'all' conceivably relevant factors and the links between them; this is counterproductive, since it is both impossible and, where the goal is to explore the future, unnecessary to design a model so comprehensive that it reflects reality in all its nuances. A conceptual model should *abstract* from reality, not *reflect* it.

A second reason for rejecting as counterproductive a complex model aiming to cover the whole field of mental health care is that such a model inevitably includes many variables and correlations which, though of value in theoretical terms, cannot be concretely expressed or empirically underpinned. What was needed was a scenario model which could offer a simple indication of the variables and correlations that can be varied and could generate a range of future scenarios. It also needed to be able to serve as a sort of 'table of contents' for the baseline analysis. The variables, links and possible causal relationships grouped in the model must be covered by the baseline analysis.

The *basic model* used is shown below. In essence the same model was applied to each of the four themes, with at most slight modifications being made to take account of the specific nature of a given theme (see the baseline analyses in chapters 5-8).

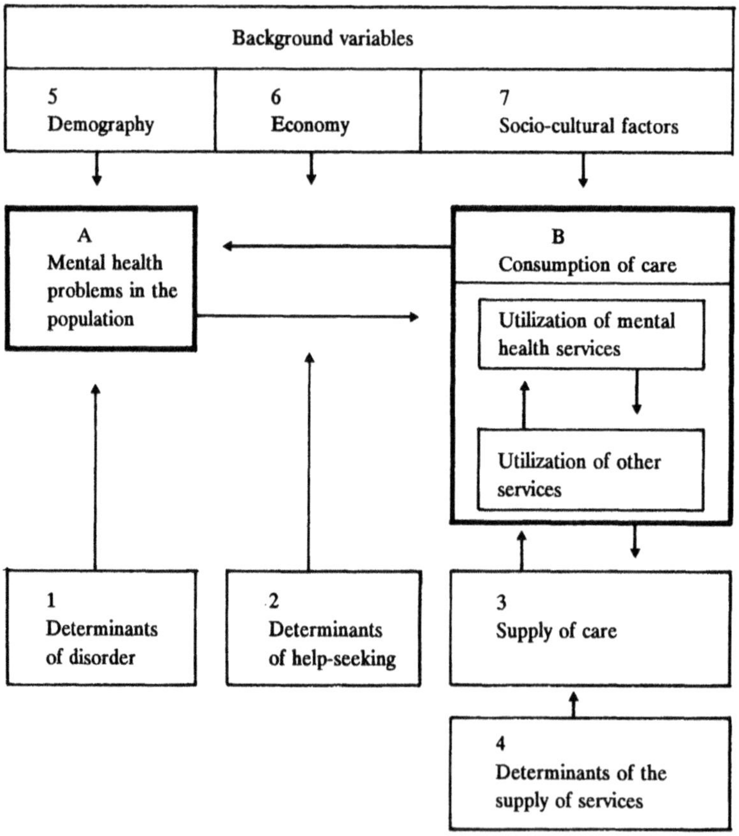

Notes

The model focuses on the correlation between mental health and illness (A) and the utilization of care as a result of mental health problems (B). Mental ill-health leads under certain conditions to the utilization of services (reflected in the arrow pointing from A to B); at the same time the work of care-providers, to the extent that it has a curative effect, has an impact in the other direction (from B to A), in that it results in some diminution in mental ill-health. The other variables indicated in the model (the determinants) affect the strength of this correlation.

Altering the strength of the various determinants allows us to construct different *exploratory scenarios* for the future of mental morbidity (A) and the utilization of care (B), while replacing the present situation in boxes A and B with a series of desired future situations enables us to design *target-setting scenarios* showing how the determinants need to change (and what the chances of altering or influencing them are) if those future situations are to be achieved.

The considerations which played a part in the design of the model were as follows.

1. The link between the occurrence of mental health problems and the utilization of specialized services is much less direct than in the case of e.g. cancer, accidents or cardiovascular disease; we return to this point in chapter 3. The impact on service-utilization of factors such as individuals' inclination or otherwise to seek help and family doctors' referral practices is at least as great as that of mental health problems themselves.
2. Much consumption of care in connection with a mental health problem takes place outside the regular institutions of mental health care. Of particular importance here are the primary health services and home and family care, welfare and judicial provision (in the case of problems affecting children and adolescents) and rehabilitation programmes aimed at the reemployment of those incapacitated by mental disorders. The utilization of services in these related sectors is covered in this project.
3. Service availability is a major determinant of the extent to which and places where professional help is sought by and for people with mental health problems and of the manner in which services are used. In the mental health field not only does the demand for services generate their supply, the converse is also true: availability influences service-utilization.
4. Influence, through policy action or preventive measures, can be brought to bear at various points in the model. It should be noted, however, that the scope for influencing the determinants of mental

health problems varies widely as between the four themes studied.

5. The model needs to be fleshed out for each of the four areas covered. Depending on the situation within each area, there will be greater or lesser scope for quantifying the variables and the links between them and greater or lesser grounds for varying certain variables within the scenarios. In concrete terms this meant that in compiling the scenarios the emphasis came to fall on alternative developments in morbidity in one area and on variations in future service-utilization in another.
6. The determinants included in the model were as follows:
   - *Determinants of disorder:* factors which give rise to a mental health problem. In each of the four areas covered the following determinants were analysed (where appropriate):
     1. biological (including hereditary) factors,
     2. the physical environment,
     3. the social environment,
     4. lifestyles.
   - *Determinants of help-seeking behaviour:* factors which determine the extent to which help is sought, the institution approached and the type of help sought in connection with a mental health problem. The determinants considered were these:
     1. the role of social networks (home care),
     2. the role of referring doctors and other professionals,
     3. financial factors,
     4. proto-professionalization.
   - *Supply of care*: the quantitative and substantive scope to provide care by specialized mental health institutions and other facilities.
   - *Determinants of the supply of services:* factors which determine the extent and substance of the professional care available. The factors considered were:
     1. public policy on the organization and resourcing of services,
     2. technical developments in treatment and care.
   - *Background variables:* the demographic, economic and socio-cultural context in which the model functions. Background developments affect the other variables in the model but are themselves autonomous, i.e. not susceptible to direct control or influence. Use was made in each case of Central Bureau of Statistics forecasts dating from 1988 (intermediate variant) for demography and Central Planning Bureau (CPB) forecasts dating from 1985 (intermediate variant) for economic prospects.

7. The model does not include *prevention* as a separate variable. Prevention, unlike the other variables in the model, is not present

necessarily and by definition: instead it should be seen as a concrete strategy, a *modus operandi* which can be adopted as required with a view to affecting the model's central links between A (morbidity) and B (services). Prevention and its effects can be located at a number of points in the model. An important distinction here is that between primary prevention (activities which remove the causes of disease) and secondary prevention (measures to minimize the severity of such mental health problems as do nevertheless occur). Primary prevention can be seen as a 'negative determinant' of disorder and as such should be included under 1., the determinants of disorder. Secondary prevention should be located notably under 2., the determinants of help-seeking; it includes for example activities aimed at strengthening a patient's social environment and other strategies for avoiding hospitalization.

2.6 *Delphi*

The construction of scenarios depends on information. This was obtained partly through the baseline analyses and partly by consulting a large number of experts on the four themes covered. Of particular importance in scenario construction is the diversity of views held by the various people concerned with each theme as to:

- probable and possible developments in the areas concerned (of importance for the exploratory scenarios),
- desirable developments in the areas concerned (of importance for the target-setting scenarios).

The procedure used for the purpose of consulting experts in the various fields was the Delphi method. While many variants are in use, the basic approach is as follows.

Delphi can be seen as a "paper-borne conference" at which a carefully selected panel of experts or key figures, not in direct communication one with another, reaches a consensus on an important issue on which information is as yet inadequate. This is achieved through the use of a series of questionnaires compiled by the researcher specially for the issue concerned. In the successive rounds of the process each panel member is given feedback (on an anonymous basis) on the responses received to earlier questionnaires and on the extent of agreement among the experts. As participants are confronted with and respond to each other's views in this way the coordinator seeks to formulate a well-founded position with which as many of the experts as possible can agree. Investigation and consultation are thus combined in a step-by-step process of arriving at a judgement.

While consensus is the aim of the Delphi method it cannot always be achieved in practice, and where views and values differ fundamentally it is better to accept the position and formulate the main standpoints in as clear and well-argued a fashion as possible. This has the advantage of bringing out the various sources of conflict, standpoints and reasonings, thereby allowing informed and rational debate to take place and making clear the positions from which the final choice must be made.

This last point is an important one in connection with scenario construction. The standpoints on which consensus exists can be translated into a *reference scenario*, i.e. one which combines the developments which the experts collectively consider to be most probable. The standpoints on which no consensus exists (they can be minority positions, provided that they are well-founded) then provide the starting points for the design of *alternative scenarios* differing from the reference scenario.

In the Delphi process it is vital that participants set out the arguments on which their views rest.

The scenario model - the basis for Delphi

The experts were asked to restrict the expression of their opinions to the variables and correlations making up the scenario model, which provided the scenario project's analytical framework and was therefore not intended to be debated or altered. The members of the panel were asked to indicate, giving reasons, what changes might be expected in the relationships within the model, how likely such changes were, how significant they would be and what consequences could be expected.

It was neither necessary nor desirable (given the need to avoid excessively long questionnaires; few panel members were all-round experts) that all participants should give their views on all the variables and links within the model. This applied particularly to the "demography" and "economy" background variables, whose development over time was to be seen as autonomous. The trends postulated for the period 1990-2010, based on Central Bureau of Statistics and Central Planning Bureau forecasts, formed the context within which the panel members were asked to formulate their views.

The appendix at the end of the report sets out the assumptions which panel members were expected to take into account in developing their expectations in all four areas covered.

Procedure

The Delphi process comprised a preliminary stage followed by three rounds of questions.

- *Preparatory stage:* it was at this stage that the four panels of experts were assembled. The panel for each theme consisted of 25-30 people with various areas of expertise, experience or interest. Participants represented *inter alia* the world of science, care-providers (mental health, primary and other), clients/patients, government, industry and education. In all 110 experts took part.
- *First round:* the first round served mainly to generate material for the design of the exploratory scenarios. Participants were not yet asked at this stage to indicate what future situations they considered desirable; this would later be relevant to the target-setting scenarios. The questionnaire included open-ended questions, to emphasize the "brainstorming" nature of this round, as well as closed questions. To allow a quantiative estimate to be made of the extent to which panel members regarded certain developments as probable and the direction and strength of the effects of those developments some of the questions involved predetermined answer categories on a three-point scale (improbable, somewhat probable, very probable).
- *Second round:* this round had a twofold purpose, namely
  1. to allow the panel to comment on the reference scenario constructed on the basis of the answers obtained in the first round, and
  2. to generate the policy measures needed to achieve the goals set in advance by the researchers for the year 2010, with an indication of any possible side-effects.

  The emphasis in the first Delphi round was thus on developments in the autonomous variables in each field, while the second focused on policy. Panel members' response in the second round was high, ranging between 85% and 95% for the various themes.
- *Third round:* this was a face-to-face round, with panel members being invited to discuss with one another the exploratory and target-setting scenarios constructed on the basis of their answers. The purpose of this round was to improve the quality of the scenarios and to make a start on one of the project's aims, namely to initiate among those concerned a debate on the future of mental health and its care.

2.7 *Scenario construction*

This section briefly outlines the procedures followed with a view to translating the results of the Delphi exercise, in as reliable and verifiable a fashion as possible, into exploratory and target-setting scenarios. The method was followed in full in the case of the themes of dementia, schizophrenia and occupational incapacity due to mental disorders; the theme of emotional and behavioural problems in children and adolescents lent itself less easily to such an approach, however, and was therefore treated somewhat more generally.

Reference scenario

For each of the four themes a scenario was compiled on the basis of the developments in prevalence and service-utilization and their determinants which were considered most likely by the Delphi panel concerned; this was the reference scenario. The textual-analysis programme ASKSAM was used to process the panel members' qualitative responses; their quantitative responses were processed using SPSS. An assessment procedure developed for the purpose was used to determine which developments were the subject of consensus among the members of a panel and which were more controversial.

The substance of each reference scenario was based on the views only of those panel members who regarded themselves as reasonably or highly expert in the various specific aspects of each theme. To ensure that the four reference scenarios were as comparable as possible a checklist was used of topics which had to be covered, as a minimum, in all the themes. This general list was then supplemented with more specific topics for each theme.

The checklist also served to show which developments or variables were the subject of divided opinions among the experts. These more controversial possibilities then provided the starting point for the compilation of *alternative exploratory scenarios*. Supplementary criteria were needed to decide which developments or variables were worth incorporating into alternative scenarios; these were *credibility*, *political relevance* and the *likely impact on prevalence and/or the utilization of care*.

Alternative exploratory scenarios

The scenario model makes a general distinction between autonomous developments and policy measures. It was decided to base the alternative exploratory scenarios departing from the reference scenario as far as possible on variations in the *autonomous developments*, treating public policy as a constant. It must of course be borne in mind that the line separating autonomous and non-autonomous developments is not a sharp one and that any such division is in some degree arbitrary.

Policy measures become the focus of attention in the target-setting scenarios (see below). The consideration underlying this approach was the difficulty of determining the likelihood of a particular measure or coherent package of measures - policy - being implemented in the future. The range of possible policy interventions in the area of mental health and its care is so great that it would be somewhat arbitrary to formulate a number of alternatives, to present them to the panels and subsequently to incorporate them in scenarios. The panels were thus also not asked their views on the extent to which particular policies were likely to be adopted.

As this implies, the assumption was that policy under the two alternative scenarios was identical with that applying under the reference scenario (see appendix 1). Given the diversity of the four themes covered it was reasonable to expect the content of the alternative exploratory scenarios to differ; in the case of the alternative scenarios, unlike that of the reference scenario, not too much effort was therefore made to achieve congruence. In one area, for example, developments in treatment would be relevant and could give rise to an alternative scenario, while in another it might be developments in the area of care by family and friends. It was important not to lose sight of the special nature of each field as a result of a drive for congruence.

As noted, a procedure was developed for the purpose of identifying, in as reliable and verifiable a fashion as possible, the developments or variables on which opinion was divided in the panels in the first round of the Delphi process as to (a) their probability, (b) the direction of their effects as regards both prevalence and the utilization of services in the future, and (c) the strength of those effects. Also any thwarting 'low probability-high impact' developments suggested by the panels were examined. For each of the four themes this method produced a list of developments on which panels were not agreed. The additional criteria mentioned above were then used to decide which were to be incorporated into an alternative exploratory scenario.

Target-setting scenarios

The point of departure for the target-setting scenarios was the situation regarding prevalence and the utilization of care in the year 2010 as described in the reference scenarios for the four themes.

Objectives were then formulated as alternatives to the situations which would obtain if the references scenarios proved correct. While the reference scenarios might be deemed the most likely, assuming no change in policy, they did not by any means necessarily represent the most desirable outcomes.

The objectives were formulated by the researchers, in consultation with the scenario committee, on the basis of credibility and policy relevance in terms of alternative situations, set out as concretely as possible, regarding prevalence and the nature and extent of consumption of care. The specific objective for each theme was formulated on the basis of the data and developments emerging from the baseline analyses and the responses and suggestions made by the panel members. Possible objectives were submitted to the panels in the second and third Delphi rounds, allowing them to be checked for their relevance and credibility.

The target-setting scenarios focused on the concrete *policy measures* needed to achieve the objectives formulated for 2010, and on their side-effects. In answering this question it was assumed that autonomous trends, not susceptible to influence by public policy (notably in the demographic and economic fields), would follow the same paths as in the reference scenario. The scenarios dealing specifically with care-utilization made a further assumption, namely that prevalence (or rather, trends in prevalence over the next twenty years) would also be as in the reference scenario. The only variations introduced in the target-setting scenarios concerned policy, including both policy concerned specifically with mental and general health and their care and policy in other relevant areas (housing, education, etc.).

Concrete objectives

In the case of the exploratory scenarios it was intended that the particular nature of the themes concerned should be reflected in divergent alternative scenarios. For the same reason the objectives in the four areas were also not formulated in the same way. For each theme different stresses were needed. The following options presented themselves, taking account of the central question addressed in the study:

- a *prevalence target:* here only one option made sense, namely the formulation "point prevalence should be ... percent lower in 2010 than under the reference scenario". This is comparable with the targets set under the World Health Organization's Health for All-programme. The exact percentage target for the reduction in prevalence would be set separately for each theme. This kind of objective was not however equally relevant to all the themes, given the extremely limited scope for altering prevalence rates over the period covered (especially in the case of dementia and schizophrenia).

- a *care target:* here too only one option made sense, namely "the quality of care should be improved in such a way that the quality of life of dementing/schizophrenic patients etc. in the Netherlands is considerably better than under the reference scenario". This formulation was chosen because a target of the type 'more care' or 'less care' - unlike in the case of prevalence - would have little meaning; it was therefore necessary to formulate a target in terms of *better* care.

For those who, despite preventive measures, education etc., nevertheless fall ill, care needs to be available of the highest standard. The quality of care is not an empirical concept to be determined objectively, however, and a criterion was thus needed to indicate when the quality of care could be deemed to be of the highest standard. It was therefore decided to define as "care of the highest standard" services which optimized the quality of life of the group concerned; in other words, a high quality of care is a condition for a high quality of life. This formulation allowed account to be taken of both quantitative and qualitative aspects of services and their utilization, including both the volume of care consumed and its nature (outpatient, residential).

The particular objectives for the four theme areas are set out in chapters 5-8.

3 Mental health

3.1 *Mental health and mental health care*

"Health relates to the optimal functioning of the organism. There are two reasons why optimal 'mental' functioning cannot be defined unambiguously. First there is a quantitative problem: we do not know all the ways in which people can function mentally and therefore can never know whether particular mental processes or behaviours are 'optimal'. Second, the notion of optimal mental functioning involves moral judgements, and science has nothing to say about the validity of such judgements" (Van den Hout 1988).

While it may be possible to speak of 'proper' or 'optimal' functioning in relation to an organism (including the human body) and hence of a particular state of health, depending on the capacities of that organism, this is not possible in the case of mental functioning, at least not in the same way or on the basis of comparable characteristics. This does not imply that we cannot talk about 'suboptimal' mental functioning, however, where internal psychological barriers mean that someone can do less than what "normally speaking" - i.e. compared with others in the same circumstances - ought to be possible for such a person, and where a particular political or normative choice is made in respect of good mental functioning it is actually possible within limits to work towards its realization.

The selective optimization of mental health is the province of primary prevention, health protection and promotion, while 'suboptimal' mental functioning is the province of mental health care, defined as "the system of professional arrangements for the care, treatment and support of those whose behaviour, feelings or thoughts show such disorders that these aspects of personhood can no longer be deemed to be integrated with one another or that contact with other people is severely impeded, while their internal freedom to alter that situation is limited" (Gezondheidsraad (Health Council) 1986).

The implication is that mental health care is socially organized in the form of care units (not specified in the definition) which are associated with one another in some degree and which are based on a procedure characterized both by personal expertise and experience and by scientific knowledge and mutual scrutiny ('system of professional arrangements'). The definition also contains an indication of the group on which mental health care is targeted and of the specific function of such care in resolving the problems which are its object.

While no precise and positive definition of mental health can be derived from the above definition of mental health care, it does take further the description of 'suboptimal' functioning. The Health Council opted for the functional view of disease (physical and mental) expressed in the Netherlands by Van Dijk (1973); this focuses not on the disease itself but on its consequences for the individual. The presence of certain limitations in the individual's functioning is taken to indicate the presence of disease, irrespective of the patient's own apperceptions or of the objective attributes of the disease. For disease to be present there must always be significant:

- diminution of the individual's freedom and autonomy of action,
- insufficiency of and deficiency in physical and mental functions,
- disorganization and disorientation in the relations between the various functions,
- maladjustment to the needs of the current moment and current surroundings,
- limitation of the individual's sense of time and the future,
- impediments to personal development.

It is clear that in this model organic diseases are seen mainly as having *consequences* for the individual's freedom and autonomy (they restrict his or her freedom), while mental disorders *themselves constitute the restriction* on freedom and autonomy: they manifest themselves as a restriction, compared with the freedom of action which the individual previously enjoyed and which other persons of similar age, background and circumstances enjoy.

Not all limitations on mental functioning are the concern of mental health care: they must be relatively serious, they must persist over a relatively long period, and they must not be what would be deemed normal and transient responses to a particular event. They must also be associated with subjective suffering by patients or objective nuisance to others. Views of what is really 'clinically relevant' in respect of mental (and indeed physical) disorders can shift, as can patients' perception of the relevance of treatment to their condition. Such views and perceptions, while independent of whatever possibilities exist for assessing the actual presence of a disorder, are major determinants of both the demand for and the supply of care.

In the broadest sense *mental health care* can be seen as any form of care offered in response to a demand for help with psychological problems, albeit it is usual immediately to specify such care in terms of expertise. Professional help with mental problems is offered by a very wide range of practitioners and institutions. The limits of mental health care in a *functional* sense (the provision of care) are much wider than its limits in *institutional terms*, i.e. the set of facilities, agencies and professional practitioners whose primary task is the provision of help with mental disorders. The institutional boundaries of mental health care are in turn wider than its boundaries as a *structure*, i.e. that sector of health care formed by recognized care facilities which are responsible, in conjunction one with another, for the provision of mental health services.

In functional terms the work of e.g. family doctors, social workers, telephone helplines, Youth Advice Centres and priests, to the extent that they concern themselves with psychological problems, can be seen as mental health care, and many psychological problems - indeed, the great majority (80-90%) - never come to the attention of the more specialized care services.

Institutionally psychogeriatric nursing homes, the Outpatient Alcohol and Drug Abuse Clinics (CAD), medical day nurseries, forensic-psychiatry units, psychologists in private practice and refuges for mental patients, given their primary concern with psychological problems, can all be included in the category of mental health care; structurally, however, they fall outside it, since they do not form part of the planning and resourcing system for mental health care or do not regard themselves as coming within that sector.

Institutional boundaries can always change. Provision for the mentally ill and the mentally handicapped has evolved into two separate care systems, for example, and a somewhat similar process is now taking place in connection with intramural psychogeriatric care (physical and psychogeriatric nursing homes as separate care sectors). In other cases we see split responsibilities (e.g. between the health and justice ministries in respect of the Outpatient Alcohol and Drug Abuse Clinics and the forensic-psychiatry service), different planning regimes (e.g. in respect of medical day nurseries and much of the remaining provision for the young), or the lack of any planning and resourcing system (e.g. in the case of psychologists in private practice).

The Health Council (Gezondheidsraad) concluded in 1986 that "the general concept of mental health care cannot be precisely defined", since more or less fortuitous historical developments of a social, political and professional nature have meant that some forms of care have evolved as mental health care, or have come to be seen as forms of such care, while others have not. The Health Council itself designed a classification for mental health care on the basis of the extent of psychiatrists' involvement in particular types of care.

Chapter 4 of this report suggests a classification starting from mental health care as a structure, supplemented with (as seen from within the structure) vital elements of mental health care as an institution.

On the international side mental health care in the Netherlands is marked by the following features:

- full institutional and structural incorporation into the health care system and funding as health care,
- a large measure of internal differentiation and specialization, with many different facilities and services,
- an increasing coordination of provision at the level of the health regions,
- a view of mental health care which implies a guarantee of its availability to individuals as of right and seeks to make the relevant facilities and services geographically, financially and socially accessible and available,
- a high level of professionalization.

Such information as is available indicates that the incidence and prevalence of mental disorders in the Netherlands does not differ significantly from that in other developed countries (see below), but the proportion of the population receiving professional care and treatment is probably greater. This is true both of the more support (care)-oriented facilities (nursing homes, sheltered housing, psychiatric residential units) and of the more cure-oriented service provided e.g. by the psychotherapy departments of the Regional Institutes of Ambulatory Mental Health Care (RIAGGs) or the treatment wards of mental hospitals.

3.2 *Public mental health*

Publick mental health, at the level of the community rather than the individual, can be defined in epidemiological terms as the extent and distribution of mental illness, invalidity and mortality in the population. Ten years ago such a definition would in practice have caused difficulties, since at that time little information was available on the epidemiology of mental disorders. Much more is now known in this field, in the Netherlands and elsewhere, and there is every reason to assume that the problems of knowledge which still exist (notably the lack of empirical measurement instruments for the less serious mental disorders and of information the longer-term course of disorders, psychiatric invalidity and mortality) will be resolved by the year 2010. The epidemiological connotation of both physical and mental health implies not only a need for knowledge (on the extent and distribution of diseases) but also a technical goal and a social challenge: reducing morbidity and mortality and improving health standards and the quality of life. While epidemiology does not itself provide the material for this purpose, it does function as an instrument of navigation.

The Dutch equivalent 'volksgezondheid' of the English-language term 'mental health' (which itself replaced the earlier and somewhat unfortunate term 'psychohygiene') came into use after the Second World War. Mental health was the theme of an international movement for the rehabilitation of societies and individuals dislocated by the war and heavy stress was placed on educational measures aimed at the community at large and in particular at children and families (Van Lieshout 1985). This situation gradually changed, and the promotion of mental health at community level came to form part of a general welfare policy promoted and funded by central government, while the promotion of individual mental health became part of the work of the extramural-care institutions; as a concept 'mental health' came increasingly to overlap with 'mental health care'. In practice this meant that much individual help of a clearly curative nature and limited preventive intent was provided under the heading of mental health care, while the gradually developing welfare services (social work, crisis centres, community centres etc.) came to stress the elimination of disadvantage, the advancement of disadvantaged groups and the promotion of awareness of structural problems in the organization of society.

The concept of mental health once had an unmistakable ethical connotation. Indeed, that was the intention from the start: "with one foot in humanism and the other in science", as Trimbos characterized the secular-rational but also moral nature of the movement for mental health (Trimbos 1959). The purpose was to promote the personal well-being of the individual in the community, with the help of general measures based on the results of scientific research and legitimated by a more or less general notion of what was 'good' for mental health.

Mental health - again as a collective rather than an individual concept - could thus be defined in very broad terms as "the complex of measures which the community takes with a view to optimizing the state of the mental health of the community, of the people, of the peoples of the world, for the good of the human individuals forming that community" (Barnhoorn 1955). The mental health movement thus wished not only to improve the mental health of individuals but also to create a mentally healthy society by bringing about changes in social relations.

Looking back it is striking to what extent the movement for mental health already lacked any religious or transcendental connotation, even where religion was seen as part of a mentally healthy existence. The perspective was both entirely secular and marked by great optimism not only that social improvement was possible in principle but also that an effective welfare technology was available in practice. In fact the whole movement was founded on the idea that the necessary knowledge and means were available and that a knowledge of mental health entailed a moral duty to benefit people by manipulating the causal links now known to exist in this field. That such 'knowledge' of what was psychologically healthy and good was largely determined by the views current in certain groups in society regarding the healthy and the good was not adequately appreciated. With hindsight it is also evident that no effective welfare technology was in fact available.

While the movement for mental health as such has disappeared, the desire and drive to improve mental health still exist. This is evident for example from the aim adopted by the Dutch government, in the WHO framework, in its policy statement 'Nota 2000' of strengthening the health-promoting behaviour of individuals and institutions. An important role is played in this connection by research into and manipulation of the determinants of sickness and health. Linking the epidemiological definition of mental health with the aim of 'Nota 2000', we can define mental health in qualitative and epidemiological terms as that social situation in which social relations and social structures, the physical environment and biological factors, individual lifestyles and finally mental health care itself are of such a nature that as mentally healthy a life as possible is and remains attainable by the largest possible number of people. There is now less emphasis than in the past on the means to be used or the achievement of concrete goals; what matters more is the identification of shortcomings and problems and the making of comparisons between past and present, here and elsewhere, more and less healthily functioning groups and so on. Here again the special nature of mental health is brought out: "science provides no basis for an unambiguous definition of mental health, still less for any direct path to its achievement... While optimal functioning cannot be defined, sub-optimal functioning due to psychopathological factors can nevertheless be pinpointed" (Van den Hout 1988). A sub-optimal state of affairs, diagnosed through a process of comparison, can constitute a reason and motivation for taking steps to improve it, both at the level of the individual concerned and, more structurally, at that of a typical array of problems in a particular society.

3.3 *Mental health problems in the general population*

Little recent research material is available in the Netherlands on which to base an accurate and reliable picture of the incidence (the number of new cases arising during a particular period) or the prevalence (the total number of cases over a particular period) of mental health problems in the Dutch population. The most recent and relevant epidemiological survey of national significance was the Nijmegen Regional Project, the data for which were collected in 1983. For the rest we must have recourse to foreign - mainly American - research results. In what follows such foreign research will be cited on a number of occasions, but with the restriction that only such results will be mentioned as are likely also to apply to the Netherlands.

3.3.1 *Prevalence*

As has already been noted, the heading of mental health problems covers a very wide range of conditions, circumstances and diseases. It is therefore impossible to give any one exact, research-based figure for the prevalence of mental morbidity in the Netherlands.

The Nijmegen Regional Project (Furer & Tax 1987) divided the broad field of mental health problems into two (overlapping) categories, namely psychiatric disorders and psychosocial problems.

Psychiatric disorders were determined by a combination of respondents' subjective views and the clinical (objective) judgement of the psychiatrist. The subjective views were obtained using the General Health Questionnaire (GHQ), completed by all respondents, while the clinical judgement was based on a standardized psychiatric interview - the Present State Examination (PSE) - carried out with a sample of the respondents (Hodiamont 1986; Furer & Tax 1987). The one-month prevalence of serious psychiatric morbidity (neuroses and functional psychoses) was put at 7.3%, with a relatively large 95% confidence interval of 5.5-9.2%. If the conditions not picked up by the PSE (addictions, personality disorders etc.) are also included estimated prevalence rises to 10-12%. We can assume this estimate to be on the low side, since the Regional Project covered only Dutch-speakers aged 18-64 not currently in hospital (general or mental), prison or some other institution (see also Bijl & Mastboom 1986); certain at-risk groups which can be assumed to show higher levels of psychiatric morbidity were thus not included. On the other hand prevalence among children and adolescents is somewhat lower (see chapter 8), so that taking everything into consideration these prevalence figures probably represent a good estimate of morbidity in the Dutch population as a whole.

Research by Myers *et al.* (1984) indicates that one-month psychiatric prevalence runs at about one-and-a-half time the monthly figure. This means that *in any one year at least 15% of the population - 2.2 million people - experience an episode of psychiatric problems*. Table 3.1 gives a picture of the types of problem found. Despite the - for the Netherlands - large scale of the Regional Project survey (3245 respondents), the prevalence rates for separate diagnostic categories proved to be insufficiently reliable owing to the very small numbers of people with a psychiatric condition turned up by such an exercise. For this reason the table gives American data, namely the DSM-III diagnoses determined in a population aged 18 and over in the authoritative and very extensive survey (covering over 18,500 people) carried out by the American National Institute of Mental Health (NIMH) (Regier *et al.* 1988). Anxieties and affective disorders (notably depressions) were relatively common. The survey did not cover all the disorders included in DSM-III, omitting such phenomena as paranoia, dissociation, psychosexual disorders, eating and sleep disorders, all personality disorders except the antisocial personality, and adjustment and behavioural disorders.

Table 3.1 **One-month prevalence of DSMIII disorders**

DSMIII disorder	**Prevalence (%)**	**DSMIII disorder**	**Prevalence (%)**
All disorders listed	15.4	Anxieties	7.3
All disorders except cognitive disorders, addicitons and antisocial personality	11.2	- phobias	6.2
Addictions	3.8	- panic disorder	0.5
- alcohol abuse/dependence	2.8	- obsessive-compusive disorder	1.3
- drug abuse/dependence	1.3	- somatoform disorders	0.1
Schizophrenic disorders	0.7	Antisocial personality disorder	0.5
Affective disorders	5.1	Serious cognitive disorders (including dementia)	1.3
- manic episode	0.4		
- major depression	2.2		
- dysthymic disorder	3.3		

Source: Regier *et al.* 1988.

The Nijmegen Regional Project demonstrated yet again that most people from time to time show symptons which point to diminished mental wellbeing and increased stress. The commonest syndromes, affecting four people in ten, were tension and worry; three out of ten experienced irritability, and two out of ten situational anxiety and malaise in company.

Only in a limited number of people does the situation develop into what could be termed a psychiatric condition. Symptoms like tension and worry are part of everyday life and as such are not precursors of psychiatric problems.

The Regional Project identified *psychosocial problems* on the basis of the respondents' subjective perceptions of their well-being and social functioning (Bijl *et al.* 1986). Wellbeing ('in the last few weeks') was measured using the Affect Balance Scale (ABS) and social functioning using a questionnaire developed for the purpose.

The prevalence of psychosocial problems - irrespective of their severity - was put at 45%. The one-week prevalence of the serious psychosocial problems was 11%, giving an estimated annual prevalence, determined in the same way as in the case of the psychiatric problems covered by the survey, of over 16%. This means that every year at least 2.4 million people in the Netherlands experience an episode of serious psychosocial problems.

Table 3.2. shows the various areas of life in which people experience psychosocial problems; it also indicates where the Regional Project respondents located the cause of their only or main episode. This last information is important to an understanding of people's approaches to seeking help and dealing with problems and to the effective deployment of care.

There is some overlap between the categories of people with psychiatric and people with psychosocial problems. Hodiamont (1986) and Furer and Tax (1987) report that 35% of people with serious psychosocial problems can also be considered to have a psychiatric problem; similarly, around three quarters of those with psychiatric conditions also have psychosocial problems of one degree of severity or another. We can cautiously estimate that 50% of those with psychiatric problems also have *serious* psychosocial problems (Hodiamont 1986, 264). This means that *around 25% of people in the Netherlands experience a serious mental health problem, whether psychiatric or psychosocial, in any one year.*

Table 3.2 **Frequencies with which various areas of life were reported as giving rise to problems and the perceived causes of those problems**

Area of life	Frequency (%)	Area of life	Frequency (%)
Worry about the future	41	Current lifestyle	8
Changes in society	37	Social environment	8
Dissatisfaction with oneself	17	Aging	8
Barriers to self-development	16	Relationship with parents	7
Religion	15	Loneliness	6
Money	13	Relationship with partner	5
Work/unemployment	12	Sexual problems	5
Contacts with others	11	Study	4
Relations with significant others	10	Relationship with own children	4
Housing	9	Leisure activities	3
		Other	10

Those concerned locate the cause of their problem in:	%
Themselves	22
People in their immediate environment	6
Society	65
Various	7
	100

Source: Furer & Tax 1987.

Another interesting finding is the fact that people with physical complaints run almost twice the risk of a psychiatric condition as people without: one in eleven people with a physical problem can also be considered to have a psychiatric condition as against one in nineteen who do not have such a problem. The risk of psychosocial problems among people with somatic complaints is just over one-and-a-half times greater than among those without. The clear implication is that there is often a cumulation of problems, and where help is sought this is an important point for the care-giving agency to bear in mind.

It is known that only a small proportion of people with mental health problems seek help or receive specialized mental health care. Goldberg and Huxley (1980) developed a filter model which clearly brings out the 'pathway to psychiatric care'. In 1983 the Groningen University Department of Social Psychiatry constructed the first Dutch version of this model, which can be fleshed out with the prevalence rates already given and the most recent data, covered in the next chapter, on new admissions and numbers of patients/clients receiving mental health care. The calculations and assumptions involved are shown in the appendix at the end of this chapter.

'Filter model': annual prevalence of psychiatric and serious psychosocial morbidity in the Netherlands per 1,000 population (all ages, excluding the mentally handicapped)

Level	Filter	One-year prevalence (per 1,000)
I General population (Mental illness in the community)		250
	I Sickness behaviour (The decision to consult)	
II Primary care (All disorders among primary-care attenders)		180
	II Recognition by family doctors	
III Primary care (Conspicuous morbidity in primary-care settings)		139
	III Decision/referral by family doctor	
IV Mental health care (All referrals to psychiatric services)		43
	IV Decision to admit	
V Intramural mental health care		7

Just over 4% of all Dutch people present for mental health care every year. This means that among the 25% with mental problems only one in six actually present for specialized care and no more than 3% are admitted to any form of residential mental institution. As the model makes clear, even with constant morbidity in the population at large the utilization of care services could fluctuate sharply through changes at the various other levels (such as changes in doctors' referral practices or the tighening or relaxation of mental hospitals' admissions policies). The primary sector's important role in helping people with mental problems also emerges clearly. The model makes explicit mention of the family doctor, but it is clear that other agencies (the community-nursing, home-help and social services) also play a significant role in respect of certain categories of patient (notably the elderly and chronically ill).

3.3.2 *Socio-demographic correlates*

Epidemiological research is concerned with the social groups at risk of suffering mental problems and with the circumstances which tend to exacerbate that risk. The distinction between risk factors and risk indicators is a vital one in this connection. An attribute or circumstance is a risk *indicator* if it correlates significantly with the occurrence of mental health problems and thus has an indicative or predictive function in respect of the problems concerned, while a risk *factor* points to an attribute which can be shown to provide an explanation of the development of mental problems, i.e. which can be deemed a cause of such problems (Bijl *et al.* 1986).

Socio-demographic attributes such as age, sex and social class can seldom if ever be regarded as the sole causal factor where mental disorders are concerned: the development of most forms of mental disorder almost always involves a complex interplay of genetic, biological, somatic and psychosocial pathogenic factors. Even as predictors of problems most demographic characteristics are of little value. It is thus surprising that, despite this, much research focuses on only the simplest bivariate links (i.e. between the occurrence of mental problems and one other demographic characteristic), ignoring any common, mediating or cumulative influences resulting from several characteristics or circumstances. The result is that reality is oversimplified and that particular groups are too easily considered to be at risk of developing mental problems. In many cases the correlations identified are apparent rather than real, disappearing when corrections are made for other factors.

The correlations outlined in this section between certain socio-demographic attributes and mental health problems are therefore not to be regarded in any way as causal links; they are no more than initial indications of possible differences in risk as between certain groups. The contradictory results obtained regarding the discriminating power of sex, age, urbanization and social class clearly show that account must be taken of other attributes (and kinds of attribute) before conclusions are reached regarding at-risk groups and circumstances which exacerbate the risk of mental problems.

Sex

While the Regional Project found no difference between men and women in the overall prevalence of psychiatric conditions, it did find a difference in the case of psychosocial problems. The literature reports divergent findings, but over many years the majority conclusion has been that women suffer more mental health problems than men (see e.g. Kessler & McRae 1981; Gove 1978; Regier *et al.* 1988; Myers *et al.* 1984).

No one explanation can be given for this phenomenon. Some authors (among them Gove 1978; Pugliesi 1989) ascribe the differences in prevalence, which they see as real, to differences in the sexual, marital and work roles of men and women, while others (e.g. Russell 1985) regard the differences rather as an artefact, a result of inadequate research techniques and the use of diagnostic systems like DSM-III which they see as coloured by subjective value judgements and excessively oriented towards the individual patient.

The NIMH survey mentioned earlier found striking differences in prevalence between men and women in particular diagnostic categories. The phenomenon was especially marked in the case of addictions, affective disorders and anxieties. The one-month prevalence of alcohol abuse is 5% among men and 0.9% among women; antisocial personality disorder is also commoner among men (0.8% as against 0.2%). Affective disorders, in contrast, are commoner in women (6.6%) than in men (3.5%); within this category major depression (affecting 2.9% of women and 1.6% of men) and dysthymic disorders (4.2% of women and 2.2% of men) are particularly common. Anxieties are roughly twice as common among women (9.7%) as among men (4.7%).

Set against these differences are the many conditions where little or no difference in prevalence is found between men and women: schizophrenic disorders, manic depression, obsessive-compulsive disorder and severe cognitive disorders (up to about the age of 80; thereafter the prevalence notably of dementia rises sharply among women).

Age

The Nijmegen Regional Project found that the overall prevalence rates of psychiatric conditions generally rose with age up to about 60, while that of psychosocial problems declined as people got older (prevalence among 18-34s was almost twice that among 60-64s). Young people also experienced the severest psychosocial problems. A review by Dohrenwend and Dohrenwend (1969) also found no consistent correlation between age and the occurrence of mental health problems in general. More recent literature too indicates that there is no unambiguous link with age. Myers *et al.* (1984), for example, report that the prevalence rate of psychiatric problems among those under 45 is around double that among those aged 45 or over. The recent NIMH study (Regier *et al.* 1988) also indicated a slight fall in overall prevalence with rising age.

With regard to particular psychiatric conditions Regier *et al.* (1988) found the following inter-age-group differences in prevalence: drug and alcohol abuse, schizophrenic disorders, manic depression and antisocial personality disorder were concentrated among the under-45s; affective disorders including major depressions and dysthymic disorders and anxieties (including phobias) were in general equally common in all age groups; and the over-65s were particularly affected by severe cognitive disorders (dementia).

Social class

Over the years a considerable volume of research has been done in different countries on the links between mental ill-health and socio-economic status; Faris and Dunham (1939) were pioneers in this field. Even though social class is probably the variable which is operationalized in the most widely differing ways, the literature consistently shows those in the lower socio-economic groups to suffer more malaise and more psychiatric problems than those in the higher groups. One of the papers published as part of the NIMH survey classified the overall prevalence of psychiatric problems into a number of specific DSM-III diagnostic categories (Holzer 1986). This survey determined socio-economic status from a combination of education, occupation and income, dividing respondents into four groups. Table 3.3 shows each socio-economic category's six-month prevalence rates for a number of important psychiatric conditions; it also indicates the relative risk of the various conditions faced by persons in each of the lowest three groups as compared with those in the highest group (a relative risk of 2.0 for a particular socio-economic group means that persons in that group run twice the risk of developing the condition in question as those in the highest group, for example, while a relative risk of 1.0 indicates that the level of risk is the same).

The prevalence of every condition is greatest in the lowest group: a high rate of cognitive disorders in particular, and to a slightly lesser extent of schizophrenia, correlates closely with low socio-economic status. Strikingly, the risk of depression in the lowest category is 'only' 1.79 times greater than in the highest.

Table 3.3 **Six-month prevalence and relative risk (corrected for age and sex) by social class**

	Socio-economic group			
	(low=) 1	2	3	4 (=high)
All DSM-III disorders except phobias and cognitive disorders				
- prevalence (%)	11.5	12.0	10.9	7.6
- relative risk	2.86	2.04	1.55	1.00
Major depression				
- prevalence (%)	2.2	2.9	2.5	1.7
- relative risk	1.79	1.92	1.51	1.00
Alcohol abuse/dependence				
- prevalence (%)	5.3	5.2	4.6	3.3
- relative risk	3.59	2.19	1.59	1.00
Schizophrenia				
- prevalence (%)	1.3	1.0	0.8	0.3
- relative risk	7.85	3.84	2.72	1.00
Severe cognitive disorders				
- prevalence (%)	5.8	1.1	0.3	0.2
- relative risk	21.15	4.88	1.60	1.00

Source: Holzer *et al.* 1986.

The Nijmegen Regional Project points to slightly different conclusions with regard to psychosocial problems: here prevalence *rises* with educational level, and among those with the highest level of education a larger proportion suffer serious psychosocial problems than among those with the lowest level. The effect of occupational level is less marked. With regard both to the prevalence rate of psychosocial problems in general and the severity of the problems suffered, people without employment (whether because they are unemployed, chronically sick or in receipt of disability benefit) stand out as the worst off.

Urbanization

While possible differences in mental health between urban and rural areas are of particular interest in view of WHO-Europe's Healthy Cities programme, here too the literature is divided. Divergent results are to be found regarding differences in the occurrence of mental problems in rural areas and cities, notwithstanding the commonly held view that problems are commoner in cities, both because urban life is alleged to be pathogenic for proportionately more people and because people with mental problems are said to gravitate towards cities.

Bell *et al.* (1981) report no difference in the scale and frequency of psychiatric symptoms between urban and rural areas; Dohrenwend (1975), in contrast, noted that eight out of ten studies which he analysed found higher prevalence rates in urban areas (albeit the differences were slight). If the general notion of mental disorder is broken down into diagnostic categories the picture is even less clear. Dohrenwend reports that personality disorders and neuroses are more common in cities and functional psychoses in rural areas. Brown and Harris (1978) found a three-month prevalence for borderline and more serious disorders of 24% among women on the Hebridean island of North Uist as against 33% in the Camberwell district of London; depression was more common in Camberwell, anxiety and phobias in the Hebrides. Blazer *et al.* (1985) concluded from the NIHM Epidemiologic Catchment Area study that major depression was twice as common in urban areas; drug abuse was also commoner in cities. Rural areas showed a higher prevalence of alcohol abuse and cognitive disorders among the elderly. No differences were found in the areas of dysthymic disorders, schizophrenia, obsessive-compulsive disorder, antisocial personality disorder and agoraphobia.

3.3.3 *Incidence*

Data on the incidence (the number of new cases occurring in a particular period) of mental health problems in the population are only to be found in foreign literature and then relating only to psychiatric disorders.

Goldberg and Huxley (1980) put the incidence of psychiatric disorders in one year at one third of the point prevalence, implying that every year 3.5% of the population of the Netherlands - 500,000 people - experience a new psychiatrically relevant episode. As for the serious psychosocial problems, the implication is that every year 3.7% - 540,000 people - are faced with a new problem episode.

The well-known longitudinal Lundby Study which Hagnell carried out in Sweden (1986) used incidence data to calculate the morbidity risk - the chance of developing psychiatric problems - in the successive decades of life. The cumulative risk of psychiatric disorder up to particular ages and the total lifetime risk were also calculated (the cumulative risk is the risk which a newborn baby faces of experiencing at least one episode of psychiatric disorder by a particular age if he or she lives that long) (table 3.4).

Table 3.4 **Incidence and risk of developing a serious psychiatric problem for the first time, by sex and age**

Age	Annual incidence (%)		Risk of developing condition in this decade of life		Cumulative risk of developing condition	
	m	f	m	f	m	f
00-09	0.00	0.00	.000	.000	.000	.000
10-19	0.03	0.10	.003	.010	.003	.010
20-29	0.31	0.24	.031	.024	.033	.033
30-39	0.20	0.16	.020	.016	.053	.049
40-49	0.16	0.45	.016	.044	.068	.091
50-59	0.26	0.31	.026	.031	.092	.118
60-69	0.50	0.46	.049	.045	.136	.158
70-79	1.19	1.48	.112	.138	.233	.274
80-89	3.63	3.22	.304	.275	.466	.474

Source: Hagnell 1986.

Up to the age of 60 the risk of experiencing a serious psychiatric disorder on at least one occasion is just over 9% among men and almost 12% among women. Given the average life expectancy in the Netherlands of 72 years for men and 79 for women, this means that the cumulative lifetime probability of serious psychiatric disorder is 25% for men and just over 27% for women. A general breakdown of these figures into neuroses, psychoses and organic brain syndromes shows the lifetime probability of psychosis to be very low (5% for men and 3% for women), and while the probability of serious neurosis is greater (7% for men and 12% for women) by far the greatest risk is associated with organic brain syndromes (notably dementia), rising sharply particularly from the age of 75.

3.3.4 *Trends*

There is no research literature focusing specifically on the Netherlands from which conclusions may be drawn as to whether the prevalence rate of mental health problems in the population at large (Level I in the filter model) has risen or fallen in recent decades. There is however extensive literature comprising findings from the Dutch regional patient registers in Assen and Maastricht (Ten Horn *et al.* 1986), so that much information is available on the numbers of persons receiving care in or from hospitals or other mental health institutions and on the pathways followed by those seeking help.

Foreign research concludes that since 1950 the prevalence of mental health problems has risen (Schwab & Schwab 1978), possible reasons being: 1. increased life expectancy, 2. a wider definition of mental illness, 3. changes in diagnostics, 4. the expansion of mental health services, among other things through the development of community care, 5. changing attitudes towards psychiatric conditions among both doctors and the public at large, and 6. changes in the methodology of prevalence studies.

While part of the observed rise in prevalence is thus 'artificial', resulting from changing views, different research methods and shifts in the boundaries between areas of work and responsibility (see also Richman & Barry 1986), part is certainly real. In particular the fact that people now live longer goes a long way towards explaining the higher prevalence of certain mental disorders - such as dementia - as compared with 35 years ago.

A WHO Europe report (1988), issued as part of the Health for All in the Year 2000 programme, assumes that the number of cases of mental disorder in Europe will continue to rise. The basis for this assumption is as follows:

1. The incidence figures for the main mental disorders are not falling, nor are they expected to fall in the near future; in combination with increasing population this implies a growing number of people with disorders.
2. The number and proportion of old and very old people in the population are rising rapidly, indicating an increase in the numbers of mental disorders, especially dementia, in this group.
3. The life-expectancy of children seriously brain-damaged at birth, and in particular those with congenital abnormalities, has improved. A contrary trend is that progress in genetic research will mean that fewer such children are born.
4. A growing proportion of the population is exposed to events and circumstances associated with increased risk of and vulnerability to disorders: long-term unemployment, high social and geographic mobility, erosion of family ties and social networks, lack of social support and social isolation. This trend will make itself felt particularly in an increase in depressive and anxiety disorders and psychosomatic syndromes.

While we can expect these four developments to affect the Netherlands, the WHO also mentions a number of other developments of a more speculative nature whose relevance to this country is more doubtful and whose impact on the prevalence of mental disorders would probably be marginal at most. They are as follows:

5. The incidence and prevalence of mental disorders associated with AIDS are forecast to rise rapidly.
6. Young people are increasingly adopting patterns of behaviour likely to lead to a rise in the incidence and prevalence of psychological and neurological disorders notably as a result of (a) the abuse of alcohol and drugs (both illegal and pharmaceutical), (b) violent behaviour, suicide and attempted suicide, and (c) irresponsible and high-risk behaviour on the roads and in sexual matters (HIV infection and unwanted pregnancy). In the Netherlands such problems appear to be concentrated in the areas of alcohol abuse, vandalism and dangerous behaviour on the roads.

7. Mental problems and disorders are expected to increase as the level of chronical physical illness rises.

In this WHO Europe report the stress is very much on individuals, their behaviour, their responses to what happens to them and their physical state. Broader factors with an impact (harmful or beneficial) on mental health, such as the physical and social environment and education and upbringing, are not covered directly; indirectly, however, they do play a part in the factors mentioned here (notably in the category of preventive measures).

While the Health for All in the Year 2000 programme seeks to achieve at least a 10% increase in the number of years through which people live without any serious illness or handicap, there is no expectation that this can be achieved other than through increased efforts in the area of prevention and intervention. The number of disorders is not expected to fall spontaneously, nor is any definitive solution forecast for particular mental disorders.

Appendix: The filter model: calculations and assumptions

The figures given in the filter model are current best estimates. The ideal would be to survey and monitor a single population with a view to determining one-year prevalence rates for the various levels; here the figures shown are taken from various studies and relate to various populations. Such a filter model was first fleshed out for the Netherlands by the Groningen University Department of Social Psychiatry (1983). The figures shown are an improvement on the Groningen figures in the following respects:

- Services for the mentally handicapped are omitted; only specialized mental health care (as noted in chapter 4) is included at levels IV and V.
- The model covers the whole population of the Netherlands, including children and the over-65s, and extends over all five levels.
- The data relate to all mental morbidity, both psychiatric and severe psychosocial. The field covered is thus wider than in the case of the Groningen model.

The data for the five levels were obtained as follows:

- Level I: see section 3.3.1.
- Level II: every year 72% of people in the Netherlands attend for primary care (CBS, Swinkels, 1988). It is assumed therefore that 72% of the Level I population consult primary practitioners.
- Level III: see Wilmink, 1989, p. 49. Family doctors judged that 77% of the patients who consulted them with 'psychological' or 'vague/-many' complaints had mental health problems.
- Level IV: one-year prevalence = number on 1 January plus registrations in the course of the year.
  Tables 4.10 and 4.11 allow us to calculate one-year prevalence rates in mental health care as a whole for the year 1990. To obtain a complete picture 86,800 outpatient registrations (at mental hospitals and the psychiatric departments of general hospitals) were added to the number of registrations shown in table 4.11. To correct for double counting (simultaneous registration at more than one institution, more than one admission to a mental hospital in the course of the year) the figures for extramural institutions were reduced by 4% and those for intramural institutions by 15%, on the basis of the findings of the Groningen University Department of Social Psychiatry (1983, pp. 20 and 46).
- Level V: calculation as for Level IV. Intramural care was defined as that provided in mental hospitals, the psychiatric departments of general hospitals, psychogeriatric nursing homes and sheltered-living facilities.

4 Mental health care

4.1 *History and development of mental health care*

Every society recognizes a distinction between those who do not wish to conform to everyday norms of behaviour and those who cannot so conform even if they wish to. The deviant behaviour of the criminal, the drunk or the clown is of a different order from that of someone who, without reason or purpose, engages in strange, dangerous or disturbing acts. Where the effect of the behaviour is the same - disturbance of public order, danger to the individual concerned or to others - the community's reaction may be the same, but the history of European societies nevertheless shows that the difference between free and unfree deviant behaviour has gradually been reflected in an increasingly clear difference of approach and regime. In the case of the insane - those who involuntarily act in unacceptable and incomprehensible ways - the chief purpose of mental health care was initially to protect society from maladjusted behaviour. In the nineteenth century there then arose a form of public mental health care with a strongly pedagogical, and later increasingly medical, emphasis.

Psychiatry and the associated care for the mentally disturbed individual developed on the basis of a social definition of 'lunacy' and a municipal or national policy of detaining 'lunatics' who disturbed the life of society. Psychiatry started in the nineteenth century with the more visible and socially disruptive forms of lunacy (as displayed by psychotics, epileptics and the behaviourally disturbed mentally handicapped), gradually extending its field to include the individually perceived but socially inconspicuous forms of suffering (depression, anxiety, compulsion, psychosomatic symptoms, neuroses) and later coming increasingly to concern itself with the problems of the maladjusted personality and finally also with the shared suffering which develops and finds expression in reactions and interactions (marriage and family problems, difficulties in education or at work, problems of upbringing).

Nineteenth-century psychiatry was an institutional psychiatry with a strong emphasis on custody and asylum: the guarding and protection of patients, often over a period of many years. Admission to a 'mental hospital' was by definition admission under duress; voluntary admission was practised only in the case of small private institutions for 'sufferers from nervous disorders'. In the second half of the century the asylums developed, in the footsteps of medicine, into hospitals, as efforts were made to establish a systematic classification of mental disorders and to understand their causes and course (Kraepelin).

By the end of the century a limited arsenal of treatments was available and the outline was becoming visible of a psychological theory describing the links between individual development and the genesis of certain mental disorders (Freud). The development and practice of mental health care has continued to rest chiefly upon the foundations laid by Freud and Kraepelin, together with a third support in the form of psychopharmacology (from the start of the 1950s onwards) and a fourth in that of the use of the social group as a therapeutic instrument.

After about 1920 a start was made on developing facilities for the care of psychiatric patients before admission and after discharge. At that time interest was growing in the possibility of preventing mental disorders and promoting the mental health of the population. The same period also saw growing interest in mental development and the specific problems of children. Later attention focused on the mental health problems of addicts, the elderly, delinquents and groups with specific characteristics (ethnic minorities, women, refugees, homosexuals, victims of violence). These developments continued and intensified after the Second World War, producing an increasingly differentiated system of extramural and semi-mural care on the one hand and a variety of activities and programmes aimed at prevention and health promotion on the other, both within and outside the system of mental health care in the narrow sense.

While psychiatry is one of the oldest medical specialties (and currently the second largest among them) the role of the psychiatrist or, better, the doctor in mental health care long remained a marginal one. The transition from a 'custodial' psychiatry with warders to a 'therapeutic' psychiatry with nurses and therapists was a gradual one, and the position of the clinician in mental health care has never been uncontroversial. In the scientific and therapeutic fields psychiatrists and psychologists have often been simultaneously colleagues and rivals, and the major field of psychotherapy has never been a medical monopoly: the work of sociotherapists, psychiatric nurses and activity supervisors is also very important in the daily lives of many patients, particularly those in mental hospitals. Mental health care, more than any other care sector, is marked by multidisciplinary approaches and teamwork at the level of treatment as well as diagnosis.

In substantive terms the development of mental health care and psychiatry in the Netherlands has largely followed American and British models. This is true both in the diagnostic field (the general acceptance of the American DSM-III system) and in the therapeutic field (the development of new forms of psychotherapy and treatment and support methods and to a lesser extent of psychopharmaceutical drugs). It is true also as regards developments in biological psychiatry, psychiatric epidemiology and social psychiatry. The traditional orientation towards German psychiatry disappeared because of the experience of Nazism, and indeed German psychiatry itself now looks primarily to the United States.

Mental health care has always had a special relationship with the *state*: even in the earliest years of the Kingdom of the Netherlands the state accounted the care of psychiatric patients one of its special responsibilities, and this always remained the case, even when the stress shifted from public to individual oriented mental health care. In the last twenty years the state has brought about the development of regional mental health care networks, laid a firmer financial base and instigated a movement towards a more differentiated care system with an accent on alternatives to hospitalization. Government policy as set out in the 'Nota 2000' statement adds a further focus on the promotion of mental health itself and measures to that end in various fields.

4.2 *Changes in the volume and composition of care*

Subsequent sections detail the main quantitative trends in mental health care in the Netherlands, looking at numbers of patients treated, at the capacity of the care system and at costs. The figures are taken from the reviews published annually since 1980 by the Netherlands Institute of Mental Health (NcGv) under the title "Mental Health Care in Figures" (most recent edition: Jacobs & Ketting 1990). These reviews bring together in systematic form statistics on mental health care derived from a wide range of admissions registers and surveys. With one or two exceptions data are available covering the period 1980-87.

The trends visible over this period have been linearly extrapolated, allowing for population growth, to the year 2000. The figures for psychogeriatrics also take account of the increasing numbers of old and very old people in the population. The purpose of these extrapolations is simply to answer the question: how will mental health care look in 2000, in quantitative terms, *if the trends of the last decade continue through the 1990s*?

The results for the period 1988-2000 thus have only reference value and should not be seen as prognoses. True prognoses are impossible in this area, since changes in the volume of care are largely the result of political and policy decisions rather than of autonomous processes.

Bearing in mind that the purpose is to identify trends, the period 1980-87 is a very short one. However, for a number of reasons it is impossible to look further back in time, the main one being of course the shortage of quantitative data on major sectors of mental health care before 1980. A second reason is that the major organizational changes which took place over that period, such as the establishment of the Regional Institutes for Ambulatory Mental Health Care (RIAGGs), mean that such data as are available cannot be formed into coherent longitudinal pictures. A third reason is that the function of some institutions of mental health care has changed markedly: over the past twenty years, for example, the care of the mentally handicapped and the elderly mentally infirm has gradually been moved out of the general psychiatric hospitals, so that there is no sense in comparing today's psychiatric hospitals with those of twenty years ago. In part they are now quite different institutions.

Two further comments are needed by way of introduction to the data. First, the total volume of mental health care is rising rapidly, despite a policy of allowing only some sectors to grow while others (notably the mental hospitals) are cut back. In fact little slimming-down has taken place: there has been a slight reduction in the capacity of psychiatric hospitals and psychiatric wards in general hospitals, but moderate to strong growth has marked all other sectors of mental health care.

There then arises the question whether this trend indicates a continuing increase in mental health problems in the Netherlands: are people in this country growing steadily more mentally unhealthy? We shall not seek to answer this question here, since it is considered at length in the last chapter of this report. The question is posed simply to set the right context for the data; three points need to be borne in mind in particular.

First, the population of the Netherlands is continuing to grow (between 1980 and 2000 by 11.5%), so that if mental problems occur at a constant rate all absolute mental health care parameters must also go on growing.

Another important autonomous factor is the aging of the population: mental problems and disease symptoms are commoner among the elderly, so that the 34% rise in the number of over-65s which will occur between 1980 and 2000 will produce a sizable increase in care requirements.

While these two factors, taken together, generate an absolute increase in the number of mental problems, they do not mean that Dutch society is growing mentally more unhealthy. This is also true of the third point to be borne in mind. As we saw in the last chapter, only a small fraction of mental health problems in fact give rise to a demand for care, implying - in principle at least - that a rising consumption of care might mean simply that treatment is being sought for an increasing proportion of a constant number of mental problems. The ratio between the number of problems for which professional help is sought and the occurrence of problems in the population at large is in fact such (one in five or ten) that only a small rise in clients' inclination to seek help or care-giving agencies' inclination to provide it could result in a huge increase in care consumption. Theoretically, indeed, an increase in the utilization of services is compatible with a fall in mental morbidity: the two are independent of one another to the point that changes in the volume of care consumed can never be taken as a direct indication of changes in morbidity.

Against this background the sharp growth in the utilization of mental health services found by simply extrapolating current trends is far less improbable than may appear at first sight.

The second point that needs to be made concerns the extrapolated cost of mental health care. The calculation started from the actual costs incurred in each sector in 1987; the costs for preceding years were then adjusted using cost-of-living figures, in accordance with the method used by the Social and Cultural Planning Office (1989). The next step was to determine the inflation-adjusted costs per bed (in the extramural sector per staff member) over the period 1980-87, which were then linearly extrapolated for the period 1988-2000. The figures thus obtained were then multiplied by the extrapolated capacity figures (which allowed for population growth). *The sums thus relate to costs corrected for population growth and are expressed in constant (1987) guilders. They will therefore need to be increased to take account of future inflation.*

4.3 *Demarcation of the mental health care field*

As the last chapter noted, the field of mental health care cannot be demarcated unambiguously: a number of different criteria might be applied, relating among other things to the type of care provided, resourcing and policy. The review which follows covers only those forms which can be accounted mental health care in institutional terms, namely those provided by general and specialized psychiatric hospitals (APZs and CPZs), psychiatric units in general hospitals (PAAZs, including the university psychiatry clinics), psychogeriatric resting homes, psychogeriatric day-treatment facilities, sheltered-living facilities, the Regional Institutes of Ambulatory Mental Health Care (RIAGGs) and the Outpatient Alcohol and Drug Abuse Clinics (CADs).

While these institutions and types of care between them cover the great majority of institutional mental health care there are also other forms, of which the most important are these:

1. *Convalescent homes* providing short-term psychosocial care (the average length of stay is about two months). At the start of 1988 there were 18 such institutions, with a total capacity of 585 beds; their operating costs totalled just over 26 million guilders. The Ministry of Welfare, Health and Cultural Affairs decided in mid 1988 to withdraw grant from eight of them, leaving only 384 beds funded under the Exceptional Medical Expenses Act.
2. *Medical children's homes* providing treatment and care for children aged up to 15 whose physical and/or mental health is compromised or under threat. There are twelve such homes, with an aggregate capacity of 671 beds; the average length of stay is around a year and the total annual cost is 47 million guilders.
3. *Medical day nurseries* offering day treatment for children aged from eighteen months to six years. There are 28 such centres, with a total treatment capacity of 1960 places. The average duration of treatment is one-and-a-half years, and in 1988 the total cost amounted to 113 million guilders.
4. *Psychiatric outpatient departments* in general psychiatric hospitals and the psychiatric units of general hospitals. In the data given below the cost of the treatment is included in the total costs of general psychiatric hospitals. The number of people treated in in outpatient departments is very large; in 1988 consultations totalled almost 700,000.
5. *Psychiatrists (and psychologists) in private practice:* little information is available on the service they provide, so that there is no point in attempting to indicate its scale or cost.

6. *Other:* as well as the above a large number of other services can also be accounted part of mental health care, either wholly or partly. They include notably the wide range of specialized facilities (refuges, crisis centres, drop-in centres, centres for runaways and the like) aimed at particular groups. Their numbers are especially large in the areas of addiction and youth problems. The boundary between mental health care and these other forms of help, support and treatment is often difficult to determine with precision. The aggregate cost of these various services amounts to between 200 and 300 million guilders a year, i.e. around 5% of the total for specialized mental health care.

4.4 *Psychiatric hospitals*

Table 4.1. presents statistics on the volume of care provided by psychiatric hospitals over the period 1980-87, together with estimates for the years 1990, 1995 and 2000 (on the basis of the assumptions detailed in section 4.2); for the sake of concision and clarity five-year intervals have been left between the figures.

Table 4.1 **Psychiatric hospitals: capacity, patients and costs, 1980-2000**

	1980	1985	*1987*	1990	1995	2000
Capacity	24689	24450	*24530*	24528	24417	24228
Number of patients:						
- absolute on 31 December	23146	23314	*23418*	23608	23836	24008
- per 100,000 population	164	161	*160*	159	156	153
Admissions	26490	32738	*34488*	38209	44541	51094
Costs 1	1578	1937	*2016*			
Costs 2	1892	1971	*2016*	2074	2162	2241

1 = nominal costs;
2 = inflation-adjusted costs (see section 4.2 for explanation); both in millions of guilders.

The first point to note is that these data relate to all psychiatric hospitals, both general and specialized; in terms of bed numbers the general psychiatric hospitals account for 93% of the total. The table shows a very slight drop in capacity, with the number of beds falling by only about 450 (1.8%) between 1980 and 2000 on present trends. This absolute decline of 1.8% does not reflect the real change in care provision, however, since with continuing population growth through the last two decades of the century the volume of care available per 1,000 people will fall by 12%.

The numbers of patients in psychiatric hospitals show a small increase, implying a gradual rise in occupancy rates; indeed, the extrapolated figure for the occupancy rate in 2000 is almost 100%. Because of population growth, however, the number of patients per 100,000 population is set to decline from 164 in 1980 to 153 in 2000 (see third line of table).

The most striking feature of the table is the very sharp rise in the number of admissions: on current trends the number in 2000 will be almost double that in 1980. This is chiefly the result of a rapid growth in readmissions, due in turn to the accelerated discharge of patients in circumstances of restricted capacity. An increase in readmissions is the logical outcome of limiting the psychiatric hospitals' residential function while not expanding the alternatives (sheltered-living facilities, day activity centres, employment facilities etc.) at an appropriate rate. The current funding system also tends to increase admissions: for every new admission, defined as including readmissions not less than six months after discharge, a general psychiatric hospital receives 3000 guilders from the funding agency. This encourages a tendency to discharge patients within a year and a willingness to readmit them six months later.

The cost of treatment and care in psychiatric hospitals also shows an increase, of almost one percent a year, despite the slight decline in capacity.

The various trends are graphed in figure 4.1 using index figures (1980 = 100) and allowing for population growth (i.e. in each case the figures are per 1,000 people in the Netherlands in the year in question). The picture which emerges is one of sharply rising admissions, a very slight rise in costs (of 6% over twenty years), a slight fall (of 7%) in the number of patients accommodated in psychiatric hospitals and a somewhat sharper fall (of 12%) in the number of beds available.

Figure 4.1 **Psychiatric hospitals, 1980-2000 (index, 1980 = 100)**

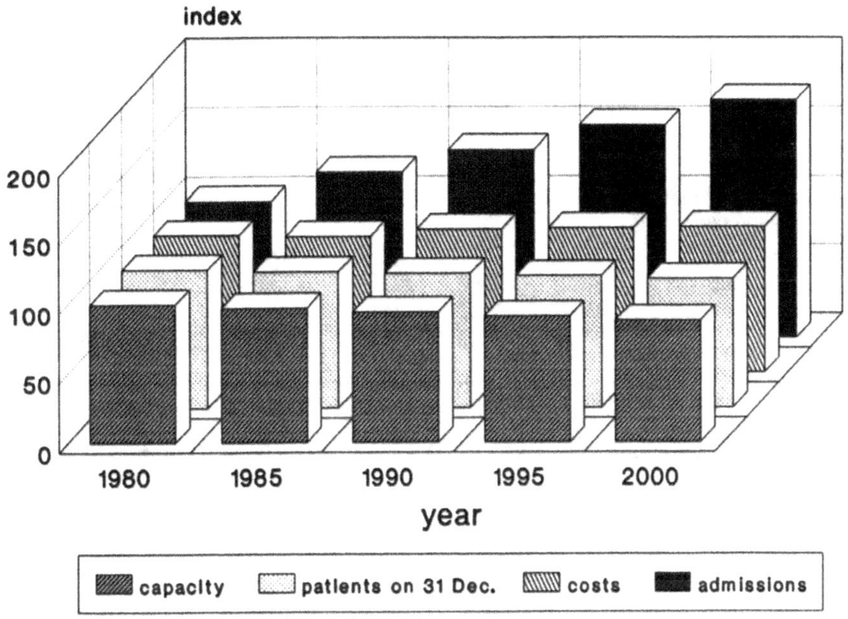

4.5 *Psychogeriatric nursing homes*

Psychogeriatric nursing homes and the psychogeriatric units of combined nursing homes provide nursing for patients affected by the mental disorders of old age. Their residents, three-quarters of whom suffer from dementia and 12% from amnestic syndrome, are generally very old; the average age is over 80 and 9% are over 90. Age on first admission averages 78.4 for men and 80.5 for women (SIVIS data 1987).

The rapid growth experienced by these nursing homes over the last ten years is explained partly by the fact that psychogeriatric care has moved out of the general psychiatric hospitals (to the extent that it was still a feature of them) and partly by the increasing numbers of old people in general and of the very old (over 80) in particular.

Table 4.2 **Psychogeriatric nursing homes: capacity, patients and costs, 1980-2000**

	1980	1985	*1987*	1990	1995	2000
Capacity	18743	21764	*22778*	24842	28074	31297
Number of patients:						
- absolute on 31 December	18000	21127	*22658*	25037	28856	32735
- per 100,000 population*	1111	1218	*1250*	1310	1410	1509
Admissions	8677	10584	*10469*	11386	12813	14229
Costs 1	1092	1527	*1662*			
Costs 2	1309	1521	*1662*	1846	2148	2464

* Of the population aged 65 or over.
1 = nominal costs;
2 = inflation-adjusted costs (see section 4.2 for explanation); both in millions of guilders.

Between 1980 and 1987 the number of beds in psychogeriatric nursing homes rose by 22%; were this trend to persist the last two decades of the century would see a total increase of 67%, to over 31,000 beds, with the number of beds available for every 100,000 people aged 65 or over rising from 1157 in 1980 to 1443 in 2000. The trend towards an increasing proportion of over-65s requiring nursing-home care probably has two main causes. First, the number of over-75s - the age group most likely to need such care - is growing more quickly than that of the over-65s in general and, second, once admitted to a nursing home psychogeriatric patients tend to live longer. The combination of these two factors has put sharply increasing pressure on the nursing-home sector in recent years, with the number of patients rising more rapidly than the number of beds; indeed, the extrapolated figures show the former exceeding the latter by 1500 by the end of the century. Another pressure indicator is the fact that annual admissions per hundred beds are set to remain roughly constant (at around 45) over the period 1980-2000, which is not compatible with the increasing average length of stay. The nursing homes will simply fill up.

Psychogeriatric nursing homes are currently subject to a national capacity norm of 1.25 beds for every 100 over-65s, giving permitted totals of 23,888 beds in 1990 and 27,113 in 2000. If numbers rise as indicated in table 4.2 around 1000 patients will be unable to find a place in 1990, rising to over 4,000 in 2000. This contrasts with the position in 1980, when there were 1,500 fewer patients in psychogeriatric nursing homes than the norm allowed. The capacity norm will have to be increased to 1.44 by the end of the century if we are to ensure that places are available for all who need them.

The cost of psychogeriatric nursing has risen sharply in recent years, and we can only assume that this trend will continue; indeed, between 1980 and 2000 the figure is likely almost to double. Of the cost increase 41% is due to the growing number of over-65s, 43% to the growing number of patients for every 100 over-65s (due in turn to the rising proportion of the very old), and only 16% to increased costs per patient.

Figure 4.2 **Psychogeriatric nursing homes, 1980-2000 (index, 1980 = 100)**

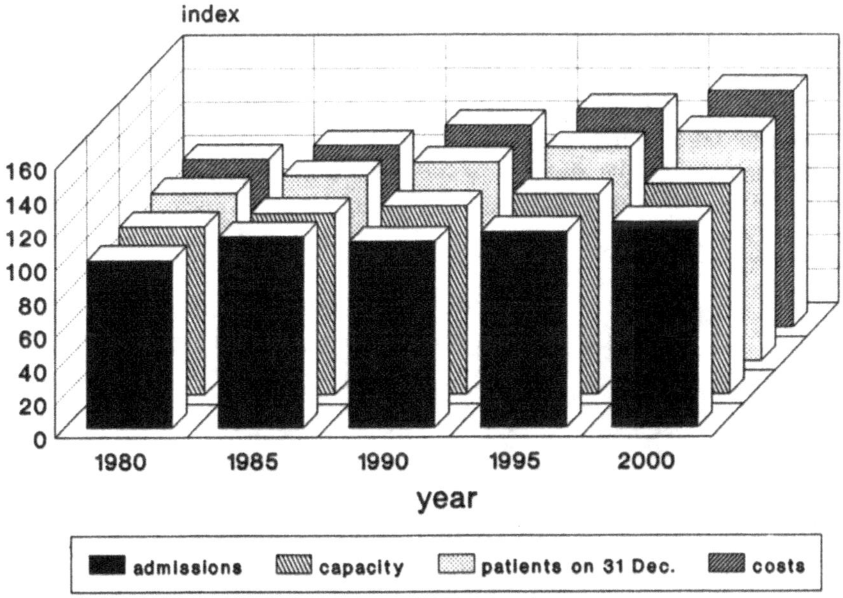

On the model set for psychiatric hospitals in the previous section, figure 4.2 graphs these various trends on the basis of index figures (1980 = 100) and with allowance made for population growth (in this case the population of over-65s). The cost per hundred persons aged 65 or over rises by a good 40% over the twenty-year period and the proportion of the over-65s living in nursing homes rises by 36%, while the relative increases in capacity and annual admissions are only 25% and 22% respectively.

4.6 *Psychiatric units in general hospitals (PAAZ)*

In 1988 there were in the Netherlands 76 psychiatric units in general hospitals (PAAZ), including the seven university psychiatric clinics. The average unit has 32 beds, used for patients who can be helped with relatively short-term treatment (the average stay is six weeks). In functional terms there is no clear boundary between the psychiatric wards of general hospitals and short-term treatment in psychiatric hospitals.

Little statistical information is available on psychiatric units, and in particular the daily treatment cost is not clear. The daily nursing cost of 275 guilders is probably a realistic estimate[1]

Only in recent years has systematic information become available on numbers of treatment places and patients treated. Until recently such statistics had to be reconstructed, with great difficulty, from scattered and disparate sources. The figures shown in table 4.3, particularly those relating to the first few years, must therefore be seen as fairly rough approximations; for the same reason too much value should not be attached to the extrapolations.

---

[1] This lack of clarity is due to the fact that psychiatric-unit costs cannot be disentangled from overall hospital costs. We have nevertheless sought to give an estimate of costs and cost changes, based on the guideline amounts for psychiatric units' various cost headings as applied in 1988 by the Central Council on Health Care Charges (COTG). This gave average daily nursing costs in a standard psychiatric unit of around 275 guilders for the base year of 1987. It was assumed that the average occupancy rate was 86% (it fluctuated between 85% and 90%) and that the unit-cost increase was the same as in psychiatric hospitals.

Table 4.3 **Psychiatric units: capacity, patients and costs, 1980-2000**

	1980	1985	*1987*	1990	1995	2000
Capacity	2618	2376	*2420*	2340	2190	2050
Number of patients:						
- absolute						
on 31 December	2359	2030	*2075*	2010	1880	1750
- per 100,000						
population	17	14		13	12	11
Admissions	20100	19200	*18350*	17600	16300	14800
Costs 1	179	198	*209*			
Costs 2	211	201	*209*	208	204	199

1 = nominal costs;
2 = inflation-adjusted costs (see section 4.2 for explanation); both in millions of guilders.

While the total capacity of psychiatric units has gradually declined in recent years it is by no means certain that this trend will continue. As so often happens in mental health care, the decline has been the result more of name changes than of bed or ward closures - some university psychiatric clinics or sections of them, for example, have been absorbed into other institutions, notably general psychiatric hospitals - and while there has been some 'tidying', in that a number of very small psychiatric units which were not recognized as such have been closed, at the end of 1989 there were no indications or plans regarding the continuation of this process. It is therefore perhaps more realistic to assume that capacity will remain broadly constant at around 2400 beds; the other indices (with the exception of costs) would then remain at their 1987 levels.

Figure 4.3's indexed data show that on current trends capacity per 1,000 population is set to decline considerably, along with numbers of admissions and numbers of patients receiving treatment. Costs are shown as declining slightly more slowly.

Figure 4.3 **Psychiatric units in general hospitals, 1980-2000 (index, 1980 = 100)**

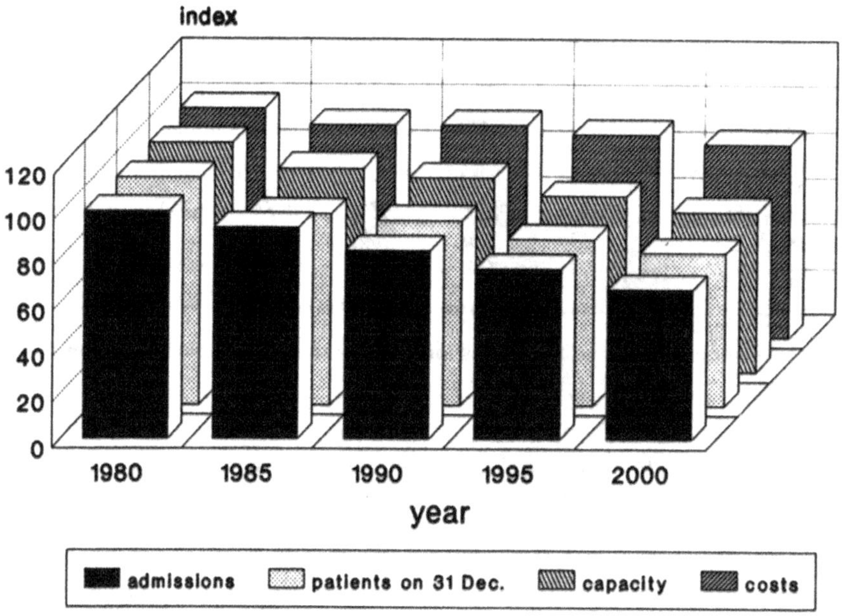

4.7 *Sheltered-living facilities*

The various forms of sheltered living provide accommodation and support for psychiatric patients and former psychiatric patients who cannot, or cannot yet, cope independently. Facilities are generally small-scale, the majority being ordinary houses. They were developed in the late 1970s, generally from other forms of provision, and more recently the government has been encouraging them to join together at regional level in Regional Institutes for Sheltered Living (RIBWs). In general the government is seeking to promote this form of care, notably as an alternative to long-stay care in general psychiatric hospitals for patients for whom no further treatment is indicated. The cost of sheltered accommodation is considerably lower than that of care in a general psychiatric hospital.

At the end of 1988 there were 130 sheltered-living units with an aggregate capacity of 3318 places.

Table 4.4 **Sheltered-living facilities: capacity, patients and costs, 1980-2000**

	1980	1985	*1987*	1990	1995	2000
Capacity	2330	2946	*3007*	3322	3857	4411
Number of patients:						
- absolute on 31 December	2310	2940	*2978*	3290	3820	4370
- per 100,000 population	16	20	*20*	22	25	28
Admissions	750	750		854	911	969
Costs 1	60	95	*102*			
Costs 2	72	95	*102*	117	144	175

1 = nominal costs;
2 = inflation-adjusted costs (see section 4.2 for explanation); both in millions of guilders.

Until a few years ago sheltered-living provision was growing much less rapidly than intended. The national capacity norm is 0.38 places per 1,000 population, implying a total in 1989 of 5626 places; in fact only 3318 places were available at the start of that year. If the current slow rate of growth is maintained total capacity in 2000 will be 4411, 1562 less than required by the norm. The pressure experienced by psychiatric hospitals, manifested in a rapid growth in readmissions, results partly from the inadequate expansion of sheltered-living facilities.

Admissions are set to rise less rapidly than the total number of residents, the latter rising by 89% between 1980 and 200 and the former by only 30%. This implies a steadily declining rate of transfers to sheltered-living facilities: where in 1980 the ratio of new admissions to total residents was 1:3, on current trends it will have fallen to 1:4.5 by the end of the century. For this reason too a more rapid expansion of sheltered accommodation would appear desirable.

In 1987 accommodation costs stood at 33,921 guilders per resident per year, as against the general psychiatric hospitals' figure of 86,088 guilders. Between 1980 and 1987 costs rose by 32% in nominal and 10% in real terms; if this trend continues the annual cost per resident in 2000 will be 39,601 guilders (1987 prices), compared with 92,495 in general psychiatric hospitals. Should the expansion of capacity shown in table 4.4 take place, then the aggregate cost of sheltered accommodation in 2000 will be 175 million guilders, equivalent to just under 8% of the cost of psychiatric hospitals.

It should be noted in this connection that many general psychiatric hospitals have given over part of their capacity to forms of sheltered living, on or off site; such facilities are not included in the figures shown here.

Figure 4.4 again shows indexed data, allowing for population growth, on current trends. 100% occupancy rates are almost universal, so that capacity figures move very closely with the number of residents. Of particular note are the substantial rise in costs and the slow rate of growth of new admissions, lagging considerably behind capacity.

Figure 4.4 **Sheltered-living facilities, 1980-2000 (index, 1980 = 100)**

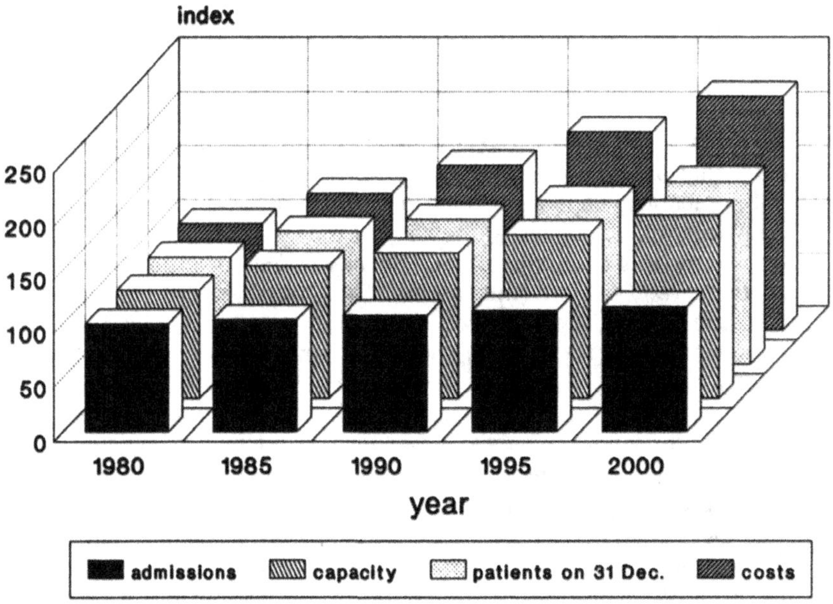

4.8 *Psychiatric day care*

In terms of intensity psychiatric day care is intermediate between intramural care and the non-residential care provided by the Regional Institutes of Ambulatory Mental Health Care (RIAGGs) and outpatient departments. Patients follow a treatment programme during the day but otherwise live at home. The day care centres normally form part of a general psychiatric hospital or psychiatric unit within a general hospital, though there are also two independent centres. Day treatment has expanded considerably over the last decade, mainly as an alternative to full-time hospitalization, and the last few years has more and more been provided on a part-time basis whereby the client is not under treatment for the whole week.

Table 4.5 **Psychiatric day care: capacity, patients and costs, 1980-2000**

	1980	**1985**	***1987***	**1990**	**1995**	**2000**
Capacity	1154	2142	*2392*	2960	3938	4959
Number of patients:						
- absolute on 31 December	910	3400	*3996*	5406	7845	10395
- per 100,000 population	6	24	*27*	36	51	66
Registrations	3500	5400	*6522*	7910	10298	12789
Costs 1	45	83	*97*			
Costs 2	54	83	*97*	112	132	144

1 = nominal costs;
2 = inflation-adjusted costs (see section 4.2 for explanation); both in millions of guilders.

The rapid expansion of psychiatric day treatment emerges clearly from table 4.4. The number of treatment places more than doubled between 1980 and 1987, and were this growth to continue almost 5000 places would be available by the end of the century; this is not very likely, however, given the national capacity norm of 20 places per 100,000 population. At current growth rates the norm would be reached in 1990, with a total of around 3000 places. In 2000 the norm would give 3134 places, far short of the extrapolated figure of almost 5000.

The number of patients is shown as rising more rapidly than the number of treatment places: this reflects the trend towards part-time day care, which allows more patients to be treated per place. Were this trend to continue there would be more than two patients for each treatment place in 2000; this is an unlikely picture, but it is difficult to see where the trend might be deflected.

The number of patients entering treatment of course also rises, albeit slightly less rapidly than the number of treatment places; i.e. on average treatment lasts longer.

The costs per treatment place of psychiatric day care have so far remained remarkably constant; indeed, the nominal rise between 1980 and 1987 of only 4% implies a real decline in unit costs of 13%. The sharp increase in capacity has of course produced a corresponding rise in total costs, and continuing growth will bring the total to 144 million guilders a year by 2000; moreover the cost per place will probably rise more quickly over the next decade than over the last, albeit no allowance is made for this factor given the uncertainty involved.

Figure 4.5 **Psychiatric day care, 1980-2000 (index, 1980 = 100)**

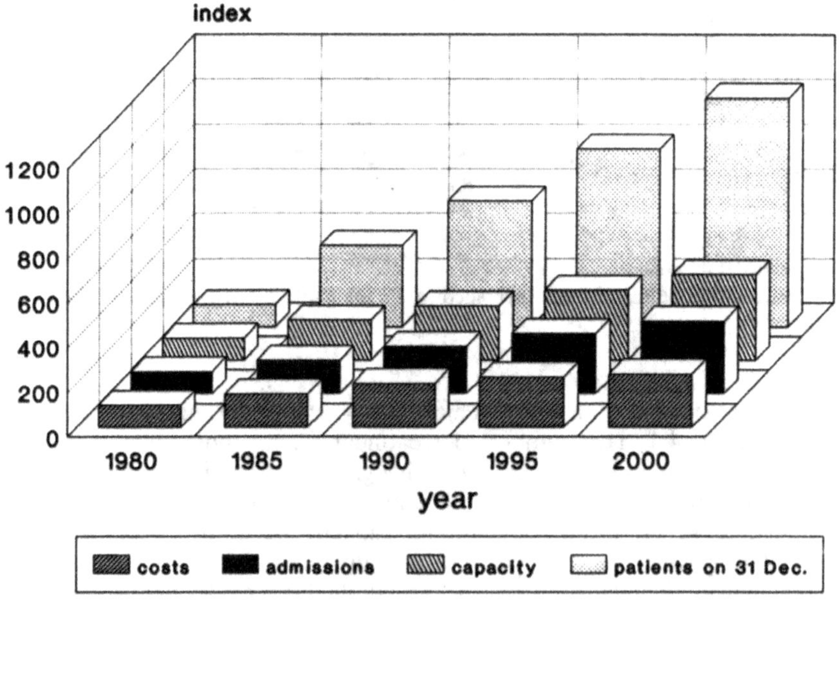

The relatively slight growth in costs, as compared with the growth in the number of patients treated, is clearly reflected in figure 4.5. Compared with other forms of care the number of patients receiving psychiatric day treatment rises much more rapidly than the other indices. The cost increase is considerably less than the growth in the number of treatment places, with the result that the unit cost declines.

4.9 *Psychogeriatric day care*

The picture for psychogeriatric day care is broadly comparable with that for psychiatric. The prevention of full-time nursing home admission is one of its main aims.

Table 4.6 **Psychogeriatric day care: capacity, patients and costs, 1980-2000**

	1980	1985	*1987*	1990	1995	2000
Capacity	642	1100	*1267*	1584	2140	2737
Number of patients:						
- absolute on 31 December	992	2237	*2535*	3318	4700	6200
- per 100,000 population*	61	129	*140*	174	230	286
Registrations	1608	2964	*3452*	4388	6040	7810
Costs 1	13	30	*35*			
Costs 2	16	30	*35*	46	67	93

* Of the population aged 65 or over.
1 = nominal costs;
2 = inflation-adjusted costs (see section 4.2 for explanation); both in millions of guilders.

Day-treatment capacity is small in relation to the total field of psychogeriatric care. The national norm of 75 places per 100,000 population was virtually reached in 1988 with 1380 places. The growing number of over-65s means that further growth is possible by the end of the century to 1630 places, considerably less than indicated by extrapolating from the trend of the 1980s.

The number of patients treated is growing faster than capacity, indicating that patients are under treatment for a steadily decreasing portion of the week. Where in 1980 there were 15 patients to every ten places, if the present trend continues there will be 23 by the year 2000.

On average patients remain in this form of care for less than a year, as indicated by the fact that the annual number of new patients is greater than the number under treatment at any one time. The average duration of treatment does however appear to be growing slightly.

The cost of psychogeriatric day care is relatively modest. In 1987 it amounted to almost 28,000 guilders per place per year, from which sum around two patients were treated; this compares with the cost of a year's stay in a nursing home, also in 1987, of 75,000 guilders for one patient. The total cost of psychogeriatric day care amounts to only 2% of that for all intramural nursing-home care; on current trends, as shown in the table, this will rise to 3.6% in 2000.

Figure 4.6 **Psychogeriatric day care, 1980-2000 (index, 1980 = 100)**

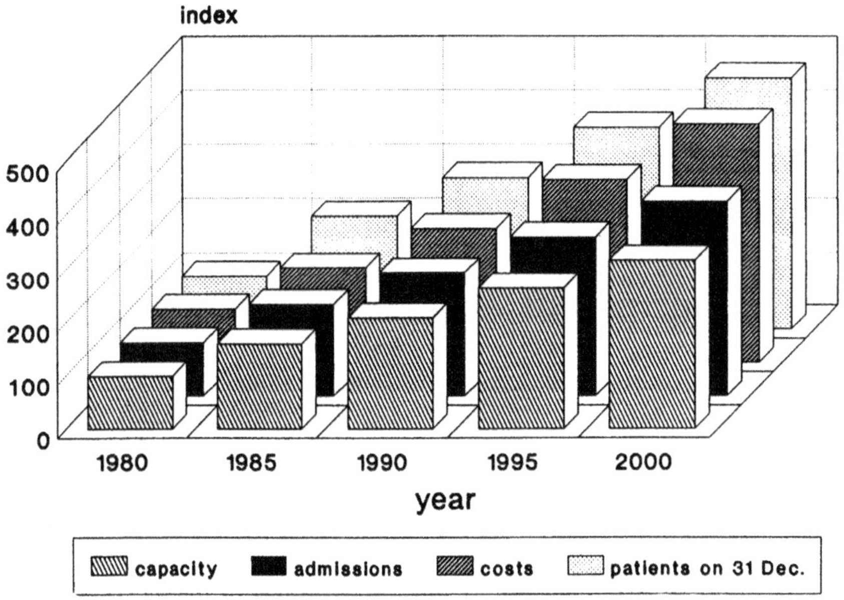

Figure 4.6, which allows for the growing population of over-65s, indicates that if current trends persist just over three times as many places will be available for every 1000 people aged 65 or over as in 1980, almost five times as many patients will receive treatment and costs will be almost six times greater.

4.10 *Regional Institutes for Ambulatory Mental Health Care ('RIAGG')*

The Regional Institutes for Ambulatory Mental Health Care (RIAGGs), which were established at the beginning of the 1980s from the merger of a range of bodies concerned with particular aspects of this field, are responsible for extramural care for all age groups in their area. The majority of the 57 RIAGGs currently in existence have separate sections for children and adolescents, adults and the elderly; some operate field teams; they also have a preventive function and provide a service to other agencies. They are funded under the Exceptional Medical Expenses Act (AWBZ); the system is one of devolved budgets, locally managed.

Since the RIAGGs' role is to provide extramural care, staffing levels are the best indicator of their scale of operations.

The RIAGGs have experienced a period of catching-up growth: their total staff (full-time equivalent) was almost one-and-a-half times greater in 1988 than in 1980, and should this trend continue it will more than double over the period 1980-2000. Even then their number will still be less than a quarter of the total currently employed in psychiatric hospitals (and only 2.5% of the total working in health care).

The number of clients receiving treatment at any one time grew very rapidly in the first half of the 1980s, even despite the problem of lengthening waiting-lists at some RIAGGs. Extrapolating the figures produces a total of 295,000 clients by the end of the century; this would be equivalent to 19 per 1000 population as against just over 11 per 1000 in 1988.

The number of new clients is rising faster than the number receiving treatment at any one time. If this trend persists 333,000 new clients will enter treatment in the year 2000.

The costs of care have been extrapolated mainly on the basis of the growth in staff and assuming the ratio of overall costs to staff numbers to remain the same as in 1987. This gives a total in 2000 of 684 million guilders, equivalent to almost a third of the cost of psychiatric hospitals in that same year; in 1988, for the sake of comparison, the cost of RIAGGs care amounted to 22% of that provided in psychiatric hospitals.

Table 4.7 **Regional Institutes for Ambulatory Mental Health Care: staff, clients and costs, 1980-2000**

	1980	1985	*1987*	1990	1995	2000
Staff	3090	3915	*4218*	4741	5630	6560
Number of clients						
- absolute ('000)[2] on 31 December	117	149	*161*	185	234	295
- per 100,000 population	8	10	*11*	12	15	19
New clients ('000)	121	157	*177*	204	261	333
Costs 1	308	389	*440*			
Costs 2	369	387	*440*	495	588	684

1 = nominal costs;
2 = inflation-adjusted costs (see section 4.2 for explanation); both in millions of guilders.

As figure 4.7 shows, the number of clients receiving treatment from RIAGGs per 1000 population will on current trends more than double between 1980 and 2000, with the number of new clients entering treatment rising more quickly still. Cost per inhabitant will increase by 66% over the same period.

[2] The change from counting 'client systems' (e.g. client plus immediate family) to counting individual clients made at the beginning of 1986 means that the data relating to the periods before and after that year are not comparable. What we have done is to redefine the pre-1986 data by assuming the growth in terms of client systems over the period 1980-85 to have persisted from 1985 to 1986, comparing the actual number of individual clients in 1986 with the number of client systems so predicted and thereafter translating the numbers of clients systems for the earlier period into individuals. It is these figures that appear in table 4.7.

Figure 4.7 **Regional Institutes for Ambulatory Mental Health Care: 1980-2000 (index, 1980 = 100)**

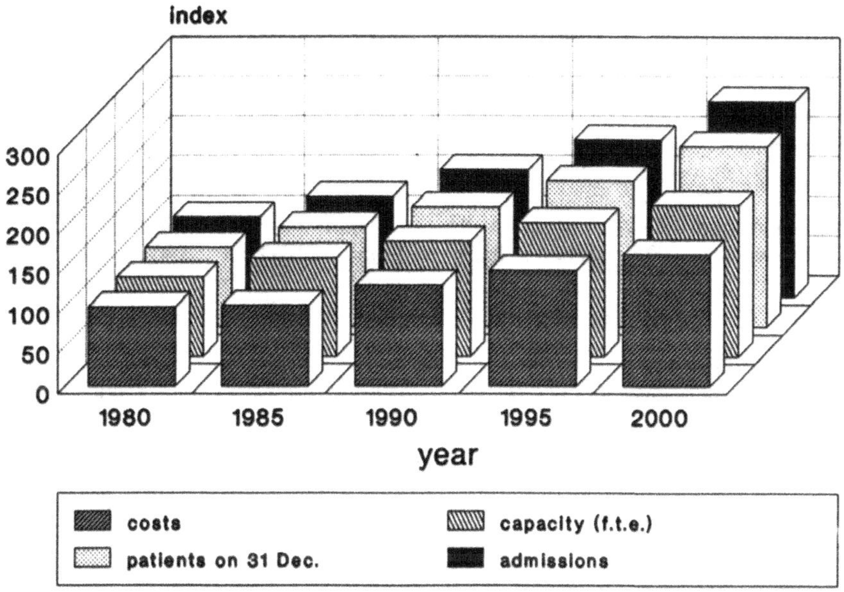

4.11 *Outpatient Clinics for Alcohol and Drug Abuse ('CAD')*

The Outpatient Alcohol and Drug Abuse Clinics (CADs) provide extramural help for addicts. There are seventeen Clinics, each with local branches. Data on the help provided have only been collected on a nationally uniform basis since 1987; the statistics for earlier years are not always equally reliable.

Hitherto the CADs have been funded from the National Budget but municipal authorities are due to take over this function in the near future. The uncertainty this involves erodes the significance of extrapolations, especially as the CADs experienced rapid growth in the period to 1985 (with the reservation that the statistics are not necessarily reliable) but have since shown an entirely stable picture in terms of staff, clients and costs. The extrapolation technique applied takes the average between the initially high rate of growth and the subsequent stabilization, producing a moderate rate of growth in the future. As in the case of the Regional Institutes of Ambulatory Mental Health Care the unit cost of staff is assumed to remain constant.

Table 4.8 **Outpatient Clinics for Alcohol and Drug Abuse: staff, patients and costs, 1980-2000**

	1980	1985	*1987*	1990	1995	2000
Staff	585	894	*927*	1085	1355	1636
Number of clients						
- absolute ('000) on 31 December	21000	24000	*24100*	26000	28000	31000
- per 100,000 population	15	17	*16*	17	18	19
New clients ('000)	11500	20000	*18500*	22000	27000	33000
Costs 1	45	72	72			
Costs 2	54	72	72	84	105	127

1 = nominal costs;
2 = inflation-adjusted costs (see section 4.2 for explanation); both in millions of guilders.

The number of CAD clients shows an increase, albeit a less sharp one than in the case of the RIAGGs. Particularly striking is the rise in numbers of new clients: if present trends continue three times as many new addicts will begin receiving treatment in 2000 as in 1980. The costs of this form of care for addicts (various other agencies also provide such care) increased from 45 to 72 million guilders between 1980 and 1985, virtually stabilizing thereafter. Noteworthy too is the fact that in *nominal* terms total costs (not just staff costs) per staff member in 1987 were practically the same in 1987 as in 1980 at 77,000 guilders; adjusting for inflation this represents a fall in unit staff costs from 92,000 guilders in 1980 to 78,000 in 1987. If the CADs' growth over the period 1980-87 were to continue through the 1990s the total cost in 2000 would be 127 million guilders, almost two-and-a-half times more than in 1980.

Figure 4.8 **Outpatient Clinics for Alcohol and Drug Abuse, 1980-2000 (index, 1980 = 100)**

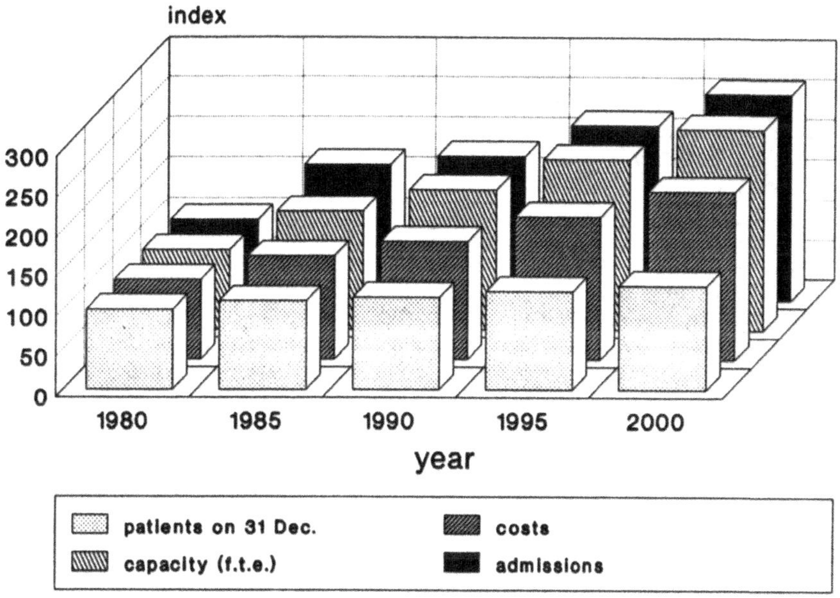

The data displayed in indexed form in figure 4.8, which allow for population growth, show the numbers of staff and of new clients rising most rapidly, followed by costs, with the number of clients receiving treatment at any one time increasing only slightly.

4.12 *Shifts within the mental health care sector, 1980-2000*

The trends and extrapolations for the various institutional categories set out in preceding sections indicate major shifts within the overall field of mental health care. This section brings out these shifts under four headings: capacity; the number of new patients/clients entering treatment per year; the number of patients/clients receiving treatment as at 31 December of each year; and costs. The changes are shown in both absolute and relative terms.

Table 4.9 **Sectoral capacity, 1980-2000**

	1980		**1990**		**2000**		**80-90**	**80-2000**
Sector	**Abs.**	**%**	**Abs.**	**%**	**Abs.**	**%**	**%**	**%**
Psychiatric hospitals	24690	46	24530	38	24230	31	-1	-2
Psychiatric units of general hospitals (PAAZ)	2620	5	2340	4	2050	3	-11	-22
Psychogeriatric nursing homes	18740	35	24840	38	31300	40	+33	+67
Sheltered living	2330	4	3320	5	4410	6	+42	+89
Psychiatric day care	1150	2	2960	5	4960	6	+140	+331
Psychogeriatric day care	640	1	1580	2	2740	4	+147	+328
RIAGG's	3090	6	4740	7	6560	8	+53	+112
CAD's	585	1	1085	2	1640	2	+85	+180
Total	**53845**	**100**	**65395**	**100**	**77890**	**100**	**+21**	**+45**

The capacities shown in table 4.9 are in terms of beds for the intramural institutions, of treatment places for day-treatment provision and of staff numbers (fte) for the extramural sector. While this last parameter is of course not directly comparable with the first two, its inclusion with them in the same table can in some degree be justified by the fact that in the intramural sector the ratio of beds to staff members is roughly one to one.

Total mental health care capacity is shown as increasing by 21% between 1980 and 1990, while the extrapolation to 2000 shows a total increase over the last two decades of the century of 45%. One quarter of that increase is needed to keep pace with population growth and a further quarter or more to cope with an aging population. The trends thus indicate real growth in mental health care capacity per 'weighted inhabitant' of just over 20% in twenty years, or one percent a year.

Figure 4.9 **Percentage capacity distribution in 1980, 1987 and 2000**

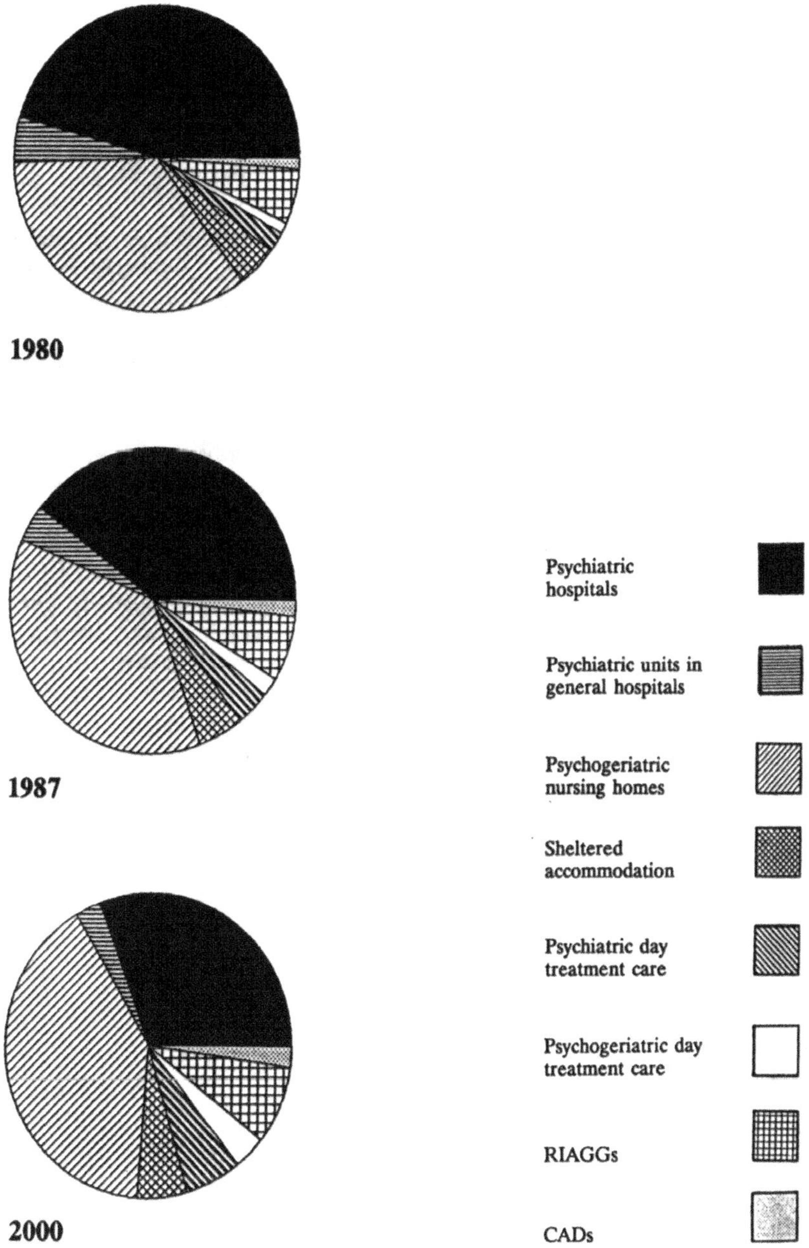

The proportion of capacity devoted to psychogeriatric care (intramural and semi-intramural) in 1980 was 36%; by 2000 it will have risen to 44%.

Outside the psychogeriatric field we see a substantial shift from intramural to semi-intramural and extramural forms of care, with the proportion of intramural care falling relatively gradually from 51% in 1980 to 34% in 2000; the share of semi-intramural care will rise from 6% to 12% and that of extramural care from 7% to 10% over the same period.

These trends notwithstanding, the major part of mental health care, at least in capacity terms, will continue to be delivered by the intramural sector, which will account for 74% of psychiatric capacity.

As previous sections showed, the number of patients/clients entering treatment in any one year is growing dramatically. If the 60% increase which occurred between 1980 and 1990 represents a continuing trend, the last two decades of the century will witness a much-more-than-doubling of the total. The RIAGGs account for the lion's share (77%) of the growth. It is emphasized that this rapid rise in the number of new registrations does not mean that the total number of patients/clients is increasing equally rapidly, since in many cases the individuals concerned are patients who have already been receiving mental health care, of varying degrees of intensity, for many years. The growth in registrations partly reflects the desire to avoid hospitalization wherever possible and to strengthen community care: where hospital stays are long new registration rates are low. Definitional changes in patient registers also play a part, which cannot be precisely determined, in the increase in the numbers entering treatment.

Table 4.10 **New registrations, 1980-2000**

	1980		**1990**		**2000**		**80-90**	**80-2000**
Sector	**Abs.**	**%**	**Abs.**	**%**	**Abs.**	**%**	**%**	**%**
Psychiatric hospitals	26490	14	38210	12	51090	11	+44	+93
Psychiatric units of general hospitals (PAAZ)	20100	10	17600	6	14800	2	-12	-26
Psychogeriatric nursing homes	8680	4	11390	4	14230	3	+31	+64
Sheltered accommodation	750	(0)	850	(0)	970	(0)	+13	+29
Psychiatric day care	3500	2	7910	3	12790	3	+126	+265
Psychogeriatric day care	1610	1	4390	1	7810	2	+173	+385
RIAGGs	121000	63	204000	67	333000	71	+69	+175
CADs	11500	6	21700	7	33000	7	+89	+187
Total	**193630**	**100**	**306050**	**100**	**467690**	**100**	**+58**	**+142**

The figures shown in table 4.10 need amplifying and correcting on two points. First, they do not include patients treated in the outpatient departments of general psychiatric hospitals or of psychiatric units in general hospitals; in 1987, according to the production agreements reached, there were some 70,000 people in this group, increasing the total by a quarter. Second, it is not known with any accuracy how many patients are treated by more than one institution in the course of a year, so that the totals shown should not be interpreted as actual numbers of people.

Figure 4.10 **Percentage distribution of new registrations in 1980, 1987 and 2000**

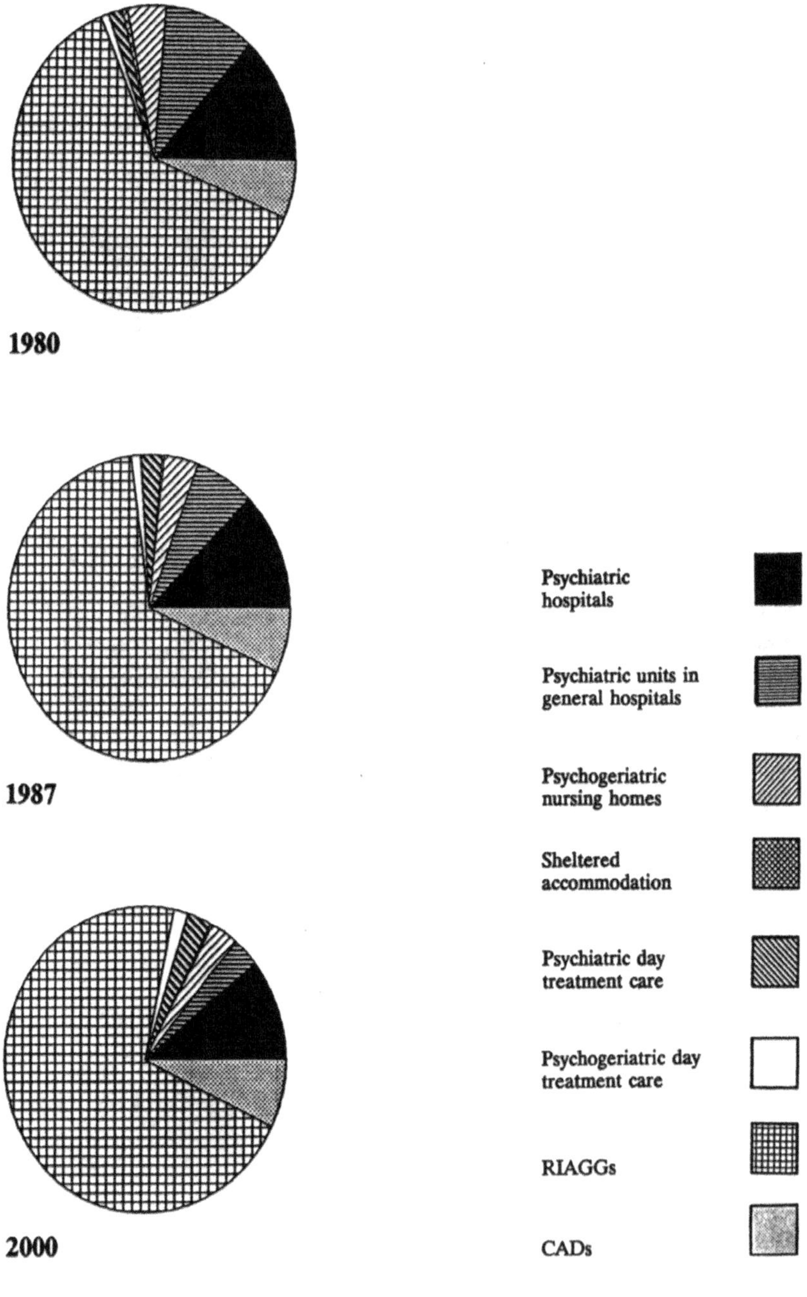

What particularly emerges from figure 4.10 is the steadily declining share of the intramural sector (general psychiatric hospitals and psychiatric units in general hospitals and nursing homes): in 1980 the intramural sector accounted for 28% of all new registrations, falling to 24% in 1987 and, on current trends, 17% in 2000.

Table 4.11 shows the numbers of patients/clients receiving treatment at the end of each year. The relative shares and shifts which emerge coincide closely with those relating to capacity in the case of intramural care.

Table 4.11 **Patients/clients receiving treatment at 31 December of each year, 1980-2000**

Sector	1980 Abs.	%	1990 Abs.	%	2000 Abs.	%	80-90 %	80-2000 %
Psychiatric hospitals	23146	13	23608	9	24008	6	+2	+4
Psychiatric units in general hospitals (PAAZ)	2359	1	2010	1	1750	(0)	-11	-26
Psychogeriatric nursing homes	18000	10	25037	9	32735	8	+39	+82
Sheltered accommodation	2310	1	3290	1	4370	1	+42	+89
Psychiatric day care	910	(0)	5406	2	10395	3	+494	+1042
Psychogeriatric day care	992	1	3318	1	6200	2	+234	+525
RIAGGs	117000	63	185000	68	295000	73	+58	+152
CADs	21000	11	26000	9	31000	8	+24	+48
Total	**185717**	**100**	**273669**	**100**	**405458**	**100**	**+47**	**+118**
Per 1000 pop.	**13.2**		**18.4**		**25.8**		**+39**	**+95**

In the case of extramural and semi-intramural care the picture which emerges is a very different one, marked as it is by very rapid growth. This applies notably to the care provided by the RIAGGs, which shows an increase (including an element of forecast) of 58% between 1980 and 1990; indeed, very recent data indicate that the forecast for the number of RIAGG clients in 1990 (181,000) had already been virtually reached in 1988. On 31 December 1988 just over twelve in every thousand people in the Netherlands were receiving RIAGG treatment, compared with just over eight in 1980, and if this trend persists the figure will reach almost nineteen per thousand in 2000. In terms of numbers of patients/clients receiving treatment there is no significant substitution of semi-intramural or extramural for intramural care; all that we see is a relatively slight shift from general psychiatric hospitals and the psychiatric units of general hospitals to sheltered-living facilities. Per 100,000 population there were in 1980 164 patients in general psychiatric hospitals, 17 in general-hospital psychiatric units and 16 in sheltered accommodation; the corresponding figures for 1990 are 159 (-5), 13 (-4) and 22 (+36). The number receiving psychiatric day treatment shows an increase from six people in 100,000 to 36 (+30). In other words, the increase in the number of people in sheltered accommodation or receiving psychiatric day treatment is much greater (+36 per 100,000 population) than the fall in the number receiving intramural psychiatric care (-9 per 100,000). This is on top of the enormous growth in ambulatory care.[3]

If the total growth between 1980 and 1990 in the number of people receiving treatment (adjusted to allow for population growth) is taken as 100, the distribution of that 100 among the various institutions is as follows. Psychiatric hospitals and psychiatric units in general hospitals show a growth of -1, sheltered accommodation +1, day treatment 6, psychogeriatric nursing homes 8 and psychogeriatric day treatment 3; the RIAGGs account for no less than 79 of the total growth of 100, and the Outpatient Alcohol and Drug Abuse Clinics for 5.

A significant observation is that 'only' 11% of the growth in the number of people receiving mental health care relates to psychogeriatric care (excluding the RIAGGs' departments for the care of the elderly).

The overall conclusion is that in 1980 13.2 per 1000 population were mental health care clients, that the figure will have risen to at least 18.4 in 1990 and that, if the trend persists, by the end of the century the figure will have reached 25.8.

[3] A proviso must be entered at this point. The increased utilization of services with which we are here concerned can only be charted accurately with the help of a case register which permits the elimination of double counting. The two case registers which exist in the Netherlands present problems in precisely this regard, the Assen register *inter alia* because the inclusion of RIAGG data after 1981 ran into technical problems and the Maastricht register because the RIAGG for the area was one of the very few in the country to have to cut staff in the 1980s, with the result that the number of RIAGG clients fell there (and almost nowhere else) after 1984.

Figure 4.11 **Percentage distribution of patients/clients receiving treatment as at 31 December in 1980, 1987 and 2000**

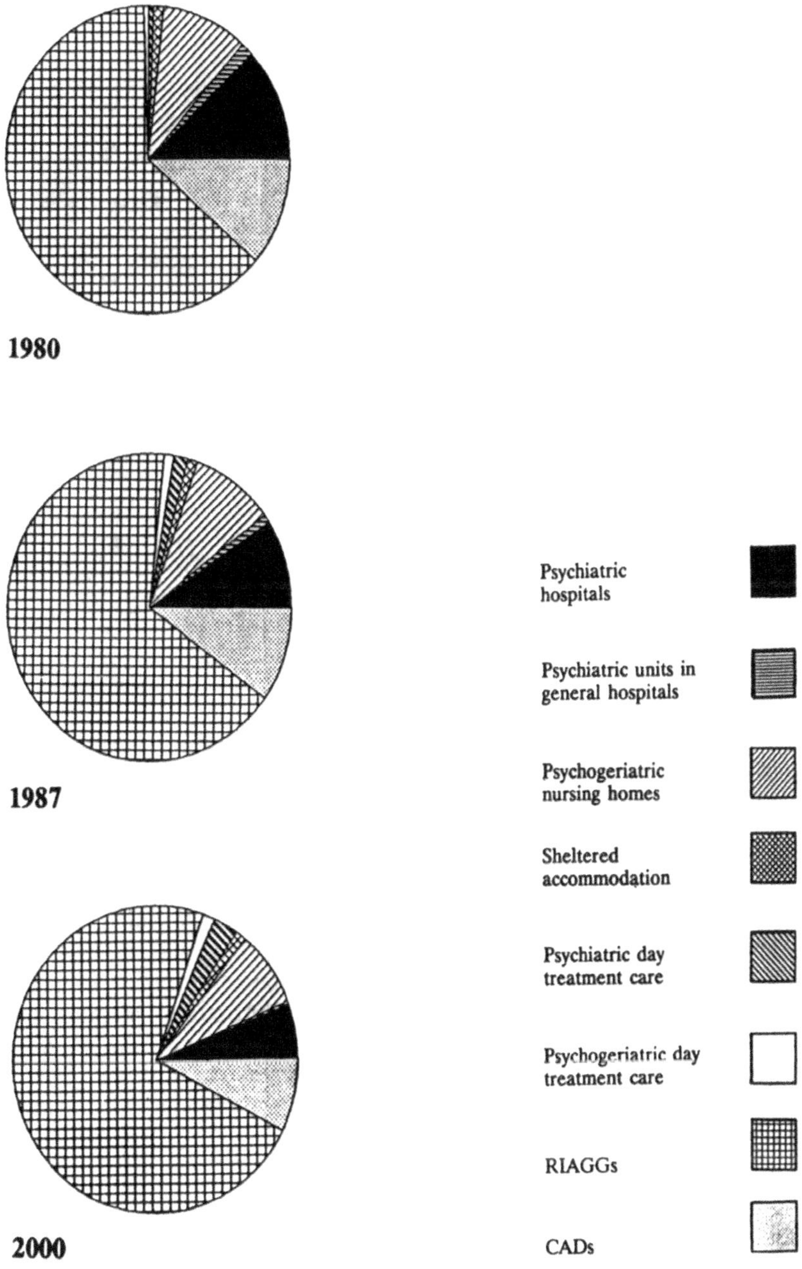

The cost of mental health care shows an increase of 25% between 1980 and 1990 and of 54% between 1980 and 2000 (constant 1987 prices).

Table 4.12 **Costs of mental health care, 1980-2000 (in millions of guilders at constant 1987 prices)**

Sector	1980 Abs.	%	1990 Abs.	%	2000 Abs.	%	80-90 %	80-2000 %
Psychiatric hospitals	1892	48	2074	42	2241	38	+10	+18
Psychiatric units in general hospitals (PAAZ)	211	5	208	4	199	3	-1	-6
Psychogeriatric nursing homes	1309	33	1846	37	2464	40	+41	+88
Sheltered accommodation	72	2	117	2	175	3	+62	+143
Psychiatric day care	1309	1	112	2	144	2	+107	+167
Psychogeriatric day care	16	(0)	46	1	93	2	+187	+481
RIAGGs	369	9	495	10	684	11	+34	+85
CADs	54	1	84	2	127	2	+55	+135
Total	**3977**	**100**	**4982**	**100**	**6127**	**100**	**+25**	**+54**

As indicated in this chapter's introduction, the figures shown are adjusted for inflation and expressed in terms of 1987 prices.

The annual rate of cost increase for mental health care as a whole over the period 1980-2000 is 2.7%; psychogeriatric nursing accounts for 54% of the total increase and psychogeriatric day treatment for a further 4%, so that over half increase is due to the increasing population of the elderly. Within the remaining 42% (equivalent to a 1.1% annual rate of increase), the psychiatric hospitals account for 16%, the RIAGGs for 15%, psychiatric day treatment for 4%, sheltered-living provision for 5% and the Outpatient Alcohol and Drug Abuse Clinics (CADs) for 3% (these figures add up to more than 42% because the declining costs of psychiatric units in general hospitals bring down the total slightly). In a period of two decades these are relatively modest shifts.

Figure 4.12 **Costs of mental health care in 1980, 1987 and 2000**

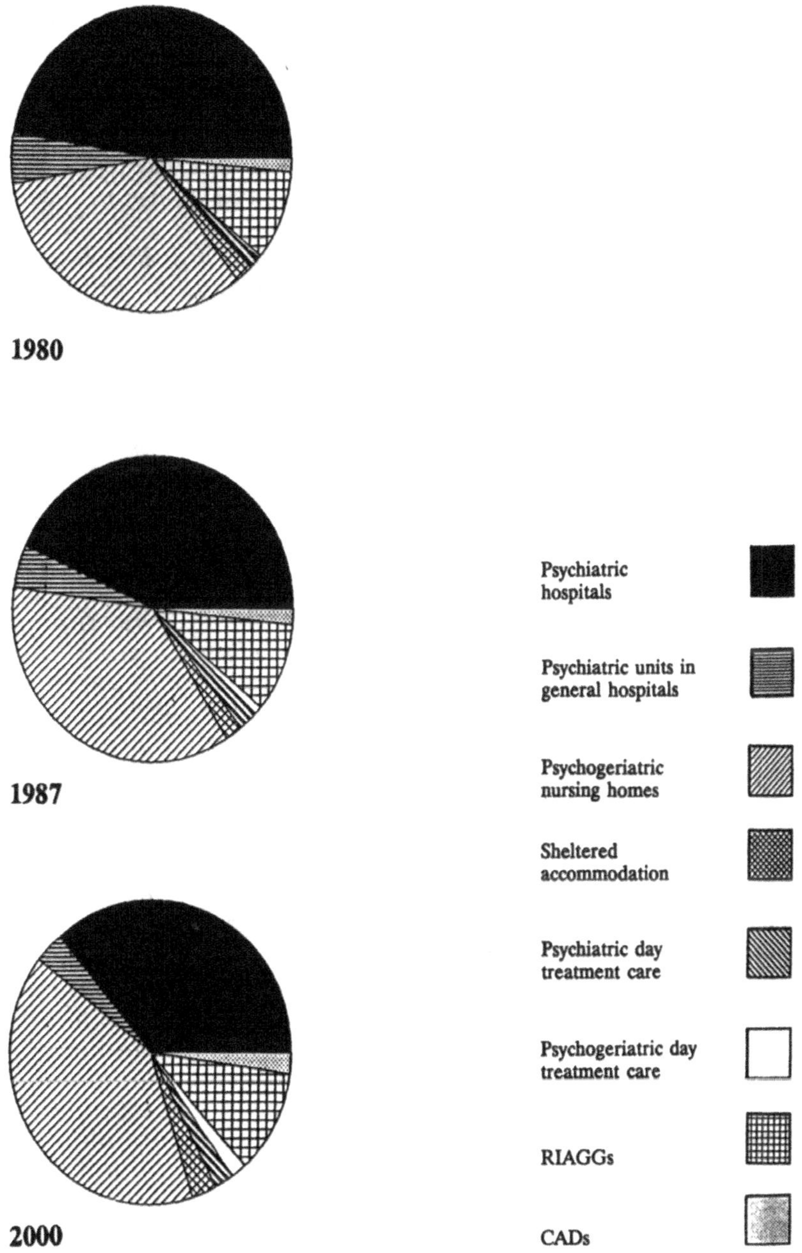

In relative terms the general picture is one of a sharp growth in psychogeriatric costs and an almost equally sharp fall in the costs of psychiatric hospitals in the context of mental health care costs as a whole. The 33% of all mental health care costs for which psychogeriatric nursing and day treatment accounted in 1980 is set to rise to 42% of the - by then much larger - total in 2000; the share of psychiatric-hospital treatment in total costs will fall from 48% to 38% over the same period. Other cost shifts are comparatively minor; the RIAGGs' share rises from 9% to 11% over the whole period, only a small increase.

All in all, if current trends are maintained there will have been in cost terms only a modest substitution of extramural and semi-intramural for intramural treatment and care by the end of the century: in 1980 the psychiatric hospitals accounted for three quarters of all mental health care costs (excluding all forms of psychogeriatric care), and in 2000 the proportion will have declined only to two thirds.

4.13 *Some conclusions*

The general picture which emerges from the data is one of continuing expansion of mental health services. More and more people in the Netherlands are making use of such services and their capacity and costs are steadily rising. Devolved budgets, locally managed, have gradually been introduced in mental health care in the course of the 1980s and the government has introduced gradually tightening capacity norms. These two factors have somewhat moderated the rate of growth, which was generally greater at the beginning of the 1980s than in recent years. The broad pattern of change is in keeping with 1980s government policy, which has been to strengthen extramural and semi-intramural care while curtailing intramural care. We see forms of day treatment expanding very rapidly, the expansion of sheltered-living provision getting under way and the extramural sector showing clear growth.

At the same time the extent of intramural psychiatric care (adjusted to take account of population growth) is gradually declining. Mental health care as a whole continues to expand substantially, however, and this is counter to government policy.

Government attempts to moderate and direct the expansion of services have regularly prompted sharp criticism from the field. Psychogeriatric nursing homes are said to be full, acute admissions to general psychiatric hospitals to be impossible because wards are full (leaving a growing number of mental patients to wander the streets), many RIAGGs to be unable to cut their waiting-lists despite financial and staff growth and increasingly strict and selective policies on the acceptance of clients, and so on. In other words, mental health needs are continuing to put pressure on the system, which in practice generally responds by accommodating it (albeit sometimes with a delay), and the result is ongoing growth. This raises the underlying question: where does that growth come from? Unfortunately no-one yet has the answer. Among the hypotheses currently circulating the most important are these:

- mental health problems are increasingly seen as treatable problems,
- people are increasingly unable to deal with their own mental health problems,
- mental health problems are decreasingly accepted as 'just part of life',
- developments in society are tending to give rise to mental health problems,
- the position in which some individuals and groups find themselves in our society makes it increasingly difficult for them to cope with mental health problems.

There may well be a kernel of truth in these and other possible hypotheses but it is very difficult to determine empirically what the true position is (and even where it can be done it has generally not been). The above hypotheses are considered at some length in the concluding chapter of this report.

At the moment only the following can be determined with a reasonable measure of certainty.

1. The continuing pressure on mental health services is a reality for both patients/clients and professionals and is thus also a reality in terms of its consequences.
2. The growing utilization of services can only partly be explained (notably by reference to population growth and the growing numbers of the elderly and very elderly).
3. Only a very modest proportion (10-20%) of all the mental health problems which occur are treated by specialists, indicating that that growing pressure on services does not necessarily have any implications regarding a possible (and often assumed) increase in mental health problems.

5 Dementia

Part I Baseline analysis

5.1 *Characterization*

The term 'dementia' encompasses a wide range of disorders. It is not itself a disease but a complex of symptoms which may be due to various underlying diseases or intoxications. 'Dementia syndrome' is therefore a better term than just 'dementia', but for brevity's sake the latter will often be used in this background analysis.

Dementia, which accounts for around 50% of mental disorders in the elderly (Henderson 1986), is characterized by (APA 1987) cognitive disorders such as disorders of memory (notably for recent events), learning, judgement, orientation, use of language, body awareness and abstract thought, albeit without a clouding of consciousness; there may also be affective disorders and personality changes, such as emotional lability, self-neglect, a reduced ability to control impulses and a lost awareness of appropriate behaviour. The condition is chronic, with the number and severity of symptoms generally showing a gradual increase over time. Depressive symptoms, paranoid symptoms (suspicion) and anxiety may occur initially as a reaction to the cognitive functions' deterioration, of which the patient is at this time still aware. That deterioriation gradually develops into an inability to function socially and carry out everyday tasks.

Dementia syndrome is an organic psychosyndrome, the mental changes it involves being associated with organic changes in the brain such as degeneration, damage and/or the loss of brain tissue or with changes elsewhere in the body which affect brain function.

Dementia can have several dozen causes. Of these the most important are Alzheimer's disease, accounting for 50-60% of cases, and cerebrovascular disorders (as in the case of multi-infarct dementia), accounting for a further 20% (Katzman 1986; Tanja & Hofman 1985). Other conditions of the brain (such as tumors or brain damage) and conditions elsewhere in the body which affect brain function may also produce a dementia syndrome: in some 13% of cases, for example, there is intoxication by medications or alcohol (Gilleard 1984; Tanja & Hofman 1985). Other causes are metabolic disorders and infections.

Table 5.1 reviews causes of dementia (Health Council (Gezondheidsraad) 1988; Frederiks 1985; Van den Bosch 1988).

Table 5.1 **Causes of dementia**

Category	*Example/note*
- Degenerative brain conditions	Pick's disease: senile dementia of the Alzheimer type (in the over-65s)
- Cerebrovascular accident	Multi-infarct dementia
- Combinations of the above	Probably frequent
- Intoxication	Medications, alcohol (Korsakoff's syndrome), metals, industrial chemicals
- Metabolic/endocrine disorders	Vitamin-B12 deficiency, functional disorders of the liver and kidneys, hypothyreoidism, hypoglycemia
- Infectious diseases	Neurosyphilis, AIDS, meningitis, Creutzfeldt-Jacob disease
- Inflammatory	Vasculitis
- Post-traumatic and post-anoxic	Following operations
- Genetic	Huntington's disease
- Degenerative	Parkinson's disease
- Brain tumors	Meningioma
- Chronic subdural hematoma	Possible without obvious trauma
- Hydrocephalus	At normal pressure

The chances of recovering from dementia or of preventing further deterioriation depend on the treatability of the underlying cause. Treatable causes include most notably intoxications, metabolic disorders, endocrine disorders and certain infections; chronic subdural hematoma, normal-pressure hydrocephalus and certain tumors are amenable to surgery. A dementia syndrome whose cause is treatable is said to be reversible; such cases are put at no more than 10% of the total (Gezondheidsraad (Health Council) 1988). In the vast majority of cases, however, treatment is either impossible or can at most slow the progress of the disease or improve patients' condition or functioning without producing recovery (Fredericks 1985; Gezondheidsraad (Health Council) 1988).

5.2 *Occurrence of dementia*

5.2.1 *Incidence*

As yet no epidemiological study has been carried out in the Netherlands to determine the incidence, course and prevalence of dementia. Data on *incidence* - the number of new cases appearing annually in the population - are to be found only in foreign literature and are scarce even then.

Mortimer *et al.* (1981) report an annual incidence of senile dementia (Alzheimer type) and cerebrovascular dementia in an open population of 1.4% in persons aged over 65. If this is also true for the Netherlands it means that there will be over 27,000 new cases in 1990, rising to around 35,000 in 2010.

The well-known Swedish Lundby study (Hagnell *et al.* 1983) distinguishes senile (Alzheimer-type) and multi-infarct (cerebrovascular) dementia, which together account for most cases of the syndrome. For each ten-year age group this study reports the following incidence figures for the severe and moderate forms (mild forms are here left out of account).

Table 5.2 **Annual incidence of severe and moderate forms of senile and multi-infarct dementia by age group and sex (% of the age group concerned) (Source: Hagnell *et al.* 1983)**

Senile dementia			**Multi-infarct dementia**		
Age group	**m**	**f**	**Age group**	**m**	**f**
60-69	0.5	1.7	60-69	3.2	0.4
70-79	6.8	4.3	70-79	4.3	11.6
80-89	15.4	17.3	80-89	15.0	8.9
Cumulative risk (%) to age of 9	21.5	22.2	Cumulative risk (%) to age of 90	21.5	19.8

In both men and women incidence rises very sharply with age, it being estimated that one in five of those who reach the age of 80 in good health will thereafter develop severe dementia (Mortimer *et al.* 1981; Schluss *et al.* 1981; Hagnell *et al.* 1983; WHO 1986). Of importance in the present context is the fact that in most cases persons with severe dementia require continuous and full care. As table 5.2 shows, the cumulative lifetime risk of developing dementia is also more than 20%.

The literature is divided with regard to overall incidence and prevalence differences between men and women, with some studies finding little or no difference, others indicating higher incidence and prevalence among women and yet others - notably from Scandinavia -

pointing to higher prevalence among men (this may be due to the effects of alcoholism, which has a significant impact on the psychiatric picture in the countries concerned) (Ineichen 1987). For the two commonest forms - senile dementia Alzheimer-type (SDAT) and cerebrovascular dementia - Kay and Bergman (1980) found that:

- under the age of 75 cerebrovascular dementia is commoner than SDAT among men and both are rare among women;
- over the age of 75 SDAT is as common as or commoner than cerebrovascular dementia in both sexes;
- SDAT is a disease which normally affects the over 75s; for women this is also true of cerebrovascular dementia, but it can occur earlier than that in men.

A number of the less common forms of dementia - the presenile dementias - can occur at an earlier age: the high-risk age for Huntington's disease, for example, is 35-40 (Matsuyama & Jarvik 1980). Other early-onset forms are Pick's disease, Creutzfeldt-Jacob disease, Korsakoff's disease and Alzheimer's disease. Post-traumatic dementia, e.g. resulting from brain damage sustained in road accidents, can occur at any age.

Socio-economic factors. Little research has been conducted specifically into possible links between social class or socio-economic circumstances and the development of dementia, and such results as are available are not unambiguous. Kay *et al.* (1964, 1970) found no link; Gurland (1981) and Weisman *et al.* (1985), in contrast, found the highest prevalence rates to be associated with the lowest levels of education. Hagnell *et al.* (1981) noted a fall in prevalence over a period of 25 years in Lundby (Sweden), inclining to ascribe this change to improvements in old people's nutrition, social conditions and physical health in that time.

Urbanization. Most dementia studies have been carried out in urban areas, and such research as has been conducted in both rural and urban areas has produced widely differing results (Ineichen 1987). No data are available on differences, if any, in the occurrence of dementia in rural and urban areas in the Netherlands.

5.2.2 *Course*

The course of a dementia syndrome depends on the treatability of the underlying cause. The non-reversible syndromes (90% of cases) generally show a gradual deterioration over the years, sometimes in stages, but the picture can remain stable for long periods. The duration of the condition ranges from a few months to twenty years or more (Diesfeldt *et al.* 1986). Its course is affected among other things by intercurrent diseases, of which the risk is greater than is normal at the same age.

The life expectancy of patients with a dementia syndrome is less than that of their contemporaries, particularly in the case of those in whom the syndrome appears relatively early (before the age of 75) (Gilleard 1984; Ineichen 1987). Tanja and Hofman (1985) cite research indicating that the life expectancy of senile dements averages 2.6 years as against 7.8 years for healthy people of the same age. Boelen and Zwanikken (1975) report that senile dementia leads to death within an average of five years. In their Dutch study Diesfeldt *et al.* found that on average around five years elapsed between the appearance of the first symptoms and the time when admission and continuous care become necessary, and a further 2.5 years between that time and death (in many cases due to a concomitant illness) (Diesfeldt *et al.* 1986). Given the difficulty of diagnosis (which is often retrospective) it is not surprising that different studies have found varying life expectancies for dementing patients.

5.2.3 *Prevalence*

The STG-study of health and aging (STG 1985) calculated on the basis of foreign literature (data from Kay & Bergmann 1980) that the number of severely and moderately severely dementing persons amounted to 6.9% of the population of over-65s (6.4% among men and 7.3% among women). 'Severe and moderate dementia' refers to the stage at which sufferers are unable to care for themselves and therefore need continuous help from other people. More recent literature indicates, however, that these estimates are too high (Ineichen 1987; Preston 1986).

When studying epidemiological literature it is important to check that the results from different studies can genuinely be related to one another. This means among other things that the age classifications of the populations studied do not differ, that the same diagnostic criteria are applied, that the populations studied are comparable (in terms of where they live, whether at home or in an institution) and that the same measure of prevalence or incidence (e.g. point prevalence or one-year prevalence) is used.

In his review article Ineichen (1987) gives the following point-prevalence rates. Table 5.3 shows the results of recent studies of dementia *without regard to the severity* of the condition, while table 5.4 is based on recent studies in which *severe* forms of the dementia syndrome were distinguished.

Table 5.3 **Studies of the overall prevalence of dementia**

Author	Date of publication	Country	Age group	Size of populat. investi-gated	Preva-lence %
Sternberg & Gavrilova	1978	USSR	60+	1020	24.6
Weissman et al.	1985	USA	65+	2588	16.1
T. Helgason	1973	Iceland	74-76	2462	11.9
Cooper & Sosna	1983	W. Germany	65+	519	11.4
Gilmore	1977	Scotland	65+	300	9.3
Kay et al.	1970	England	65+	758	8.8
Maule et al.	1984	Scotland	62-90	487	8.6
Gruer	1975	Scotland	65+	762	8.3
Broe et al.	1976	Scotland	65+	808	8.1
Campbell et al.	1983	New Zealand	65+	559	7.7
Weyerer	1983	W. Germany	65+	295	7.5
Gurland et al.	1983	USA	65+	445	5.8
Shibayama et al.	1986	Japan	65+	3106	5.8
Nilsson	1983	Sweden	70	404	5.2
Bollerup	1975	Denmark	70	619	5.0
Shinfuku et al.	1984	Japan	65+	9218	4.5
Clarke et al.	1986	England	75+	1203	4.5
Persson	1980	England	70	392	4.3
Bergmann et al.	1979	England	65+	800	3.1
Gurland et al.	1983	England	65+	396	2.5

Source: Ineichen 1987.

Table 5.4 **Studies of the prevalence of severe dementia**

Author	Date of publication	Location	Age group	Size of population investigated	Type of population	Prevalence of severe dementia (%)
Weyerer	1983	Bavaria	65+	295	Whole community	7.5
Kay *et al.*	1964	Newcastle	65+	758	Living at home	6.2
Cooper & Sosna	1983	Mannheim	65+	519	City districts	6.0
Gurland *et al.*	1983	New York	65+	445	Living at home	5.8
Shinfuku *et al.*	1984	Tokyo	65+	9218	Various samples	4.5
Clarke *et al.*	1984	Melton Mowbray	75+	1203	Whole community	4.5
Broe *et al.*	1976	Glasgow & Kilsyth	65+	808	Living at home	3.8
T. Helgason	1973	Iceland	74-76	2642	Whole community	3.6
Sternberg & Gavrilova	1978	USSR	60+	1020	Not indicated	3.6
Weissman *et al.*	1985	USA	65+	2588	Living at home	3.4
Bergmann *et al.*	1979	Newcastle	65+	800	GP patients	3.1
Gurland *et al.*	1983	London	65+	396	Living at home	2.5
Campbell *et al.*	1983	Gisborne	65+	559	Whole community	2.4
Bollerup	1975	Copenhagen	70	619	City districts	1.6
Persson	1980	Gothenburg	70	392	Whole community	1.5
Gilmore	1977	Scotland	65+	300	Not indicated	1.0
Nilsson	1983	Gothenburg	70	404	Whole community	1.0
Maule *et al.*	1984	Edinburgh	62-90	487	GP patients	0.6

Source: Ineichen 1987.

As table 5.3 indicates, the proportion of over-65s suffering from some form of dementia, from mild to severe, cannot be determined unambiguously: the research results diverge too widely, from 2.5% in one English study to 16.1% in one American study.

The six studies mentioned in table 5.4 covering general populations of more than 500 people aged 65 or over indicate an average prevalence rate for severe dementing syndromes of 4.3%.

For the Netherlands this means that over 80,000 people aged 65 or over are currently suffering from severe dementia (i.e. require continuous assistance from other people) but still not living in a specialized care institution; in addition there are currently more than 19,000 elderly sufferers from severe dementia in nursing homes and psychiatric hospitals. The total estimate is thus around 100,000, equivalent to 5.4% of all over-65s.

Some forms of dementia also occur in under-65s, and while we lack exact epidemiological data we can assume that the numbers involved are relatively small (no more than perhaps 2,500 patients).

Caution is needed in interpreting overall prevalence figures. These show a progressive course with age, so that if the average age of one of the groups investigated is higher than that of another, then - even where the age-specific figures per age group are the same - the result will be divergent overall prevalence rates for the group as a whole. This is true also of incidence rates.

Before soundly based statements can be made regarding future trends in the numbers of demented patients the overall prevalence figure of 5.4% therefore needs to be broken down into specific age groups.

Having examined several dozen studies of dementia Jorm *et al.* (1987) concluded that the prevalence of moderate and severe forms of the syndrome doubled every 5.1 years from the age of 60 onwards; combined with data from Kay and Bergmann, which are broken down by sex, this produces the following picture (table 5.5).

For the Netherlands these percentages imply the following numbers of elderly dements, assuming that the age- and sex-specific prevalence rates do not change in the future (table 5.6).

Table 5.5 **Prevalence rates for moderate and severe forms of dementia syndrome by five-year age group**

Age group	Prevalence % (m+f) (a)	Prevalence % (m) (b)	Prevalence % (f) (b)
65-69	1.4	3.0	0.4
70-74	2.8	3.1	2.0
75-79	5.6	6.1	6.1
80+	14.0*	10.1	16.0
In the Netherlands, all groups aged 65+	5.4	4.9	5.8

* Estimate
Source: (a) Jorm *et al.* 1987; (b) based on data from Kay & Bergmann 1980.

Table 5.6 **Moderate and severe forms of dementia in the Netherlands in 1985, 1990, 2000 and 2010 (x 1,000 patients)**

Age group	1985	1990	2000	2010
65-69	8.2	9.6	10.5	12.6
70-74	11.6	11.5	13.6	14.9
75-79	21.6	23.2	27.9	28.8
80+	52.1	61.5	74.1	87.9
All groups aged 65+	93.7	105.8	126.1	144.2

Source: Population Forecast: Central Bureau of Statistics (CBS) Statistical Bulletin 1988 no. 50.

Tables 5.7 and 5.8 break down the overall prevalence rates by sex. In the future as at present around two thirds of the dementing elderly will be women. It should be noted here that up to the age of 75 there are twice as many male as female sufferers, but the absolute numbers are small when set against the numbers of patients aged over 75. Three quarters of sufferers aged over 75 are women, reflecting women's greater life expectancy, now and in the future.

Table 5.7 **Moderate and severe forms of dementia among women in the Netherlands in 1985, 1990, 2000 and 2010 (x 1,000 patients)**

Age group	1985	1990	2000	2010
65-69	1.2	1.3	1.4	1.6
70-74	5.5	5.4	6.2	6.5
75-79	13.4	14.4	17.0	17.0
80+	39.7	47.8	58.6	69.1
All women aged 65+	59.8	68.9	83.2	94.2

Table 5.8 **Moderate and severe forms of dementia among men in the Netherlands in 1985, 1990, 2000 and 2010 (x 1,000 patients)**

Age group	1985	1990	2000	2010
65-69	7.1	8.5	9.1	11.0
70-74	6.1	6.1	7.4	8.4
75-79	8.2	8.8	10.9	11.8
80+	12.4	13.6	15.5	18.8
All men aged 65+	33.9	37.0	42.9	50.0

The number of old people with dementia in the Netherlands will rise by more than 35% over the next twenty years, from 105,000 currently to 144,000 in 2010; in both relative and absolute terms the increase will be greatest among the over-80s. This great increase in the number of sufferers from severe dementia, and particularly the sharp rise in the number aged 80+, has major implications for the care of the elderly. Section 5.5 considers the effects of rising prevalence on the demand for help by and for elderly sufferers.

5.3 *Aetiology and possible changes in prevalence*

The previous section included a calculation of the numbers of senile dements in 1990, 2000 and 2010 based on the assumption that the age-group prevalence rates for men and women will not change in the future; this section considers whether that assumption is justified.

The prevalence of dementia (the total number of sufferers at any one time) is determined by its incidence (the number of new cases arising), course (duration) and outcome (recovery or death).

The incidence of dementia will change as and when something can be done about its causes. As yet little is known of the aetiology of dementia, partly because the syndrome covers a wide range of disorders. All these symptoms have a common root, namely a disease of the brain, since all dementia results ultimately from a failure of the central nervous system. Something is nevertheless known about some of the causes (the picture is summarized in table 5.1); in fact most is known about the aetiology of the less common forms of dementia, while the causes of the commonest, senile dementia of the Alzheimer type, are still unknown. In the case of the second commonest form, multi-infarct dementia, it is assumed that hypertension and cerebral embolisms play an important part in pathogenesis (Tanja & Hofman 1985; Sloane 1980; (Gezondheidsraad (Health Council) 1988).

Most of the research into Alzheimer's disease has focused on the role of heredity. While the mechanisms involved remain largely unclear it is not disputed that genetic factors play a part in the aetiology of this form of dementia (Matsuyama 1983; WHO 1986, Davies 1986; Small & Greenberg 1988; Gezondheidsraad (Health Council) 1988; Henderson 1986). Recent research has indicated a slightly increased risk of dementia among the blood relatives of patients who develop Alzheimer's before the age of 65; there is little if any increase in the risk to relatives where the onset is later (Davies 1986). Researchers are also seeking biological markers which would enable Alzheimer patients to be identified at an early stage (Small & Greenberg 1988; Owen & Whatley 1988); they are encouraged in this task by the example of Huntington's disease, where the gene involved has now been located. Genetic research is also under way into the links between SDAT and Down's syndrome on account of their striking neuropathological similarities (Heston *et al.* 1981; Davies 1986). Many *post mortem* studies have been carried out in the areas of neuropathology (morphological changes, changes in brain tissue, etc.), neurochemistry (neurotransmitter research, studies of the cholinergic system, a certain analogy with Parkinson's disease, the role of neuropeptides, etc.) and immunology (viral infections, antibodies etc.) (Roth 1985; WHO 1986). Many possible causes of SDAT are thus under investigation, and while the research is producing a large volume of knowledge (albeit fragmented among the various specialisms) there is no immediate prospect of an aetiological breakthrough.

Given that the prospects of prevention or of finding causes of Alzheimer's diseases which can be treated or otherwise influenced are therefore also slight, we can assume with considerable confidence that the incidence of the condition (the rate at which new cases appear every year) will remain constant over the next twenty years.

Research in other countries has shown the incidence of *multi-infarct dementia* to have fallen (Hagnell *et al.* 1983); the explanation may lie in the generally observed decline in the incidence of cerebrovascular accidents, due among other things to improvements in the prevention and treatment of hypertension. It is not clear whether a further fall in the incidence of multi-infarct dementia can be expected in the future; here too our aetiological knowledge is inadequate.

Other forms of dementia which could show an increase in the future include Korsakoff's syndrome (resulting from excessive alcohol consumption) and dementia due to AIDS; dementia due to brain traumas (resulting from road accidents) may also increase. These forms can all arise at an early age, and while the numbers of patients are still relatively small there are indications that increased alcohol consumption among the young is leading to a rise in the number of young sufferers from Korsakoff's syndrome. As for AIDS-related dementia, much will depend on how quickly the human immunodeficiency virus (HIV) spreads through the population and how much the lives of AIDS patients can be prolonged.

In the area of the *course* of dementia as in that of its incidence no great changes are expected over the next twenty years. Given that the causes are largely unknown or untreatable no change is likely in the average duration of the condition. The proportion of reversible or curable dementias (currently around 10%) is unlikely to rise much for the same reason. We can however expect some slight reduction in the risk of death from intercurrent diseases in dementia patients, who will therefore on average live slightly longer.

Conclusion

Since neither the incidence nor the course of dementia is likely to change much (except perhaps in the case of a small number of relatively rare forms), its future prevalence will depend mainly on the changing makeup of the population. As was noted in section 2.3, epidemiological research has produced sex- and age-specific prevalence data. The occurrence of dementia thus correlates with age and sex, though this does *not* mean that age and sex are causal factors.

The numbers of elderly dements shown in tables 5.6, 5.7 and 5.8 were derived from the most recent population forecasts (CBS 1988) coupled with the age- and sex-specific prevalence figures given in table 5.5. The expected rapid increase in the number of demented patients can mainly be ascribed to rising average life expectancy in the Netherlands and the consequent increase over the next twenty years in the numbers of the very old.

5.4 *Diagnostic and therapeutic prospects*

5.4.1 *Diagnosis*

A recent report on psychogeriatric syndroms by a Health Council committee (Gezondheidsraad (Health Council) 1988) emphasizes the importance for the patient and those around him or her of careful diagnosis, stressing in particular:

- differentiation from normal aging processes,
- differentiation from other syndromes involving pathological memory disorders which require a different approach,
- early identification (or exclusion) of a treatable cause and decision on causal therapy,
- early identification of attendant somatic and psychiatric syndromes and decision on symptomatic treatment,
- decision whether psychological treatment and on support for carers and family members is indicated,
- decision on appropriate care (avoidance of unnecessary hospitalization).

Diagnosing a dementia syndrome and deciding what action to take is not always straightforward: it can be very difficult to distinguish symptoms of dementia from memory disorders due to normal aging, other psychogeriatric symptoms (notably depression and delirium) and combinations of somatic and psychiatric symptoms: follow-up investigation is needed to confirm the preliminary diagnosis and certainty is often achieved only through neuropathological examination after death. As used in this section 'diagnosis' refers to the clinical diagnosis reached in the case of living patients on the basis of their and their relatives' medical histories, tests and the observation of patients' behaviour.

The recognition of a possible dementia syndrome and its provisional diagnosis normally takes place in general practice. But there is evidence that currently many patients with dementia do not begin to receive help until too late, if at all (Gezondheidsraad (Health

Council) 1988; Cooper & Bickel 1984). The system for picking up patients with a dementia syndrome at an early stage is inadequate, in part because many relatives of elderly people fail to notice incipient dementia or take no action because they think nothing can be done; in addition, when a doctor is consulted regarding a possible dementia syndrome (often there is some vague behavioural problem or memory loss) he or she generally has insufficient specialized knowledge of the condition and no reliable tests to hand with which to reach a firmer diagnosis. At the same time it is likely that numbers of elderly patients are wrongly considered to be incurably demented (and are approached as such) when in fact their condition is a treatable one such as depression (Gardner 1984; Van den Bosch 1988).

When the general practitioner has established the probable diagnosis, specialist examination is needed to determine the type of dementia and possible treatable causes.

Compared with the limited diagnostic tests available to the family doctor, the *specialist* has a relatively wide range of possibilities. Ideally the patient's whole situation over a period of time should be taken into account to maximize the likelihood that the correct diagnosis will be made and the best form of treatment or care selected (Gardner 1984; Gezondheidsraad (Health Council) 1988); history taking (anamnesis) and examinations are therefore needed covering physical, social, psychiatric and psychological factors (CBIT 1989).

- Physical investigation: a number of causes of a dementia syndrome, inside and outside the brain, can be identified or excluded. Neurological examination has an important role to play here (Frederiks 1988), and the technical arsenal available for this purpose is extensive: EEG, ECG, computed tomography (CT scan), MRI or NMR (magnetic resonance imaging, nuclear magnetic resonance), SPECT (single photon emission computer tomography), and laboratory tests (blood and urine). An important point here is that many of these tests are non-invasive and cause the patient little distress.
- Social investigation: this is of particular importance with a view to determining future care needs. Bearing in mind the progression of the condition and the nature of its symptoms it is necessary to determine whether and to what extent patients can continue to be cared for in their own surroundings, with professional help if necessary.
- Psychiatric examination: this is needed on the one hand to distinguish the cognitive disorders associated with dementia syndrome from those associated with other conditions (depression, schizophrenic defect, etc.) and on the other because a dementia syndrome is often complicated by other psychiatric symptoms

(anxiety, aggressive behaviour, nocturnal agitation) (Rubin *et al.* 1988). Careful differential diagnosis is of great importance with a view to determining appropriate treatment and care.

- Psychological/neuropsychological examination: psychological tests can provide information on the nature and severity of patients' loss of psychological and cognitive functions, important in connection with the kind of support and treatment to be offered. Various standardized observation scales have been developed in the Netherlands for the assessment of behaviour (Diesfeldt & Jolles 1988; Jolles 1988), and in some parts of the country there are 'memory clinics' carrying out diagnostic work with patients suffering from memory problems and other cognitive disorders (Verhey *et al.* 1987).

5.4.2 *Therapeutic interventions*

The diagnostic arsenal is larger than the therapeutic. Most patients cannot be treated *causally* because the commonest cause of the condition is the untreatable Alzheimer's disease. Between 10% and 30% of the causes of dementia are treatable, however, though this does not necessarily mean that the condition is reversible. The number of reversible cases of dementia is put at 10% of the total (Gezondheidsraad (Health Council) 1988); reversibility depends on the nature of the cause and the length of time it has been present (Frederiks 1985). The main causes of treatable forms of dementia are shown in table 5.9.

It is not known how many dements actually recover following treatment.

In the vast majority of patients with a dementia syndrome only symptomatic treatment is possible, aimed at improving sufferers' condition and functioning. In a proportion of cases this involves treating concomitant physical or psychiatric symptoms which may have an adverse effect on patients' functioning (such as dehydration, malnutrition, anemia, hypoxemia, electrolytic disorders, cardiovascular problems and depression).

Table 5.9. **Treatable causes of dementia**

* *Primary (causal) treatment*	* *Secondary (symptomatic) treatment*
- Depression (pseudodementia)	- Dietary deficiency
- Intoxications (medications, alcohol)	- Dehydration
- Metabolic causes (e.g. vitamin-B12 deficiency)	- Decompensation
- Endocrine causes (e.g. hypothyroidism)	- Hypoxaemia
- Infections (e.g. neurosyphilis)	- Anaemia
- Vascular causes (e.g. multi-infarct dementia)	- Electrolytic disorders
- Other (e.g. neurosarcoidosis)	- Intercurrent infections
	- Other internal causes
	- Social factors
Neurosurgical treatment	
- Certain brain tumors	
- Chronic subdural haematoma	
- Normal-pressure hydrocephalus	

The following measures are also necessary to maintain or improve patients' condition and functioning:

- the patient should remain as active as possible and social isolation should be avoided;
- deterioration in sight or hearing should be remedied;
- medication should be as far as possible avoided. Many drugs produce confusion even in elderly people not suffering from dementia (such as digitalis, antihypertensiva, hypnotica and sedativa, psychotropic drugs and anticholinergic drugs). Anxiolytic, antipsychotic and antidepressive drugs may however sometimes be indicated;
- in deciding whether surgery is indicated account must be taken of the risk, which increases with age, that an operation may lead to permanent cognitive functional disorders;
- the patient's family and care-givers must be given attention and where necessary help (Gezondheidsraad (Health Council) 1988).

For the current position in the area of *pharmacological* treatment we cite the recent Gezondheidsraad (Health Council) report (1988):

"Most cases in the 'dementia syndrome of unknown cause' category involve Alzheimer's disease. Over time many drugs have been tried on patients with this condition, often on the basis of incorrect aetiological assumptions. [The Swaab and Fliers article (1986) reviews the position at length; RB.]

"The incorrect belief that narrowing of the blood vessels of the brain led to the condition resulted in the administration of vasodilators and anticoagulants, which proved ineffective. Antidepressiva, neuroleptica and anxiolytica also have no effect on the cause of the condition and moreover have adverse side-effects (in the form of states of confusion). They can however be very effective in treating the behavioural disorders which can develop as a part of a dementia syndrom, sometimes enabling admission to hospital or nursing home to be postponed. The administration of vitamin B12, alone or in combination with zinc, or of other vitamins has also proved ineffective, as have the 'psychogeriatric drugs' intended to improve the brain metabolism.

"Drugs which are related to or weaken or reinforce the working of neurotransmitters have been administered with a view to restoring or stimulating neurotransmitter systems which have degenerated. There are for example drugs which have been thought to simulate the cholinergic transmitter system when it has deteriorated as a result of Alzheimer's disease (Perry 1988), but research has shown that so far at least this strategy has failed to produce results (Swaab, Fliers 1986).

Research has also been done into the effect of neuropeptides, notably the hormones vasopressin and ACTH or related preparations. The results do not yet point to any significant improvement in memory functions" (Gezondheidsraad (Health Council) 1988).

Swaab and Fliers (1986) conclude that "'therapeutic' drugs are at present more often the cause of pseudodementia than they are the cure of Alzheimer's disease". While some of the available pharmacological therapies can improve patients' condition to some extent there is as yet no indication that they arrest or reverse the progress of the disease; indeed, it is by no means clear that there are drugs which can even slow the rate of deterioration. Changes in the diet and social surroundings of Alzheimer's patients can be as effective as drug therapies (Held *et al.* 1984; Mirmiran *et al.* 1986).

Systematic research into the effects of the *psychological* treatment of dementia remains scarce (Diesfeldt & Jolles 1988). Research involving normal elderly adults has shown that the results they achieve in numerous cognitive tasks can be considerably improved on a fairly long-term basis; a broad range of treatment options are available (among them psychotherapy, functional training, discussion groups, memory groups, reality orientation training, activity therapy and so on); as yet there is only limited experience of their use, however, so that it is not clear what scope there is for delaying or reducing by the use of psychological treatments the development of the cognitive limitations associated with a dementia syndrome.

5.5 *Utilization of care by demented elderly, now and in the future*

Statistics on the utilization of services by the severely demented elderly are scarce. The systematic recording of patient data (including DSM-III or ICD-9 diagnoses) mainly takes place in intramural-care institutions such as general and psychiatric hospitals and nursing homes; the use made of other agencies, notably the various forms of primary care (general practice, community nursing, home help), community mental health care (the RIAGGs) and residential homes for the elderly can currently only be estimated.

Caution is always needed in interpreting data on the utilization of services by the demented elderly, first because diagnosis is not straightforward and often requires long-term assessment and second because old people often suffer from several conditions, both mental and physical, at the same time (co-morbidity). Often only one principal diagnosis is noted when patient data are recorded, and it is to some extent therefore a matter of chance what diagnoses appear in the statistics. Finally, quantitative data on service-utilization generally tell us nothing about the quality either of the care provided or of patients' lives - something of great importance in the case of a generally chronic and untreatable condition like dementia.

5.5.1 *Non-residential care*

General practice

The family doctor is generally the first health professional on whom dements and their care-givers call for help. A modal general practice with 2500 patients includes 18 severely demented elderly patients; the number will have risen to 21 by 2010. Every year there are four or five new cases, of which the family doctors encounters or identifies only two. General-practice morbidity records indicate that a family doctor diagnoses dementia for the first time in 6.3 patients per 1000 people aged 65 or over every year (annual incidence) (Lamberts 1984; Van Hoogen *et al.* 1985). Overall this means that every year some 12,000 new dementia cases (i.e. 45% of all new cases arising in the Netherlands) are recognized by general practitioners every year. There is some evidence that dementia is often not recognized in general practice (Ten Horn 1987).

The nature of the condition is such that the scope for treatment in general practice is limited. An important function is the early identification notably of treatable physical causes of mental deterioration. De Graaff and Hupkens (1985) urge the use of a checklist or dementia protocol to assess the somatic background of observed behavioural disorders in the elderly.

Home-help and community-nursing services

The home-help and community-nursing services are an important source of help for elderly people suffering from the milder forms of dementia for whom admission to a hospital or nursing home is not or not yet indicated. The available data provide information on the help given to old people in general but not on that specifically aimed at the demented.

We can assume that two thirds of the severely demented elderly do *not* receive intramural care in a hospital, nursing home or residential home (see section 5.2), implying that some 65,000 are cared for at home by family, friends and agencies like the home-help and community-nursing services. A not inconsiderable number of old people (and presumably therefore of the demented elderly) live with their children or grandchildren. The 1988 Social and Cultural Report (SCP 1988) gives the following information:

- in 1987 8.2% of all over-65s lived with their children or grandchildren, as against 11.2% in 1983;
- in 1987 15.2% of all over-80s lived with their children or grandchildren, as against 12.1% in 1983.

Table 5.10 **Numbers of old people living at home and proportion receiving home help in the last four weeks of each year, 1983-87**

	1983	1984	1985	1986	1987
Number of people aged 65+ ('000)	1692	1709	1730	1772	1803
Number of people aged 65+ ('000) living at home	1512	1529	1550	1592	1623
Percentage of the living at home receiving professional home help	8.59	8.75	8.59	8.50	8.50

Source: Ministry of Welfare, Health and Cultural Affairs, Financial Overview of Care 1989, pp. 78, 84 and 105; CBS population data.

NB. It was not possible to take account in the calculations of the fact that help may be provided either for couples or for persons living alone.

A recent report by the STG-Scenario Committee on Aging (STG 1988) calculated that the proportion of over-65s receiving *professional home help* ('gezinsverzorging') has remained more or less constant since 1985 (table 5.10).

In 1987 as a whole some 180,000 people aged 65 or over living at home received home help (Ministry of Welfare, Health and Cultural Affairs 1988). A cautious estimate puts the proportion of the severely demented elderly receiving professional home help at 30%, i.e. around 20,000 people. The severely demented elderly thus represent a significant fraction (11%) of home-help clients in the 65+ age group. The proportion can be expected to rise in the future as the number of very old people increases and as old people wish and are obliged to remain in their own homes for longer.

The number of users of community-nursing services ('Kruiswerk') can be calculated on the basis of the Financial Overview of Care 1989 (Ministry of Welfare, Health and Cultural Affairs 1988) and the 1988 population forecasts of the Central Bureau of Statistics (see table 5.11).

Table 5.11 **Utilization of community-nursing services by age and number***

Age group	Contacts per 100 people		Total contacts ('000)		Average contacts per client		Total clients (est., '000)	
	1985	1990	1985	1990	1985	1990	1985	1990
65-69	200	200	1068	1258	17	20	63	63
70-79	402	404	3317	3430	18.3	23	181	149
80+	1308	1350	3087	3847	23.3	28.5	132	135
65+							376	347

* Excluding group activities, visits by clients to community-nursing units and services to residents of old-people's homes.

In 1985 around 23% of all over-65s living at home were community-nursing clients; by 1990 the figure had fallen to 20%. The volume of help given to the very old has increased in terms both of the proportion of all help and of the volume of help per client. A cautious estimate puts at 30% the proportion of the severely demented elderly living at home who make use of community nursing, i.e. around

20,000 people; they thus represent about 6% of all the service's clients. The use made of community nursing by the demented elderly, like that made of professional home help, is expected to rise over the next few years.

Extramural mental health care (RIAGG)

Within the complex of services for the elderly the role of the RIAGGs is an expanding one. The RIAGGs are increasingly involved in consultation with residential homes, decisions on treatment and care and placement in nursing homes; their role in providing social psychogeriatric care is also increasingly recognized as a contribution to maintaining the uncertain balance of some old people's lives (STG Scenario Committee on Aging 1988).

Over-65s currently account for 17% of the RIAGGs' clients; in particular the proportion of the very elderly among the RIAGGs' clients is growing.

Table 5.12 **Regional Institute for Ambulatory Mental Health Care (RIAGG) clients aged 65 or over, by age and sex, in absolute numbers and as a percentage of all over-65s in 1986 (in brackets: 1982)**

Age	Men		Women	
	Number	Percentage	Number	Percentage
65-69	1087 (1301)	0.43 (0.53)	1987 (2007)	0.64 (0.67)
70-74	1493 (1408)	0.75 (0.75)	2457 (2516)	0.89 (0.96)
75-80	1929 (1741)	1.42 (1.35)	3818 (3409)	1.70 (1.66)
80-84	1873 (1691)	2.39 (2.26)	4307 (3365)	2.81 (2.58)
85+	2479 (1856)	5.27 (4.05)	5338 (3939)	4.90 (4.47)

Source: NVAGG 1988.

Since no diagnostic data are available on their clients it is not possible to say how many demented elderly people receive care from the RIAGGs. Their main role at the moment is probably that of determining, at the request of the family doctor, the need for admission to a hospital or nursing home. Support activities aimed at the families of the demented elderly, undertaken by RIAGGs' prevention departments, are also showing an increase.

5.5.2 *Residential care*

Nursing homes

Psychogeriatric nursing homes and psychogeriatric departments of general nursing homes are the main institutions providing intramural care for the demented elderly 74% of diagnoses on admission are of dementia and a further 12% of amnestic syndrome (serious memory disorder) (see figure 5.1).

Figure 5.1 **Percentage frequencies of the ten commonest principal diagnoses on first admission to psychogeriatric nursing homes and the psychogeriatric departments of general nursing homes, 1987**

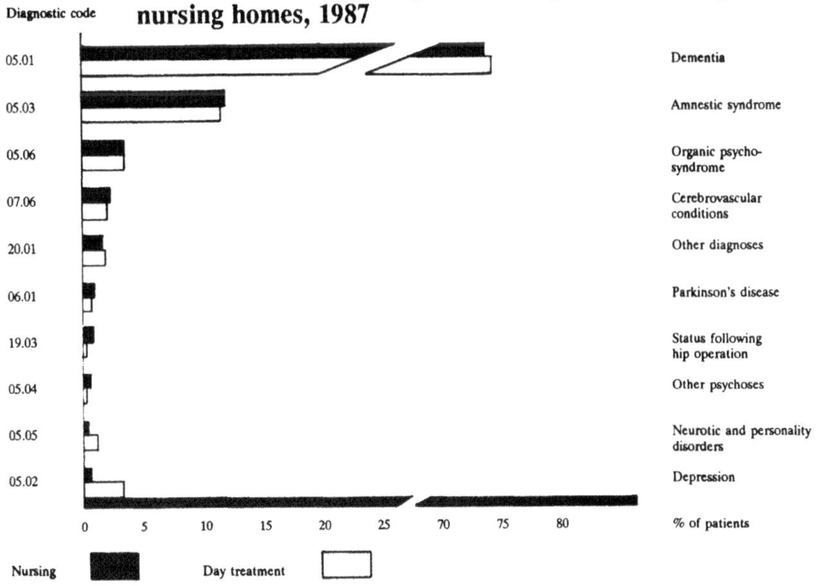

Between 1982 and 1986 the number of psychogeriatric beds rose from 19,861 to 22,319, but despite this increase the number still falls short of the norm of 1.25 beds per 100 people aged 65 or over set by the Hospital Services Act (Ketting & Jacobs 1989).

In 1985 17.3% of elderly sufferers from severe dementia in the Netherlands were being cared for in psychogeriatric nursing homes or the psychogeriatric departments of general nursing homes; by 1987 the figure had risen to 18.2%, and as the numbers of very old people continue to grow we can expect it to rise still further.

Table 5.13 shows estimates of future numbers of patients diagnosed as suffering from dementia, together with the numbers of beds required under the statutory norm. The calculations are based on the (very cautious) assumption that the percentage of demented elderly people admitted to psychogeriatric nursing homes will remain constant at 18% of the total and that the percentage of beds in psychogeriatric nursing homes occupied by patients diagnosed as demented will remain constant at 74%.

Table 5.13 **Estimated numbers of demented patients and numbers of beds in psychogeriatric nursing homes and the psychogeriatric departments of general nursing homes**

	1985	1990	2000	2010
Total number of demented over-65s	93,700	105,800	126,100	144,200
a. Of whom 18% in psychogeriatric nursing homes	16,200	19,000	22,700	26,000
Number of psychogeriatric beds required under statutory norm	21,630	23,890	27,110	30,590
b. Of which 74% in use by dementia sufferers	16,000	17,680	20,060	22,640
Bed shortfall for demented patients (a-b)	200	1,320	2,640	3,360

Even on these cautious estimates of numbers of patients and admissions the statutory norm of 1.25 beds per 100 old people is inadequate to meet future demand for care. The impending bed shortfall is all the more serious in that it is increasingly the most handicapped patients who are admitted to nursing homes. The general competence especially of psychogeriatric patients has clearly deteriorated over the years, partly because the average age of nursing-home patients has risen (see figure 5.2).

Figure 5.2 expresses patients' competence in terms of the ADL (activities of daily living) index. This is based on individuals' ability to carry out with or without assistance five activities, namely: 1, washing (upper body); 2, washing (lower body); 3, dressing; 4, toileting; 5, eating. The score can range from 0 (no help or supervision needed) to 5 (help or supervision needed with all five activities).

Psychogeriatric patients (of whom three quarters are demented) emerge as having very low levels of competence.

Figure 5.2 **Average ADL scores on first admission, 1982-1987**

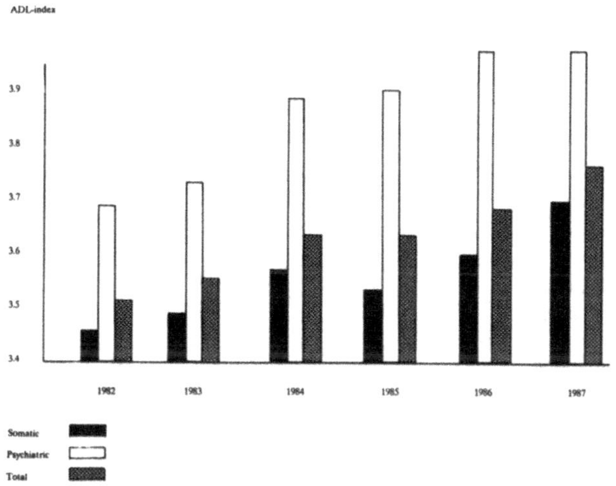

Source: SIVIS 1988.

Other intramural facilities

- *General psychiatric hospitals*
  Only a small number of elderly patients diagnosed as suffering from a dementia syndrome are cared for in general psychiatric hospitals. Since the start of the 1980s there has been a considerable shift of patients from such hospitals to, mainly, nursing homes. It is estimated that just under a thousand elderly dementia sufferers are currently in Dutch general psychiatric hospitals (PIGG 1989).
- *General, university and specialist hospitals*
  Every year just under 5,000 patients are admitted to non-psychiatric hospitals with dementia as a principal or secondary diagnosis. In most cases these patients are admitted on the grounds of, and are treated for, conditions other than their dementia syndrome. Psychiatric units in general hospitals and university psychiatric clinics encounter only a few hundreds of demented patients every year.
- *Nursing-home daycare*
  Nursing homes have a therapeutic as well as a residential function in respect of psychogeriatric patients and every year around 2,000

patients diagnosed as having a dementia syndrome receive daycare in a psychogeriatric nursing home or the psychogeriatric department of a general nursing home.

- *Old-people's homes*
  The function of old-people's homes remains primarily residential but in the course of the 1980s their nature has changed. Average age on admission has risen sharply to around 82 years, so that residents' average age is higher still. This means that the residents of old-people's homes increasingly also need nursing as a result of their declining average level of competence (STG Scenario Committee on Aging 1988) and the difficulty of transfer to a nursing home. On a cautious estimate 7.5% of the residents of old-people's homes are demented (Vink *et al.* 1988), but because no diagnosis is made on admission no reliable figures are available; in absolute terms this means that at at 1 January 1988 there were around 10,000 dements among the 134,000 residents (Ministry of Welfare, Health and Cultural Affairs 1988).

Overview

Tables 5.14 and 5.15 bring together seven years' data on demented patients admitted to and cared for in the various types of intramural institution.

Table 5.14 **Numbers of admissions/registrations per year of persons with a principal or secondary diagnosis of dementia**

	1981	1982	1983	1984	1985	1986	1987
General psychiatric hospitals	1550	1730	1740	1190	1010	1000*	800*
Nursing homes (residential care)				5452	5870	5930	6750
Nursing homes (daycare)				1890	1900	2190	2430
General, university and specialist hospitals	4720	4870	5520	5200	5090	4800	4730
Of which:							
psychiatric units in general hospitals				250	280	240	212

* Estimates.

Table 5.15 **Numbers of patients/clients with a principal or secondary diagnosis of dementia as at 31 December**

	1981	1982	1983	1984	1985	1986	1987
General psychiatric hospitals	1800	1820	1590	1220	1080	950*	900*
Nursing homes (residential care)				16060	16200	17070	17980
Nursing homes (daycare)				1180	1340	1530	1780
Old-people's homes*				10000	9950	10200	10150
Total				**28460**	**28570**	**29750**	**30810**

* Estimates.

Source: PIGG, SIVIS, LMR, FOZ, Mental Health Care in Figures 1987 (Ketting & Jacobs 1989).

Even allowing for double counting and other inaccuracies in the data, table 5.15 indicates that barely a third of all patients aged 65 or over suffering from severe dementia receive intramural care.

5.5.3 *Social developments and possible changes in the future utilization of care*

The extent of the use which elderly dements will in future make of professional care depends on more factors than just the number of sufferers in the population as a whole. By no means all of the severely demented present for professional care, as preceding sections have shown, and the ratio of users to non-users is not fixed; moreover for those patients who do receive professional care a number of options exist - extramural or intramural, institutional daycare or home care, psychiatric care, non-medical support (home help) - and here too the proportions of total care provided for which each accounts may also vary over time.

Inflows into the various forms of care relate to the nature or severity of the condition only to a limited extent, depending more on patients' individual circumstances. Future policies in such areas as housing, welfare, tax legislation and of course health care, together with social and cultural trends in Dutch society, will also affect the utilization of services in the future. While the factors which can give rise to changes in the pattern of care are very numerous they can be broadly divided into two groups, namely:

1. *demand* factors which determine when sufferers and/or their families seek professional help or care and what agencies they

approach, and
2. *supply* factors which determine the scale and nature of provision.
We shall not discuss the interactions which exist between supply and demand in health care, limiting ourselves instead to a brief consideration of a number of developments relevant to future care use.

Demand factors

- *Willingness of families to provide care:* Changes in role patterns and 'intergenerational solidarity' and increased geographical mobility, particularly among the younger generations, may mean a decline in the willingness notably of the children of the demented elderly to care for infirm relatives. Increasingly the traditional carers - generally daughters - have neither the time nor the inclination to take on the care of an elderly relative as a matter of course (in part because more women now go out to work), and this trend is not offset by any increase in care-giving by male relatives. The picture is reinforced by the fact that on average there are now fewer young people in families to each old person, that more old people now live alone as a result of the growth in divorce, and that families are often geographically scattered and are both less willing and less able to take on responsibility for day-to-day care.
- *Ability of families to provide care*: Even where the willingness to look after a parent or partner with dementia is present there may be practical problems. Many of the partners of the demented elderly, being themselves old, cannot provide the care needed and are thus forced to seek professional support. The rising numbers of very old people may therefore lead to a relative increase in the demand for care, even in cases where the patient's partner is still reasonably healthy. The children or other relatives of the demended elderly can also face financial disincentives: care-giving may entail leaving a job or changing to part-time work, for example, while accommodating a sufferer in one's home may require costly special facilities. Grants to relatives to cover the cost of home care may in future prove to be cheaper than full (intramural) professional care and could extend the length of time that the families of the demented elderly are able to look after them.
- *Expertise in the primary sector*: There is growing interest in the problems of aging and the elderly in the primary sector (general practice, community nursing, home help), and this may mean that in future relatively fewer demented patients will have to be referred to intramural facilities or that patients will not need to be admitted until a later stage in the development of their condition.

Supply factors

- *Availability*: The volume of resources which the state provides for the care of the elderly in general and of the demented elderly in particular has of course a major impact on the utilization of services. Fundamentally what is involved is a *political* choice with a number of *ethical* aspects, since resources are always limited and choices always have to be made: how much is society prepared to set aside for its older members? are there some groups of old people who should have priority, and do these include the demented? how prolonged and interventionist may the care of the demented be (i.e. what are the limits of acceptability in this field)? We can expect such issues to be increasingly debated as the numbers of old people grow.
- *Diversity:* The utilization of services depends on their diversity as well as their overall availability. Ideally care should be available for the demented elderly at all stages of their condition, geared to patients' current needs and capabilities. An overemphasis on home care, with or without professional backup, is as undesirable as an overemphasis on intramural care. The need for both intramural and extramural services can be expected to grow over the next few years; some caution is therefore needed regarding the scope for substituting extramural for intramural care.
- *Support for care-givers*: If the primary sector and the Regional Institutes of Ambulatory Mental Health Care (RIAGG) can offer adequate and above all timely assistance not only to the sufferers themselves but also to their often overburdened families, partners or friends who live with or look after them, then the utilization of services by those in this category can be reduced. The question of the 'burden on the family' is considered in greater detail in the next section.

5.6 *The burden on relatives*

Over two thirds of elderly sufferers from severe dementia in the Netherlands are cared for at home by a partner, relative or friends, often with professional assistance from the community-nursing and home-help services. This means that several hundred thousand people are currently having to deal with a demented relative on a day-to-day basis, and the number is set to rise sharply over the next few decades. Looking after a demented relative often entails considerable personal suffering and a heavy burden on the family; indeed, it can lead to great stress and even psychiatric problems on the carers' part (Engels *et al.* 1987). Whenever attention is focused on the care of the demented elderly, now and in the future, it must always extend to the problems of these 'hidden patients' (Fengler & Goodrich 1979) and on ways of giving them help and support.

Research into the problems which arise in the care of the demented elderly by their families has been conducted notably in Britain, and while studies of the burden on relatives are lacking in the Netherlands we can provisionally assume that the British findings are also relevant to the Dutch situation.

Carers living with demented relatives show relatively many symptoms of stress; indeed, most studies have found high levels of psychiatric morbidity (Gilleard *et al.* 1984; Eagles *et al.* 1987). The stress on relatives depends among other things on:

- the stage reached: incipient dementia can cause relatives more suffering, uncertainty, anger and fear than a later stage of the syndrome (Gilleard 1984);
- the patient's functional limitations and behaviour: the gradual decay of the cognitive functions and the growing emotional distance and alienation between carer and patient can give rise to problems. Attendant behaviour problems (incontinence, aggression, deterioration of personal habits, nocturnal agitation, apathy etc.) often engender stress (Gilleard 1984; Zarit *et al.* 1986);
- attributes of the carer: age, health and skill in dealing with the situation and the carer's attitude to dementia and the demented elderly correlated demonstrably with the burden experienced (Peute 1988; Gilhooly 1984);
- the nature and quality of the past and present relationship between carer and patient: the closer the link, the greater the stress. Spouses are most at risk, followed by children, other family members and neighbours (Peute 1988);
- the support which the carer receives in her/his own environment: as in the case of other psychiatric conditions (Fadden *et al.* 1987), carers may find themselves socially isolated as a result of looking after a demented relative, given the prolonged and often very time-consuming nature of the task, and where help and sympathy are lacking the burden on the carer is very much greater (Scott *et al.* 1986).

As the above summary shows, interventions intended to prevent or resolve problems faced by those caring for the demented elderly may be aimed at the sufferer himself/herself, the carer or the carer's social environment (family and friends). Moreover a great variety of interventions are possible, depending on the specific situation, ranging from the patient's admission to a hospital or nursing home to psychotherapy for the carer with a view to enhancing her/his ability to cope. In many cases financial assistance helps to make the care of a demented relative tenable in the longer term (Overman & Stoudemill 1988).

The foreign literature is predominantly positive regarding the impact of the work of the support groups, family associations etc. through which carers and relatives of the demented elderly share their experiences and emotions with others in a similar position and give each other and outsiders information on dementia and coping with sufferers (Peute 1988). In the Netherlands the Alzheimer Foundation is active in this area, while the Regional Institutes of Ambulatory Mental Health Care organize support groups for family members.

This background analysis was completed in November 1989.

Part II Dementia Scenarios, 1990-2010

5.7 *Exploratory scenarios*[1]

5.7.1 *Scenario 1: Reference scenario*

Incidence and prevalence

The reference scenario envisages a rise from 5.3% to 6.0% in the proportion of over-65s with severe dementia syndromes over the next twenty years, giving around 150,000 sufferers in 2010 as against around 100,000 in 1990. Almost 60% of these demented elderly will be over 80.

By far the most important factor in the increase is the aging of the population. Life expectancy will continue to grow, thanks partly to technological advances in the area of somatic medicine, and in the absence of any breakthrough in the prevention or treatment of the main forms of dementia (particularly of the Alzheimer type) the chances of developing the condition in old age will be considerable. Some progress will be made in slowing the dementing process in old people by medication, adding to the rise in the numbers of very elderly sufferers.

Dementia will continue to be seen as a primarily biological condition whose genesis and course does not normally depend on and cannot be influenced by other factors. In the long run ecological factors such as air, ground and water pollution may lead to an increase in the number of dementia cases.

While improvements in early diagnosis (and in particular in differential diagnosis) will give some scope for cutting the incidence of certain relatively rare reversible forms of dementia over the next twenty years, the impact on the total number of cases will be negligible. Preventive measures will allow some slight further reduction in the incidence of dementia due to cerebrovascular disease but this will be offset by the growth in the number of cases due to alcohol abuse.

Both the range of diagnostic facilities and the demand from a more knowledgeable and articulate public for early diagnosis will grow, producing an increase in the number of elderly patients with recognized dementia. In other words, more cases will be identified but the scope for treatment and cure will not expand proportionately.

While measures to reduce the number of dementia cases (through prevention and information campaigns concerned with alcohol abuse and through the promotion of multidisciplinary research into the causes of and ways of dealing with dementia syndromes) will have some slight impact, their effects will become visible only in the (very)

---

[1] The basic assumptions of the exploratory scenarios are set out in Appendix 1.

long term; moreover only the number of *new* patients will be cut, however, not the standing patient population.

Services and their utilization

Over the next twenty years the intensity of care provided per patient will increase. The growing focus on dementia in the media and among carers and the resulting 'proto-professionalization' of the relatives of demented patients will lead to a sharp increase in the demand for both intramural and extramural care.

The public will increasingly demand screening tests for dementia and fear of dementia will put growing pressure on general practitioners to offer such tests. Given their inadequate specialist knowledge and limited diagnostic resources GPs will however refer individuals for such screening to more specialized facilities such as memory clinics and the geriatric departments of Regional Institutes for Ambulatory Mental Health Care (RIAGG) and general and psychiatric hospitals.

Patients in whom dementia has been diagnosed will also make greater use than at present of intramural and extramural services. This has various causes.

When they become sick or otherwise infirm a growing number of elderly people will need and want to be nursed at home as far as possible and for as long as possible, but such home care will increasingly be provided by (or at least with support from) professional care-givers such as the community nursing service. The main reason for this is that, while people's willingness to care for demented relatives will not decline (or grow), family and friends will not generally be in a position to take on the long-term care of sick relatives. Perhaps because they are too old themselves (as the average age of demented patients rises) or live too far away, due to the fact that in the future relatives will more often be spread all over the country. A further complication is that many demented elderly will be widows and thus have no partner to look after them. Moreover people now have fewer children, on average, who might care for them in their old age. Finally, the higher standards increasingly demanded will mean that care can often only be provided by professionals.

The confidence of the majority of elderly people and their carers in the professional services will not decline and old inhibitions about seeking help with one's own or a relative's mental problems will even weaken. This will cause difficulties. The 50% rise in the number of elderly dements over the next twenty years will be accompanied by an increase in the number of cases where nursing-home admission is indicated. Under the existing norm for numbers of nursing-home beds, however, intramural capacity will be inadequate to accommodate the growing numbers of patients and admissions will be blocked. The pressure on other intramural institutions (notably old-people's homes) and extramural care (outpatient clinics and the RIAGGs will rise as a result.

Among the extramural facilities sheltered accommodation and the institutions and departments providing daycare will have to deal with a large number of elderly dements. However, these will be only the milder cases. Little experimentation is likely in new forms of accommodation for psychogeriatric patients and the nursing home will remain the final destination of many.

Despite this considerable increase in the utilization of professional services of all types the majority of the demented elderly will continue to be cared for by relatives in their own or their relatives' home, albeit often for lack of any alternative and under far-from-ideal conditions. The continuing low social status of old people and the lack of tolerance in society for deviant behaviour will remain significant factors in this connection over the next two decades.

5.7.2 *Scenario 2: Radical professionalization*

Outline: The next twenty years will see a major decline in families' willingness and ability to care for demented relatives. The professionals' role will grow not only in nursing homes but also, and in particular, in home care. The often overburdened relatives of demented patients will form a new target group for professional care-givers.

Incidence and prevalence

This scenario envisages trends in the incidence and prevalence of dementia paralleling those in the reference scenario: the proportion of over-65s with severe dementia syndromes will rise from 5.3% to 6.0%, giving around 150,000 sufferers in 2010 as against around 100,000 now. Almost 60% of these demented elderly will be aged over 80.

As 2010 approaches patients of a new type will be encountered, namely those developing dementia syndromes as a result of slow-acting ecological factors (as yet unidentified) such as air, water and ground pollution and food additives. The numbers will initially be small but could rise sharply after 2010.

Services and their utilization

The major differences between this and the reference scenario are to be found in the area of dealing with and caring for the demented elderly.

In this scenario the next twenty years are marked by a radical increase in the involvement of specialized professionals in caring for the demented elderly, aimed at applying the latest scientific advances to looking after patients (whose average age is rising) and at maintaining them in good physical shape for as long as possible. Care provided by family and friends will be seen as less expert and not ideal. The media will devote growing attention to dementia and its sufferers and educational activities (undertaken e.g. by associations of the families concerned) will expand rapidly. The aging of the population will be regarded by society as a major threat. While knowledge of dementia and understanding of the problems of demented patients will grow this will not produce increased tolerance of the elderly infirm; growing and being old will continue to have negative connotations in Dutch society.

People will increasingly demand to know at the earliest possible stage whether they have incipient dementia and the health-care system will respond by offering extensive screening and diagnostic facilities. In the absence of preventive, therapeutic or curative techniques attention will focus on the development of diagnostic instruments for the early detection of dementia syndrome in ever younger elderly people. Responding to the fears and anxieties of many over-55s many activities will be offered in the area of memory training as a (supposed) preventive measure against mental decay. Staff and resource shortages at institutions in the health-care mainstream could well lead to a rapid expansion of commercial clinics for the elderly. Old people, particularly those in the 55-70 age group, will represent a gap in the market. An important result of this development will be the 'stretching' of the term dementia, with more people being labelled as 'ill' or 'incipiently ill' in circumstances where today we would refer to normal aging.

The commercialization of screening for dementia and mental decay will mean that much professional advice and assistance are reserved to the better-off elderly.

Professional care-givers' involvement in the care of the demented elderly will also increase markely; professionals' skills in caring for infirm elderly people will increase; and the public's belief and confidence in the technical prowess of medical science will remain rock-solid. As a result Dutch society will not see it as unethical to entrust a demented partner or parent, wholly or partly, to professional care, and this will be done even where home care is still possible. A number of objective factors, also envisaged in the reference scenario, will make good home care of the demented difficult: patients' relatives will themselve be old, families will be geographically scattered, each old person will have fewer children, and so on. In this scenario, however, the professionals' involvement in home care will also be promoted by subjective factors, with more emphasis being placed, by both care-givers and the public at large, on the fact that ignorance and inexpert care on relatives' part may worsen the course of the condition; such cases will be thought far from rare, so that the professional supervision of home care will be seen as an urgent necessity.

Taking all these trends into account both the willingness and the ability of relatives and friends to care for a demented patient will decline. 'Consumerist' attitudes will be more marked, with the families of the demented elderly claiming they have a right to care and individual patients being entrusted (or abandoned) to professional care more frequently and at an earlier stage.

A similar trend will mark the primary-care sector. General practitioners, confronted by increasingly articulate and expert relatives of demented patients, will be pressured to refer them to more specialized institutions for the care of the elderly, both commercial and non-commercial.

This scenario envisages a greater role for professionals at all care levels the next twenty years. Increasing competition and a lack of statutory compulsion will, however, greatly limit the development of inter-level cooperation. The demand for care will rise more rapidly than in the reference scenario, affecting both extramural and intramural institutions; with government policy remaining unaltered this will produce lengthening waiting lists. The rapid growth in early screening for the elderly will concentrate much of the extra pressure on extramural institutions (RIAGGs, outpatient departments etc.) Cautious attempts will be made to avoid admitting sufferers to hospital or nursing home and to help them instead to go on living for as long as possible in small groups or communities with professional support and supervision; it will mainly be the milder cases that can make use of such schemes. The pressure on nursing homes will remain great, partly because patients will on average live slightly longer. Old-people's homes will offer some relief, and in terms of both care provided and clients accommodated the difference between the residential home and the nursing home will steadily narrow as the former increasingly provides nursing services.

Increasing professionalization will mean that fewer and fewer patients have to spend their final years poorly cared-for at home or with their children, since the scenario's side effects include an increase in the numbers seeking help at an early stage for a relative showing signs of mental decline.

5.7.3 *Scenario 3: Strengthening informal care*

Outline: Concern will be focused on the quality of life of those who are growing old. Dementia-related care will concern itself with the total network of family members and will seek to maintain and make use of the particular home situation of the individual patient wherever possible. The nursing homes will increasingly concentrate on the most severely affected sufferers.

Incidence and prevalence

This scenario envisages trends in the incidence and prevalence of dementia paralleling those in the reference scenario: the proportion of over-65s with severe dementia will rise from 5.3% to 6.0%, giving around 150,000 elderly sufferers in 2010 as against around 100,000 now. Almost 60% of them will be aged over 80.

A feature of this scenario is that over the next twenty years euthanasia is both discussed and indeed practised with growing openness: for a growing proportion of the elderly and their families euthanasia will be seen as a real and acceptable possibility, allowing life to be terminated should severe dementia develop, and several thousand instances can be expected annually by the year 2010.

Services and their utilization

This scenario puts the focus of care for dementia sufferers on the quality rather than the number of years of life remaining to them.

Dutch society will be increasingly aware of the important role played by elderly people's immediate surroundings in both the genesis and course of psychogeriatric symptoms and the care of the demented elderly. The focus of dementia-related care will shift radically from the individually orientated approach to sufferers now current towards one which stresses the caring capabilities and limitations of immediate relatives (the social network) and takes more serious account of such carers' needs.

Aging and all its disagreeable signs will be accepted more as a matter of course and the taboo on mental health problems will gradually weaken, with such problems being seen as a fact of life which can strike anyone. One effect of this will be a growing understanding of and interest in psychogeriatric patients and their total mental, physical and social functioning and a weaker emphasis on the rigid subdivision of patients by their condition (dementia, depression etc.).

Against this background individuals will increasingly accept a measure of responsibility for the welfare of a mentally deteriorating or even dementing relative. The views of the next generation of old people and their relatives on what constitutes a decent and worthwhile life will have crystallized more clearly than ever before, and as people grow more aware and articulate they will be increasingly inclined to claim rather than request the kind of care that will guarantee optimum quality of life. It will be generally accepted that the life of psychogeriatric patients, including the demented, should not be prolonged at whatever cost and that it should be possible to bring life to an end in a dignified manner. The view will also take root that it is in patients' own interest that those who care for them - partners, children - should be physically and mentally healthy; there will be a growing focus on the position and welfare of the carers as well as on that of the patients themselves.

With increasing frequency efforts will be made to go on caring for the demented elderly in the home situation for as long as possible. The professional home-help services and community-nursing services will have a much greater role in helping and supporting the carers but its purpose will change: excellent professional assistance will be available for home care aimed at maintaining and using elderly patients' specific home situation, the concern of the primary services thereby shifting in significant degree to the support and care of those who care for sufferers.

Unfortunately the state will not provide all the resources needed to fund the necessary growth of the primary sector, and while the shortfall will partly be covered by commercial services there will still be many people looking after dementing partners or parents at home who are unable to obtain sufficient, or indeed any, professional support. The phenomenon of 'burn-out' among carers will therefore become very common, despite a greater willingness in principle to care for elderly relatives. Given the growing numbers of physically and mentally exhausted carers the numbers of neglected and abused old people can also be expected to rise. Among elderly sufferers referred to specialist services a large proportion will be in a relatively poor condition, requiring more intensive care than the average sufferer currently admitted to a nursing home.

The growing stress on psychogeriatric patients' overall functioning will find concrete expression in a large number of experimental projects involving suitably adapted forms of accommodation. Facilities for supervised living and daycare will be created with a view partly to postponing admission to nursing home and partly to lightening the burden on families. The necessarily intensive support will come from volunteers and from professionals working in various disciplines and institutions. Since many of the patients concerned will be very elderly, often suffering from physical ailments in addition to their mental condition, professionals from the worlds of both physical and mental health care and of social welfare will be active in such community-living projects. The general lack of emphasis at national level on coordination and cooperation between care levels, disciplines and institutions will mean that such experiments are predominantly regional and small-scale in nature.

While all these developments in the areas of home care and supervised living will tend to delay somewhat admission to hospital or nursing home, they will produce only a very slight proportionate reduction in the number of cases in which intramural care is indicated. Given the aim of maintaining the quality of care as far as possible the substitution of extramural or home care for intramural capacity would be undesirable and even harmful to the health and wellbeing of the demented elderly since it would mean even longer nursing-home waiting lists.

5.7.4 *The three scenarios in brief*

Autonomous developments over the period 1990-2010	*Reference scenario*	*Radical professionalization scenario*	*Strengthening informal scenario*
• Demography Socio-economic context	CBS intermediate variant CPB intermediate variant (low growth)	Idem Idem	Idem Idem
• Socio-cultural developments: - Tolerance of mental problems/deviant behaviour/old people	Unchanged (low)	Idem	Greater
- Protoprofessionalization /articulacy of patients and their carers	Greater	Much greater (focused on care and life expectancy)	Much greater (focused quality of life)
- Inclination to seek professional help	Greater	Much greater	Reduced
- Willingness/ability to undertake home care	Unchanged	Much reduced	Unchanged
- Professionals' referral practices	More frequent referral to both intramural and extramural institutions	Much more frequent referral to both intramural and extramural institutions	More frequent referral for extramural care
- Impact of lifestyles on mental health; high-risk behaviour	Unchanged (little general concern)	Increase in preventive behaviour	Increase in preventive behaviour
- Social attitudes to health care/home care/-extramural services	Increased importance attached to both intramural and extramural health care	Idem; predominantly individualistic approach	Decrease; shift towards system-oriented approa
• Other ('new') causes of dementia	None	Ecological factors	None
• Medical advances: - Diagnosis	More reliable tests and earlier diagnosis	Idem	Idem
- Treatment	Unchanged	More drugs available to slow progress of condition and prolong life	More critical use of the emphasis on quality rat than lenght of life
- Prevention	Slight improvement in the area of alcohol and diet	Idem	Idem
- Rehabilitation	Unchanged (little scope)	Idem	More adapted accomm
• Other (ethical) dilemmas associated with aging	Emphasis on prolonging life	Idem	Greater acceptance of voluntary euthanasia
• *Government measures affecting mental health and mental health care in the period 1990-2010:* - Prevention/health education - Substitution and refinement of care - Funding - Research - Measures in other policy areas - Other	Such trends and developments as are currently visible are maintained	idem	idem
	↓	↓	↓
	Consequences for prevalence and the nature and scale of care consumption	*Consequences* for prevalence and the nature and scale of care consumption	*Consequences* for preva and the nature and scal care consumption
	↓	↓	↓
	Side effects: costs etc.	*Side effects:* costs etc.	*Side effects:* costs etc.

5.8 *Target-setting scenario*[2]

The target-setting scenario assumes that those developments whose nature is primarily autonomous occur as outlined in the reference scenario.

A point needs to be made here regarding the *prevalence* of dementia syndrome. Since this is a factor which cannot be directly influenced by concrete measures, the prevalence rate in the population of over-65s is assumed to be the same as in the reference scenario, namely 6% in 2010 (150,000 people). This scenario is thus concerned predominantly with the help provided for sufferers and the utilization of services.

Target-setting scenario for dementia, 1990-2010

Objective: *To ensure that the quality of dementia-related care provided at all stages of the condition is considerably higher in 2010 than under the reference scenario.*

More specifically, the care provided must help maintain patients' quality of life at the highest possible level. Depending on the seriousness of individual patients' condition a 'high quality of life' is taken to mean that:

- they can go on living in their own home for as long as possible, and/or
- they can continue functioning socially in their own environment, and/or
- the psychological burden on their immediate family and the physical and mental suffering of the patients themselves is minimized.

Necessary measures

1. General measures

Achieving the objective will require a number of radical measures over the next twenty years in the areas of diagnosis, prevention and treatment and of the care of sufferers and their families. Before we begin distinguishing the various groups of patients and the measures needed to improve the quality of the care they receive a broad indication can be given of the areas in which action will be needed.

---

[2] The basic assumptions of the target-setting scenario are set out in Appendix 1.

- Information and education: greater public education is needed to break down the taboos associated with mental illness in general and dementia and other psychogeriatric conditions in particular. In addition more systematic information is needed by the relatives of dementia sufferers; this will require greater expertise, of different types, in the areas of education, network development etc. aimed at family members.
- A considerable increase is needed in the psychogeriatric component of training courses for primary and specialist health professionals if current gaps in knowledge are to be eliminated.
- Patients' home environments ('natural resources') need to be given greater support and reinforcement in terms of both finance and psychological resilience.
- The care of the demented demands a multidisciplinary approach: coordination and cooperation among the care levels and professional groups concerned must be vigorously pursued. In many cases the necessary changes in the structure of care will not be attainable on a purely voluntary basis and will therefore need to take place under central (government) direction. The shift towards regional structures and client-oriented delivery must remain the guiding principle.
- The substitution of extramural for intramural services and the run-down of intramural capacity must be avoided. The capacity currently planned is inadequate and must be considerably expanded.
- Research needs to be expanded. In addition to the biologically oriented research now underway, longitudinal (non-clinical) epidemiological studies and studies of the effects of the various forms of care given to patients with dementia need to be initiated with a view to filling gaps in our knowledge.
- More facilities are needed for different forms of supervised living for the demented elderly. General housing policy is of relevance here.

2. *Measures geared to the premorbid and incipient stages of dementia*

Here we focus on people who live at home, are not ill and at most are concerned that they themselves or a near relative are showing signs of incipient dementia. The following measures are needed.

- *Greater public education:*
  - on the typical features of the dementing syndrome;
  - on the risks associated with alcohol abuse;
  - on screening and diagnostic techniques;

  - aimed at altering negative attitudes to deviant behaviour and old age, with warnings against misplaced faith in memory training as a preventive measure;
  - aimed at fostering appreciation of the often isolated position of the demented and their families/carers, with greater attention being devoted to the (often unavoidable) ethical problems involved in weighing the interests of dementia patients against those of their families.
- *More specific information for particular target groups:*
  - courses need to be provided aimed at improving the attitudes and skills of patients' partners/families;
  - the geriatric and psychogeriatric component of training courses for primary and specialist health workers needs to be increased, but no new specialized functions should be created;
  - primary health professionals need specific education on psychogeriatric conditions while initial training remains inadequate in this field; ethical issues (e.g. how to deal with requests for euthanasia) must be covered explicitly.
- *Greater emphasis on early diagnosis, with a view principally to:*
  - reassuring many anxious 50-60-year-olds that they (or their partners) are not suffering from dementia even if they are becoming forgetful etc.;
  - the early detection of the relatively rare forms of dementia and dementia-like conditions which are treatable.

These measures are a joint responsibility of government and the primary-care agencies. An important input can also be expected from those with direct personal experience (members of bodies such as the Alzheimer Foundation), while pensioners' associations have an important part to play notably with a view to promoting the more material interests of sufferers and their families. Attitudinal changes will be needed to this end.

Many of these measures can work only if they are implemented on the small scale, i.e. at regional level or in suitable cases local or even neighbourhood level.

3. *Measures geared to mild cases of dementia*

Here the focus is on patients who have been diagnosed as demented and who, while they can generally continue living at home, nevertheless need help. As in the case of the measures geared to the premorbid and incipient stages of the condition, here too measures are needed aimed both directly at the sufferers themselves and at their care-givers.

The following measures are needed

- *More information and training:*
  - for families/care-givers: learning to live with disturbed behaviour, acquiring caring skills. This is very much a task for the Regional Institutes of Ambulatory Mental Health Care and the community-nursing services;
  - for the primary-care sector, notably family doctors: greater skill in recognizing psychogeriatric conditions and the differences between them and greater awareness of possible interventions.
- *Changes in the form and content of care for patients and their families:*
  - case management should be instituted wherever possible, with individual patients being guided and helped around the various agencies concerned from the earliest possible stage. This will require functional coordination (the 'client-centred' approach) and greater cooperation at regional level among the agencies, secured if necessary by the use of financial sanctions. Of particular importance here are the old-people's homes, which currently occupy a somewhat autonomous position separate from the health-care system: the large numbers of demented patients living in old-people's homes mean that these institutions will also need to be involved, more than in the past, in the processes of coordination and cooperation. The fundamental attitude must be that the institutions are there for the patients, not *vice versa*;
  - a shift in the approach to care from one focusing on the patient as an individual towards greater system-orientation, taking account of the needs not just of the sufferers themselves but also of their families;
  - people must be enabled and even encouraged to look after demented relatives where they are willing to do so, and this must be borne firmly in mind by the professional carers concerned (notably in the home-help and community-nursing services). Voluntary activities, often aimed at preventing loneliness among the elderly (shopping, chatting, 'sitting with'), also need to be supported (but not taken over) by the professional institutions;
  - these activities must be resourced. Options include tax allowances (a 'parent allowance' on the lines of the child allowance) and paid 'caring leave' on the lines of maternity leave for those who wish to undertake the care of a partner or other relative. Where somatic conditions are also present provision must exist for suitably adapted accommodation;
  - the primary sector's increased role in caring for a growing number of elderly demented patients and their families implies

more training and greater capacity notably in the home-help and community-nursing services;
- day-treatment and day-activity facilities need to be radically expanded to relieve the burden on patients' home environments and postpone nursing-home admission as long as possible; for the same reason more alternative supervised-living facilities are needed for the demented elderly, partly with a view to reducing the risk of isolation;
- greater attention must be focused on protecting demented patients who live at home from their families: steps are needed to prevent the physical and psychological maltreatment of sufferers and the misappropriation of their assets;
- the quality-control of the care given to geriatric and psychogeriatric patients must be improved on the one hand by expanding inspection activities and on the other through research into the effects of the various forms of home care, daycare and alternative forms of accommodation.

Some of these measures will need to be made compulsory and can thus only be implemented under central direction; this will involve either the amendment of legislation and regulations or substantial state intervention.

4. *Measures geared to severe cases of dementia syndrome*

Here the focus is on chronically sick patients requiring constant care. Many of them have not been admitted to an institution and are looked after at home. Once again some of the measures proposed are aimed directly at the sufferers themselves and others at their caring environment.

The following measures are needed.

- *Aimed at severely demented patients not in institutions:*
  - greater efforts are needed to locate severely demented patients who live alone. The welfare and police services have a part to play here;
  - professional support where patients are cared for at home. The heavy burden involved in looking after a chronically sick and often very old person can exhaust and even 'burn out' the caring partner or other relative, and the consequences for both carer and patient can be serious (illness, maltreatment etc.). While help in the form of host ('foster') families, holiday trips and the like is very welcome it does not take away from the need for more structural measures (financial support, suitable housing).

- *Aimed at patients in institutions:*
  - a considerable expansion of nursing-home capacity (in terms of both beds and staff). The serious shortfall which now exists (and which can be expected to continue while current capacity norms remain in force) needs to be remedied so that patients can receive sufficient personal attention from staff and the need to use isolation and other coercive methods is reduced to an absolute minimum. Capacity needs to be expanded to the point that all patients in psychiatric or general hospitals for whom nursing-home care is indicated can be transferred;
  - the foregoing implies a need for more clinical geriatricians, whose training must focus more explicit attention on the care of the chronically and terminally ill. The training of geriatric nurses and others who care for the old needs reforming in the same way.
  - nursing-home admission criteria should not be further tightened; the lengthening waiting lists in which this would result could mean many patients being inadequately cared for at home or in old-people's homes;
  - greater clarity is needed in the area of regional cooperation and the division of functions between nursing homes and other institutions providing intramural and extramural care for the elderly (old-people's homes, hospitals). Case-management procedures could help bring this about;
  - the expansion of capacity should allow stricter quality standards to be applied to nursing homes. The approach used should be one which helps stimulate patients rather than allowing them to vegetate. The various aspects of the care provided should be systematically recorded with a view to the regular evaluation of activities;
  - better support is needed for the partners, often themselves very old, of elderly patients admitted to hospital or nursing home. This is primarily a task for family doctors and social workers;
  - greater attention must be focused on protecting patients in intramural care from their families: steps are needed to prevent the misappropriation of their assets;
  - research is needed with a view to determining clearer criteria for intramural admission.

5.9 *Impact on the consumption of care and financial implications of the scenarios*

The four scenarios' implications for the demand for care and hence for costs cannot be fully determined: much of the information needed is unavailable or at best incomplete. Moreover in some cases we do not as yet have adequate ways of operationalizing certain essential concepts, among them the intensification of home care included in several of the scenarios: the notion may be interesting and relevant, but how can it be satisfactorily quantified?.

Only a small number of directly attributable costs and benefits can be estimated; more indirect costs and benefits can be estimated only very roughly if at all.

This section deals with the utilization of services and the resulting pattern of costs under each of the three exploratory scenarios and the target scenario over the period 1990-2010 under the following headings:

- psychogeriatric nursing homes and psychogeriatric units in general nursing homes,
- home help,
- community nursing,
- other costs and benefits.

The methods of calculations and assumptions used are set out in the appendix at the end of this chapter.

Table 5.16 **Demented patients aged 65+ in *psychogeriatric nursing homes and psychogeriatric units in general nursing homes* under the three exploratory scenarios and the target-setting scenario (end of year)**

	Reference scenario		**Radical profes-sionalization scenario**		**Strenghtening informal care scenario**		**Target-setting scenario**	
	<80	≥80	<80	≥80	<80	≥80	<80	≥80
1990	4400	14600	4400	14600	4400	14600	4400	14600
Total	19000		19000		19000		19000	
2000	5200	21100	7800	23400	5200	17200	5200	18700
Total	26300		31200		22400		23900	
2010	6000	27000	12000	32400	6000	18000	6000	21600
Total	33000		44400		24000		27600	

The Hospital Services Act (WZV) norm (of 1.25 psychogeriatric beds to every 100 people aged 65 or over) coupled with a constant 75% rate of occupancy by demented patients produces the following numbers of 'dementia beds': 1990, 17900; 2000, 20300; 2101, 22900.

In none of the scenarios is planned bed capacity sufficient to meet future demand; indeed, under the reference and radical-professionalization scenarios the *total* number of planned psychogeriatric beds is insufficient to accommodate demented patients alone in 2010.

Table 5.17 **Annual costs of caring for demented patients in *psychogeriatric nursing homes and psychogeriatric units in general nursing homes* under the three exploratory scenarios and the target-setting scenario (in millions of guilders, 1987 prices, index: 1990 = 100)**

	Reference scenario	Radical professionalization scenario	Strenghtening informal care scenario	Target-setting scenario
1990	1394 (100)	1394 (100)	1394 (100)	1394 (100)
2000	1929 (138)	2289 (164)	1643 (118)	1753 (126)
2010	2421 (174)	3257 (234)	1760 (126)	2025 (145)

Table 5.18 **Demented patients living at home and receiving *home-help service* and the costs thereof under the three exploratory scenarios and the target-setting scenario (in millions of guilders, 1988 prices, index: 1990 = 100)**

	Reference scenario		Radical professionalization scenario		Strenghtening informal care scenario		Target-setting scenario	
	Number	Cost	Number	Cost	Number	Cost	Number	Cost
1990	22800	137 (100)	22800	137 (100)	22800	137 (100)	22800	137 (100)
2000	30000	181 (132)	29300	177 (129)	34200	206 (150)	33600	203 (148)
2010	36400	219 (160)	34400	207 (151)	46400	280 (204)	45000	271 (198)

Table 5.19 **Demented patients living at home and receiving *community-nursing service* and the costs thereof under the three exploratory scenarios and the target-setting scenario (in millions of guilders, 1988 prices, index: 1990 = 100)**

	Reference scenario			**Radical professionalization scenario**			**Strenghtening informal care scenario**			**Target-setting scenario**		
	Number	Cost		Number	Cost		Number	Cost		Number	Cost	
1990	22800	44	(100)	22800	44	(100)	22800	44	(100)	22800	44	(100)
2000	30000	58	(132)	29300	56	(127)	34200	66	(150)	33600	65	(148)
2010	36400	70	(159)	34400	66	(150)	46400	89	(202)	45000	87	(198)

Other costs and benefits
While certain costs and benefits cannot easily be quantified, if at all, they must nevertheless be taken in account in assessing the various scenarios. They include:
- the cost of family doctors' increased workload (more screening for the elderly, greater help and support for families, etc.). Assuming the annual incidence of dementia to remain constant at 1.4% of all over-65s the number of new cases every year will rise from 27,000 in 1990 to 34,500 in 2010;
- the cost of referring demented patients to extramural facilities;
- the cost of diagnostic procedures, memory training etc. undertaken by commercial care institutions;
- the cost/benefit of regional trials of case management and other forms of cooperation and coordination between nursing homes, the primary sector, extramural mental health care etc.;
- the cost of 'parent allowances' and 'caring leave' for those undertaking the care of a demented partner or other relative;
- the cost/benefit of increased/reduced drug use by patients resulting from e.g. extended life expectancy and of alternative care strategies.
- the cost/benefit of curriculum changes and further training in relation to psychogeriatrics for workers in the primary sector and old-people's homes;
- the cost/benefit of expanding nursing facilities for psychogeriatric patients in old-people's homes;
- the cost/benefit of research and education programmes relating to aging and dementia;
- the cost/benefit of increased employment in the field of psychogeriatric care;

- the cost of supporting and caring for demented patients aged under 65 (dementia resulting from AIDS, Korsakoff's syndrome or trauma).

Careful analysis is needed of these costs and benefits to determine whether the target scenario in fact produces the sort of financial gain compared with e.g. the reference scenario which the tables suggest.

Appendix: Assumptions and methods of calculation

1. *Numbers of demented patients in psychogeriatric nursing homes and psychogeriatric units in general nursing homes*

The prevalence figures under all four scenarios are as follows (the age-specific prevalence is based on the baseline analysis):

Age	1990	2000	2010
< 80	44000	52000	60000
≥ 80	61000	78000	90000
Total	**105000**	**130000**	**150000**

On 1 January 1990 18% of dements aged 65 or over (= 19,000 patients) were in psychogeriatric nursing homes or the psychogeriatric units of general nursing homes (calculated on the basis of nursing-home data in SIVIS 1988). It is estimated that this total includes 10% of sufferers aged under 80 (= 4,400 patients) and 24% of sufferers aged 80 or over (= 14,600 patients). Each scenario makes assumptions as to changes in these percentages over the next twenty years:

- Reference scenario: <80, the proportion of sufferers in nursing homes remains constant at 10%; ≥80, the proportion rises from 24% in 1990 to 27% (21,100 patients) in 2000 and 30% (27,000 patients) in 2010.
- Radical-professionalization scenario: <80, the proportion rises from 10% in 1990 to 15% in 2000 and 20% in 2010; ≥ 80, the proportion rises from 24% in 1990 to 30% in 2000 and 36% in 2010.
- Strengthening informal care scenario: <80, the proportion remains constant at 10%; ≥80, the proportion falls from 24% in 1990 to 22% (17,200 patients) in 2000 and 20% (18,000 patients) in 2010.
- Target-setting scenario: <80, the proportion remains constant at 10%; ≥80, the proportion remains constant at 24%.

2. *Costs of nursing-home care for the demented elderly*

The costs are expressed in terms of 1987 prices. From Jacobs and Ketting (1989) we can calculate that the running costs of psychogeriatric nursing homes and psychogeriatric units in general nursing homes in 1987 totalled 1662 million guilders for a patient population of 22,658, equivalent to 73,352 guilders per patient. Total costs under each scenario can then be calculated on the basis of the patient numbers determined in accordance with the preceding section.

3. *Numbers of demented patients receiving community-nursing and home-help services*

Here the calculation starts from the numbers of sufferers living at home (i.e. not in a hospital, nursing home or old-people's home) and receiving help from their families; only they are entitled to community-nursing and home-help services. The assumption is made that despite the reduction in places currently underway the absolute number of demented patients in old-people's homes remains constant at 10,000 (the position in 1990), implying a relative increase. By subtracting these from the total number of demented patients in the country (calculated in accordance with section 1) we arrive at an estimate of the number living at home. The picture under the four scenarios is as follows.

	Reference scenario	**Radical profes-sionalization scenario**	**Strenghtening informal care scenario**	**Target-setting scenario**
1990	76000	76000	76000	76000
2000	93700	88800	96100	100000
2010	107000	95600	112400	121400

The number of patients living at home thus rises considerably under all four scenarios.

Each scenario makes assumptions as to the proportion of sufferers receiving help from the community-nursing and home-help services. The baseline analysis estimated that in 1990 30% of sufferers living at home received assistance from the home-help service and 30% from the community-nursing service; the numbers of patients receiving help were thus assumed to be the same for each service. The various scenarios' assumptions regarding the proportion of sufferers receiving help were as follows:

- Reference scenario: a rise from 30% in 1990 (22,800 patients) to 32% (30,000 patients) in 2000 and 34% (36,400 patients) in 2010.
- Radical-professionalization scenario: a rise from 30% in 1990 to 33% in 2000 and 36% in 2010.
- Strengthening informal care scenario: a rise from 30% in 1990 to 35% in 2000 and 40% in 2010.
- Target-setting scenario: as under the 'strengthening informal care' scenario.

4. *The cost of community nursing and home help*

The Financial Overview of Care (FOZ) 1990 shows:
- running costs (excluding vaccination programmes) of the community-nursing service in 1988: 835 million guilders,
- running costs of the home-help service in 1988: 1679 million guilders.

Given that 80% of community-nursing contacts involve persons aged 65 or over it was assumed that 80% of the service's operating costs were also attributable to this client category; with a total of 347,000 clients aged 65 or over (see the background analysis) the unit running cost was therefore 1925 guilders. The total cost of community nursing for elderly dements was then calculated on the basis of the numbers of service-users as determined in section 3.

In the case of home-help the proportion of clients aged 65 or over is 75%; this category was therefore assumed to account for 75% of the service's running costs (1,266 million guilders). With a total of 210,000 clients aged 65 or over the unit running cost was thus 6029 guilders. The total cost of community nursing for elderly dements was then calculated on the basis of the numbers of service-users as determined in section 3.

6 Schizophrenia

Part I Baseline analysis

6.1 *The concept of schizophrenia*

Schizophrenia is among the more serious forms of mental dysfunction; indeed, 'serious mental dysfunction' is often given that name. Certainly those who have been diagnosed as schizophrenic live lives marked by a considerable degree of mental suffering and major limitations in their personal and social functioning, often having difficulty in maintaining their autonomy and individuality. They consume a disproportionate amount of intramural care and their families often share in the mental suffering involved. Recovery occurs in only a minority of cases and can take many years.

The term fell somewhat into disuse in the 1960s and 1970s, following strong criticism, but in the 1980s schizophrenia has been revived as a scientifically accepted concept. It does however still encounter resistance, notably in the patients' movement.

Criticism of the schizophrenia concept came from various quarters: the 'anti-psychiatrists' (Laing, Esterson 1974; Cooper 1967; Szasz 1976), established psychiatrists (Kubie 1971; Kuiper 1976) and behavioural scientists (Bannister 1986; Sarbin, Mancuso 1980). The critics objected that:

- the wide variations in views, definitions, diagnostic practices and theoretical foundations covered by the single term 'schizophrenia' make worthwhile communication impossible;
- the diagnosis 'schizophrenia' is not sufficiently reliable;
- the validity of the concept is shaky, its predictive and construct validity slight. The conditions for validity (e.g. reliability) are not met and indications for validity (e.g. etiological specificity) are lacking;
- schizophrenia is a heterogeneous concept, it being generally accepted that it comprises a collection of unrelated symptoms;
- the results of research are disappointing, contrasting as they do with the enormous scale of the activities undertaken to clarify the causes of schizophrenia;
- the term has negative connotations, being for some people more a moral judgement than a neutral medical diagnosis.

Over the past fifteen years some of these criticisms have been met. The concept of schizophrenia has been further operationalized by means of research criteria (such as the New Haven Index, the St Louis criteria and Catego) and international standardization of its classification was achieved with the ICD and the DSM. The reliability of the diagnosis has thereby been considerably enhanced while greater standardization has enabled more internationally comparable research to take place. Increasingly the view has taken hold that schizophrenia has been reduced to a hard core of symptoms recognized in all countries. It is these developments that have helped the concept to regain its scientific status.

Wide diagnostic variations nevertheless persist. Gottesman *et al.* (1987) submitted case descriptions from an earlier twin study (Gottesman & Shields 1972) to a range of diagnostic procedures and research criteria; their original panel of six assessors having identified 69 cases of schizophrenia in a sample of 57 pairs of twins, other procedures were found to produce widely differing results (see table 6.1).

Table 6.1 **Numbers of identified schizophrenics according to various assessors and assessment systems (N=114)**

Clinical assessment	Result	Research criteria	Result
J. Welner (Danish 'spectrum')	81	Research Diagnostic Criteria (RDC)	54
P. Meehl	79	St Louis (broad)	53
UK hospital records	70	Catego S,P,O	52
Six assessors	69	RDC (narrow)	49
E. Slater	62	Tsuang/Winokur	49*
K. Abe (Japanese)	56	St Louis (narrow)	46
J. Birley	50	DSM III	44**
J. Welner		Abrams/Taylor	39
(Danish 'traditional')	42	Carpenter *et al.*	33
E. Essen-Möller (Swedisch)	34	Catego S	17
		First Rank Symptoms	17
		Crow, Type II	3***

Source: Gottesman *et al.* 1987.
* Minimum estimate.
** Excluding schizoaffective, schizophreniform and paranoid syndromes.
*** Crow's (1985) two-syndrome concept, here without Type I (which approximates to the schizophreniform syndrome).

The clinical judgement of diagnosticians generally proves to give a higher percentage of cases than diagnosis on the basis of research criteria. The data also bring out the fact that there are 'broad' and 'narrow' definitions of schizophrenia; more problematic, however, is the absence of an unambiguous hierarchy, in that the broader definitions do not necessarily encompass the narrower ones (Van den Bosch *et al.* 1988; Stephens *et al.* 1982). There thus exist more than one schizophrenia, depending on the assessor or assessment system involved.

Current views of schizophrenia are relative and pragmatic in nature: it is no longer seen as a single disease but rather as a somewhat vague and heterogeneous condition with arbitrary boundaries and recognized as deficient in validity. It is thus an open-ended, provisional concept whose nature is hypothetical (Van den Bosch *et al.* 1988). The concept is still developing and further adjustments are likely. Others go further. Bentall *et al.* (1988) interpret the current state of affairs regarding schizophrenia as a paradigm crisis in which the development of knowledge stagnates because the wrong questions are consistently asked; in their view the paradigm which determines how schizophrenia is seen and studied requires not adjustment but replacement. Constructively, Bentall *et al.* make alternative suggestions and give empirical results: one possible line of development is to focus thinking and research on individual symptoms, such as hallucinations, as they occur among patients and among 'normal' people (Bentall & Slade 1985). Romme's auditory-hallucinations project (1989) could be seen as a variation on this approach. Another line might be to regard schizophrenic symptoms more positively and less as manifestations of a disease requiring treatment (Muilwijk 1988).

Here we follow the line taken by Van den Bosch *et al.*, accepting schizophrenia as a vague and not entirely adequate concept for lack of a better alternative. When making pronouncements on the condition we must bear in mind that deficient diagnostic validity makes it uncertain that such pronouncements do indeed mean what they are supposed to mean; indeed, we cannot even be sure that the real world includes an entity which we can call schizophrenia.

6.2 *Characterization and definition*

In the scenario project it was decided to use the ninth version of the International Classification of Diseases (ICD-9) as the frame of reference. This applies to the consideration of schizophrenia as elsewhere, even though in practice preference is often given to the DSM-III description. The main differences between the two definitions will be indicated.

ICD-9 (code 195) defines schizophrenia as a group of psychoses characterized by:

- disorders of thought, perception, mood, behaviour and personality,
- delusions and hallucinations (mainly auditory),
- clear consciousness and intact intellectual powers,
- a course that is not necessarily deteriorating or chronic.

The symptoms, which need not all appear together, are often qualified as bizarre, freakish or abormal.

DSM-III gives a more extended and specific definition of schizophrenia which narrows the concept by requiring that:

- the disorders must have manifested themselves in the patient's life for a continuous period of at least six months,
- there must be a perceptible decline in the level of social functioning.

Schizophrenia symptoms are divided into positive (active) and negative (passive). The positive symptoms are delusions, hallucinations, incoherence and bizarre behaviour; the negative symptoms, such as withdrawal, apathy, weak affect and poverty of thought, are given the name 'defect' where they persist.

Both positive and negative symptoms can involve extreme forms of behaviour: living in a world of visions and being impervious to human contact, proclaiming that one is God or withdrawing to one room for years on end. It may well be that such behaviours are perceived as more extreme in western societies which no longer have room for seers, prophets or hermits.

The manifestations of schizophrenia are very variable: they can develop suddenly or insidiously; they may be of short duration or permanent; the course may be a chronic psychosis (permanent positive symptoms), a recurring psychosis or long-term defect without psychotic symptoms; there may be alternation with other (e.g. depressive) syndromes; the extent to which the condition disrupts daily life and is experienced as severe can vary widely; and outcomes can range from full recovery to permanent hospitalization.

While it is tempting to see the symptoms of schizophrenia as determined by an ongoing disease process, cases are known in which severely regressed schizophrenics proved able to play a leading role when sudden disaster occurred (Strauss *et al.* 1989). A more familiar phenomenon is that of the disturbed and apathetic chronic patient who nevertheless shows surprisingly normal and active behaviour on excursions. Such examples illustrate the assertion of Strauss *et al.* (1989) that negative symptoms can be precisely the expression of active coping behaviour. This underlines once more the importance of not approaching schizophrenic symptoms in reductionist fashion but rather of recognizing their complexity. Biological, mental and social factors, interacting with one another, are always involved.

6.3 *Occurrence of schizophrenia*

6.3.1 *Incidence and prevalence*

While studies of the incidence and prevalence of schizophrenia are not easily comparable owing to the different diagnostic criteria used, it is generally accepted that the lifetime prevalence is about 1% (Cutting 1985): one person in a hundred is likely to experience one or more schizophrenic episodes in his or her life.

It is also often assumed that schizophrenia occurs to the same extent in different countries and cultures and at a rate which is constant over time, but the data show this not to be the case. Prevalence rates (six-month and one-year) in different countries range between 1 and 12 per 1000 population and incidence rates between 0.1 and 0.5, with wider fluctuations not infrequently reported. Reviewing 79 prevalence studies Torrey (1987) concluded that, methodological and diagnostic differences notwithstanding, tenfold prevalence variations must be deemed to exist. Torrey (1989) reports both falling and rising trends over time.

The ratio of incidence to prevalence lies between 1:10 and 1:20. This reflects schizophrenia's often long-term nature (for every new case there are, on an annual basis, 10-20 existing cases) and indicates the limits to the efficiency of primary prevention: it would take many years before even highly effective preventive measures, even were they available, could produce a perceptible drop in the prevalence of schizophrenia.

Only very limited data are available on the incidence and prevalence of schizophrenia in the Netherlands. Giel *et al.* (1980) found an incidence of 0.11 per 1000 population for patients receiving intramural or extramural treatment for the first time. The Netherlands Schizophrenia Foundation (Slooff 1989) reports that around 3500 new cases arise every year, giving an incidence of 0.23% per 1000.

The most reliable data on the prevalence of schizophrenia in the population at large are provided by the Nijmegen Regional Project. Hodiamont (1986) found a one-month prevalence in the region's population of 6 per 1000, subject to a wide but unspecified margin of error; the figure relates to the non-hospitalized population aged 18-65, excluding non-Dutch-speakers and persons with no fixed abode. If certain assumptions are made this can be converted into a prevalence figure for the country as a whole.[1] Adding together the extrapolated figures for the population at large, the figures for schizophrenic patients in psychiatric hospitals and the estimated numbers of schizophrenic homeless persons gives a total of around 67,000 people diagnosable as suffering from schizophrenia (with a range of perhaps 20,000 either way). This gives us an estimated one-month prevalence figure for schizophrenia (Catego criteria, class S) in the Netherlands of around 7.5 per 1000 18-65s.

This figure coincides reasonably closely with that of the Netherlands Schizophrenia Foundation (Slooff 1989), which puts the number of schizophrenia cases in the population at about 100,000 or 6.7 per 1000. This figure was produced by working from the morbidity risk, assuming this to be around 1% in the Netherlands as elsewhere (Slooff 1989, personal comment). This estimate gives a somewhat lower prevalence, albeit account must be taken of the fact that an age correction for the young and old (among whom schizophrenia is less common) would produce a higher figure for the population of 18-65s.

Only a small minority of the schizophrenia-vulnerable are in psychiatric hospitals. At a rough estimate[2], of those 100 persons who could be diagnosed as schizophrenic at any given time:

---

[1] The calculation involves a number of assumptions and estimates. It was assumed that Hodiamont's regional figures could be generalized to the country as a whole (to which there appears to be no major objection) (Hodiamont 1988, personal comment); it was further assumed that the figures for non-Dutch-speakers were the same as for Dutch-speakers. The extrapolated figure for the number of cases of schizophrenia in the Netherlands in 1983 (when Hodiamont's study was made) then emerges as 54,230.
An estimate was made of the number of homeless people in the Netherlands and of the number of such people diagnosable as schizophrenic. On the basis of data reported by Smit (1986), Knulst (1987), Heydendael and Nuy (1983) and Nuy and Heydendael (1987) it may be estimated that there are between 90,000 and 120,000 homeless people in this country, of whom 33-50% are suffering from some form of psychiatric disorder and 10-25% could be diagnosed as schizophrenic. This gives us a total of between 3,000 and 15,000 homeless people with a vulnerability to schizophrenia. Taking the average of these estimates (9,000) gives a prevalence figure for schizophrenia among the homeless of 8.6%, not far from the 11.5% found by Koegel *et al.* (1988) among a representative sample of the homeless of Los Angeles.
Allowance was also made for 3993 patients aged 18-65 diagnosed as schizophrenic in general psychiatric hospitals (PIGG 1983) and a further 150 in the psychiatric units of general hospitals and university psychiatric clinics (estimate based on PIGG, LMR and NcGv data). This gave a total of 67,370.
After this baseline analysis had been completed lower estimates were published of the numbers of homeless (VNG/SGBO 1990); they did not however necessitate any fundamental change in our calculations. Further research in this area is essential.

[2] In addition to the information given in this section this estimate takes account of the following: for every chronically sick patient receiving intramural care there are five in extramural care (Wiersma *et al.* 1988); American studies indicate a ratio of treated to untreated prevalence of 50-100% with a median of 83% (Babigian 1985); our Delphi-panel experts estimate that schizophrenia is not recognized in 20-30% of cases.

- 6 are in intramural care,
- 30 are in extramural care,
- 26 are recognized cases but not, or no longer, in care,
- 13 are homeless,
- 25 have never been diagnosed or received care.

This picture raises a number of issues. The majority of schizophrenics are evidently not receiving care: does this constitute neglect? Around a quarter of cases are not recognized as such and can thus hardly be said to be patients; evidently such persons manage to live with their symptoms and do not see them as grounds for consulting a doctor. The question is: how? Little is known about those who have been recognized as schizophrenic but are not (or no longer) receiving care: what is the quality of their life? Are they deteriorating or can they cope? How much of a burden are they on those around them? Finally, is there perhaps a risk that stressing the clinical study of schizophrenia will give a distorted picture of the problem as a whole?

6.3.2 *Background variables*

Schizophrenia is found to be linked with a number of background variables: individuals' socio-economic status, sex, age, race, living conditions and environment (urban/rural) and the state of the economy. These are of course correlations and not causal links.

Schizophrenia is commoner in the lower social classes than in the higher. There is an association here with a number of other attributes: the prevalence of schizophrenia correlates directly with urbanization (cities with a population of over 100,000), race (ethnic minorities in situations of disadvantage), poor living conditions, poor working conditions and unemployment. Among the status factors Babigian (1985) considers social isolation to play a more important role than low income (or poverty).

To explain the links between schizophrenia and socio-economic status there are the rival hypotheses of social stress ('poor living conditions cause schizophrenia') and social drift ('downward mobility is the result of schizophrenia'). In many cases the slide down the social ladder resulting from psychosis or admission to a psychiatric institution is very evident: in their sample Wiersma *et al.* (1983) found downward mobility not only after the onset of schizophrenia but also in the preceding period, indicating that premorbid functioning also causes socio-economic slippage. Some epidemiological data are however difficult to reconcile with the drift hypothesis (Albee 1985); Warner (1985) describes historical fluctuations in the prevalence of schizophrenia which prove to be associated with the state of the economy. The processes of social drift and social stress both appear to play a part.

Schizophrenia also correlates with age, generally making its first appearance fairly early in life (between the ages of 14 and 35 in 68% of cases). Assuming this to be fixed association, a somewhat lower incidence can be expected in the Netherlands as the average age of the population rises.

While schizophrenia is equally common in both sexes it tends to develop earlier in males than in females. Goldstein and Kreisman (1987) attribute this to differing patterns of expectation whereby boys come into conflict with their parents' norms and values at an earlier age than do girls.

Mortality among schizophrenics is high, higher than the average for the population as a whole for most of the causes of death (Babigian 1985).

Such statistical associations tell us little about possible causes, but whatever the causes are there is cumulation in major cities: a build-up of schizophrenia cases can be expected in old districts with poor social conditions, large ethnic-minority populations, high unemployment and diminished social cohesion.

6.3.3 *Causes of schizophrenia*

There is considerable uncertainty as to the causes of schizophrenia. Since 1896, when Kraepelin postulated the organic cause of 'dementia praecox', schizophrenia has continued to be seen as a primarily biologically determined disease. In recent decades the clash between the medical and social models has resolved itself into the compromise of multicausality, with schizophrenia being thought to result from a multiplicity of factors of a psychological, biological and social nature, albeit it was on biological research that the greatest efforts were focused (Janssen 1982). Today biological factors are again seen as primary, with psychosocial factors precipitating or accelerating the expression of a biologically determined condition. Even so nothing is yet known with any certainty regarding the biological causes of schizophrenia (Weiner 1985).

Current thinking on the causes of schizophrenia is based on a model in which the disease is viewed as a vulnerability or predisposition which can manifest itself as an outbreak of symptoms under the influence of environmental factors. This model combines biopsychosocial factors. Figure 6.1 depicts the model developed by Warner (1985), which is itself adapted from the vulnerability/stress model of Strauss and Carpenter (1981).

Figure 6.1 **Warner's vulnerability model (1985)**

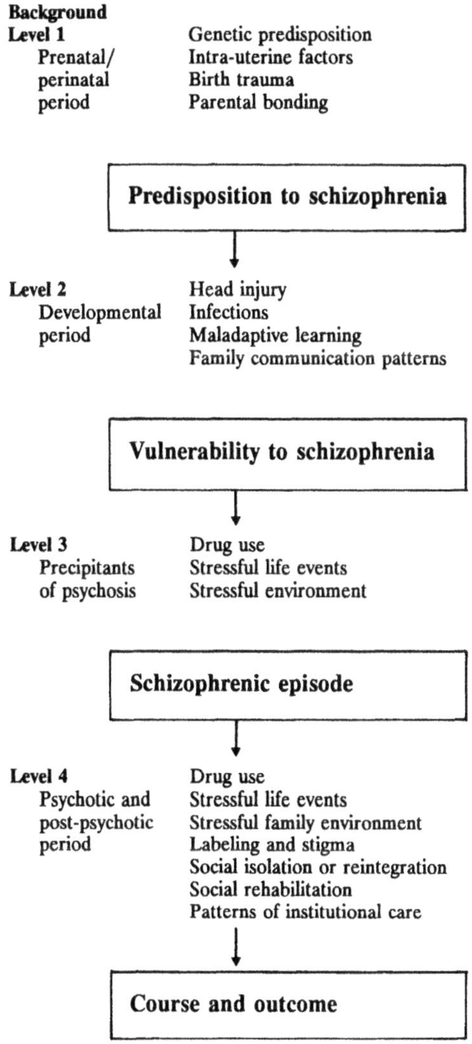

The model involves a predisposing factor itself determined by genetic and/or environmental factors; brain damage sustained at birth and bonding difficulties in early childhood may play a part here alongside the genetic component. The predisposition to schizophrenia may become a vulnerability as a result of somatic and/or psychosocial factors affecting the child's development. The characteristics of such vulnerability are a reduced capacity for information processing and hyperreactivity to stimuli, leading to a reduced ability to cope with (notably social) problems. Social stress factors and e.g. drug abuse may unbalance a vulnerable individual and cause decompensation, giving rise to positive symptoms such as delusions, hallucinations and incoherent thinking. The course and outcome of schizophrenia thus depend on the extent of vulnerability and on various environmental factors, among them social support, the backup given during rehabilitation and the pattern of institutional care (see section 6.6).

The vulnerability model represents a multicausal but nevertheless still largely heuristic integration of current knowledge as set out in standard works (see e.g. Kaplan & Sadock 1986). A genetic predisposing factor has been demonstrated in twin and adoption studies (Kendler 1986), albeit its significance is often exaggerated.[3] Mednick *et al.* (1971) among others have argued that complications during pregnancy and birth increase the risk of schizophrenia. Empirical support has been found for the view that disturbed family interaction plays a part in the genesis of schizophrenia (Goldstein 1985), though earlier hypotheses of this kind, such as the 'double bind' (Bateson *et al.* 1956) and the 'schizophrenogenic mother' (Fromm-Reichmann 1948), have been questioned or rejected. It has been suggested that 'expressed emotion' plays a part in the genesis as well as the course of schizophrenia (Asselbergs 1989). Stress factors are disproportionately frequent in the childhood of schizophrenic patients (Mirsky & Duncan 1986). Both painful life events (Brown & Birley 1968) and adverse living conditions (Albee 1985) cause stress, which can promote an outbreak of schizophrenic symptoms. A lack of social support makes people more vulnerable to stress (Liem & Liem 1978); the same is true of those with insufficient coping capacity or "hardiness" (Kobasa *et al.* 1982).

Social factors (including care factors) play a major part in determining the course of the condition and our knowledge of the factors which influence it is growing. These are discussed in the next section.

Though the vulnerability model is based on a multicausal view of

---

[3] Those who take the view of Cutting (1985) ("schizophrenia is largely genetically determined") or Slooff (1989) ("genetic factors contribute about 70% to the genesis of the condition") have to explain why it so often happens that one of a pair of identical twins develops the condition and the other does not (Strömgren 1975), why the schizophrenic gene has not yet disappeared from the gene pool (given the low reproduction rate among sufferers) and why the genetic factor seems to shrink the more narrowly schizophrenia is defined (Abrams & Taylor 1983); table 6.1 illustrates this last point clearly. Methodological criticisms of twin and adoption studies (Sarbin & Mancuso 1980; Rose *et al.* 1984; Marshall 1984) also need to be answered.

schizophrenia, acceptance of it is often associated with an assumption that schizophrenia is a fairly autonomous disease process, influenced by social or psychological factors in its manifestations but not in its genesis or cure. The incidence and prevalence of schizophrenia are then seen as independent of the psychosocial factors distinguished in the vulnerability model.

6.3.4 *Course and outcome*

Schizophrenia has long been associated with a very poor prognosis. Deterioration is often seen as characteristic of the condition, to the point that where cures occur it has sometimes been concluded that the diagnosis must have been mistaken.

According to Cutting (1985) the outcome of schizophrenia is good (full recovery) in 25% of cases, poor (permanent hospitalization) in 25% and somewhere between the two in the remaining 50%. Zubin *et al.* (1983) found comparable ratios: 33% recovery, 33% improvement and 33% stabilization or deterioration. The mental suffering associated with schizophrenia is evidenced by the number of suicides: between 2% and 10% of schizophrenics eventually commit suicide (Torrey 1983); Slooff (1988) found a figure of 9% in his cohort at the end of seven years.

A noteworthy fact relating to the outcome of schizophrenia and patients' position on the labour market is summarized by Gmür: in times of economic prosperity two thirds of patients are eventually able to function successfully as employees, but the proportion falls to between a third and a fifth in times of recession and high unemployment. Evidently schizophrenia is a label which hides a considerable reserve of labour.

Recovery and improvement can be very fast; they can also take decades. An illustration is provided by the course study of Harding *et al.* (1987): a group of therapy-resistant patients from the "back wards" were discharged and put on an intensive rehabilitation programme. A sharp improvement took place between the tenth and the twentieth year of the study, with 50-67% of the patients eventually achieving a considerable improvement or complete recovery. These figures are all the more remarkable in that they relate to a group of chronic patients rather than a representative sample of patients on first admission.

The vulnerability model sees the course of schizophrenia as being mainly influenced by environmental factors. The empirical data are in keeping with this view and are briefly reviewed out below.

That the course and outcome of schizophrenia are worse in industrialized countries than in the developing world (WHO 1973; WHO 1979) indicates the importance of social, economic and cultural factors. The stability of society, the strength of family ties and the extent of the accessibility of social roles (including the work role) all appear to play a part. In a twelve-year course study on Mauritius Murphy and Raman (1971) found that 59% of patients eventually achieved full recovery. Torrey (1987) notes that the proportion of patients in the worst-outcome category is comparable in different countries; the difference would appear to lie in the greater likelihood of recovery in developing countries.

The recurrence of psychotic symptoms is associated with stress, which may result from painful life events (such as the loss of a job or a relationship). The impact of such stress factors depends on individuals' coping capacity and particularly on the degree of social support provided by their environment (Asselbergs 1989).

It has been shown that stressful patterns of family interaction can have a major impact on the course of schizophrenia. There is a close link between the recurrence of schizophrenic psychoses and the extent of 'expressed emotion' (EE) - excessive anxiety on the one hand, relatives' hostile and critical attitudes towards the patient on the other - in the family (Leff, Vaughn 1985). Lowering EE by supporting the family, offering psycho-education or reducing contact between patient and family are found to have a favourable impact on the course of the disease.

Labelling and stigmatization are socio-psychological processes which help perpetuate deviant behaviour and thus adversely affect the course of schizophrenia. Labelling (Scheff 1966) refers to the process whereby the individual is 'reduced' to a label (e.g. 'chronic schizophrenic') and treated accordingly, thereby making it difficult for him or her to give up the deviant role. Scheff sees labelling as the major factor in the genesis of a deviant career. The notion of stigmatization (Goffman 1963) has much in common with that of labelling but puts the emphasis on the negative connotation of labels and the operation of prejudices, such as those which flow from the 'ideology of dangerousness' (Tranchina 1979, 171). Stigmatization has damaging consequences for individuals in terms both of their self-image and self-confidence and of the attitudes of the community in terms of social distance and exclusion.

Hospitalization adversely affects the course of schizophrenia (Wing & Brown 1971) as long stays in unstimulating surroundings of 'institutional poverty' induce dependence, loss of initiative, apathy and diminishing skills; social contact with the outside world gradually declines, the way back becomes steadily more difficult and even the desire to take it disappears. Institutionalization should not however be seen as the sole factor in the poor progress made by hospital patients: the mental problems themselves can also make a contribution

(Holman & Wennink 1984).

'Rehabilitation' is a collective term for a wide range of strategies aimed at preventing chronicity, avoiding hospitalization or shortening stays, and improving the functioning of long-term care-dependent patients in the community. The effect of such strategies (including the EE approach) has been demonstrated for schizophrenia in terms of decreased psychopathology, reduced consumption of intramural care and improved social functioning (Kiesler 1982; Gmür 1986). Rehabilitation techniques are of a practical and supportive nature but their ultimate effects can also be seen as therapeutic (Strauss 1986).

It is generally accepted that strategies to influence the course of schizophrenia can make a major contribution to improving outcomes and patients' quality of life. As yet, however, there is no consensus as to whether this effect manifests itself not just in generally improved functioning but also in a higher percentage of cures and hence declining prevalence. Longitudinal and controlled effect studies are needed to clarify the position.

6.4 *Care facilities and their utilization*

6.4.1 *Prevention*

Primary prevention in relation to schizophrenia has in practice mainly been developed in the genetic and psychosocial fields. Genetic measures are aimed at preventing the transmission of the genetic factor predisposing to schizophrenia. One way of doing this is to influence fertility rates, and in the 1960s 24 US states had legislation providing for the compulsory eugenetic sterilization of (among others) mental patients (Deutsch & Fishman 1963, p. 1970). These days contraception (by the use of slow-release implants) can fulfil the same role.

A second approach involves genetic counselling aimed at preventing the conception of children at risk for schizophrenia (or at terminating pregnancies in such cases). There is still much uncertainty as to the role of the genetic factor in schizophrenia, however, and the risks are differently assessed by different experts: some (Fuhrmann & Vogel 1983) always oppose conception where either parent has ever experienced a schizophrenic episode; others (Reveley 1985) see this position as exaggerated. Genetic counselling should take account not only of genetic factors but also of psychosocial circumstances (Reveley 1985): genetic measures can very usefully operate in tandem with psychosocial measures.

Psychosocial preventive measures focus particularly on children in high-risk groups (Watt *et al.* 1984). Such groups can be distinguished on the basis of suspected genetic factors (the children of schizophrenic parents), epidemiological statistics (see section 6.3.2) or psychophysiological tests (WHO 1977). Cognitive tests concerned with attention disorders also appear to be a promising approach (Erlenmeyer-Kimling & Cornblatt 1987). Preventive interventions may involve intensifying pre- and post-natal care for mothers known to be vulnerable to schizophrenia, enhancing communication skills within the family or improving children's attention function through cognitive therapy. The effectiveness of such measures needs further study.

Secondary prevention is possible in the form of e.g. action to prevent the recurrence of symptoms. Many of the measures for the treatment and rehabilitation of schizophrenia patients discussed in the next section can be seen as forms of secondary prevention.

6.4.2 *Treatment*

Psychoactive drugs play a major part in the treatment of acute schizophrenia and in chronic cases too heavy stress is placed on maintenance medication (often using depot preparations) in preventing relapses. However, when Hogarty *et al.* (1974) compared a group on medication with one receiving a placebo they found relapse rates after two years of 48% and 80% respectively, and while the difference is considerable it indicates that only a minority of patients benefit from medication: when drugs are used half the patients still relapse, and when no drugs are used a fifth nevertheless do not relapse. Research is underway into the factors involved. Research is also underway into the optimum dosage of neuroleptic drugs (Kane 1986), partly in response to growing concern at side effects (notably tardive dyskinesia). In this light it is striking that, in some countries at least, the dosages used appear to be increasing markedly: Reardon *et al.* (1989) found that American schizophrenics received on average twice the daily dose of neuroleptic drugs in 1982 as in 1973, concluding - given that no link had been confirmed between higher doses and better results - that it was prescribing practices that had changed rather than treatment decisions. Hirsch (1989) in contrast reports attempts to achieve refinements in prescribing practices by watching for the signs of an impending relapse and adjusting medication accordingly.

Early enthusiasm for intensive psychotherapy for schizophrenia cooled considerably after initial trials (e.g. Foudraine 1971). Studies revealed disappointing results, including in the case of the Chestnut Lodge psychodynamic approach (McGlashan 1986). This does not however detract from the importance of the therapeutic relationship: its elements are as essential for the treatment of schizophrenia as for psychotherapy (McGlashan 1986a). Psychotherapy for schizophrenic patients is now primarily supportive and practically oriented.

This last is also true of group therapies. Alongside personal interaction, exploring problems and learning to cope, heavy stress is placed on the acquisition of social skills. A gradual shift is taking place towards more recreational groups able to operate as part of day-activity programmes (McGlashan 1986a).

Family therapy is very much in the ascendant in the treatment of both acute and chronic schizophrenia. The heading covers both the 'old' system-focused family therapies (Wynne, Minuchin, Palazzoli) and the new family approaches (Leff, Falloon) which have mainly developed around the EE concept and psycho-education. Compared with the 1970s there is a much greater inclination towards pragmatism and the integration of methods and theories (McFarlane 1983). Therapeutic goals are more modest and interventions are often geared to influencing the course of the condition. Important results were found by Falloon *et al.* (1982): when two groups were compared, one receiving both family therapy and medication and the other medication alone, the relapse rates after nine months were 9% and 44% respectively. Related to the family approach is the social-network approach (Baars 1984), which seeks to exploit and extend the possibilities of social support in networks.

Directive and system-focused therapies are increasingly applied in the treatment of both acute and chronic expressions of schizophrenia. They may be used as part of family approaches and also at individual level.

Forms of skill training are increasingly being developed (Liberman *et al.* 1986) and are often applied in conjunction with behaviour therapy. Training focuses on social, vocational and, to a lesser extent, cognitive skills (Brenner & Hodel 1989). Cognitive training can affect schizophrenic symptoms: patients can learn not to 'hear voices' e.g. with the help of an earplug (Van der Gaag 1988).

Rehabilitation is a collective term encompassing many treatment and support strategies aimed at influencing the course of schizophrenia (Tantam 1988). Almost all the therapies mentioned can be applied in rehabilitation, the facilities used ranging from clubs and day activity centres through rehabilitation centres, outpatient departments and sheltered accommodation to community centres and churches. The purpose of rehabilitation is practical, namely to prevent relapses, provide support in the activities of daily living and promote reintegration into society. Under this last heading heavy stress is placed on work (Harding *et al.* 1987b). In the United States a national Community Support Programme has been instituted for the purpose of integrating and implementing activities (Turner & TenHoor 1978);

under it agencies and services are given contracts at regional level for the provision of various forms of support for long-term care-dependent patients. Case management has an important part to play here in ensuring the coordination and continuity of formal and informal care (Harris & Bergman 1987).

McGlashan (1986) emphasizes that there is no single or preferred treatment for schizophrenia: several strategies need to be deployed and combined depending on circumstances, the phase of the condition and individual needs and abilities. The care relationship must be central and treatment open-ended, perhaps even life-long. In practice the various treatments are often intertwined. Particularly in those countries where deinstitutionalization is underway the accent has increasingly shifted from 'cure' to 'care', the goal of achieving a cure giving way to one of learning to live with the problem (albeit the two sometimes prove to be the same thing (Strauss 1986)).

6.4.3 *Utilization of care*

Little is known with certainty regarding the utilization of care services by schizophrenics in the Netherlands. National figures are available only for the psychiatric hospitals (see table 6.2).

The admission figures in table 6.2 may distort the picture downwards, since there is some reluctance in practice to diagnose schizophrenia (Slooff 1984). A striking feature is the small proportion of schizophrenic patients in the figures for psychiatric units in general hospitals and the large proportion in those for general psychiatric hospitals: this reflects the fact that schizophrenia, more than other diagnoses, leads to long-term care dependence. Of the patients remaining in general psychiatric hospitals for more than two years almost half are diagnosed as schizophrenic (PIGG 1987).

Little is known about the utilization of services by schizophrenics in sheltered accommodation. Given that at a rough estimate 25-50% of residents in such accommodation are schizophrenic patients, the total number of individuals concerned must lie in the range 750-1500. Unfortunately no registration data are available for sheltered-living facilities.

Diagnosis-specific data are not available on extramural mental health care, but if the statistics given by Wiersma *et al.* (1988), which indicate that there are five extramural patients for every hospitalized chronic patient, are representative of the country as a whole, then we can estimate that around 30,000 long-term care-dependent schizophrenics are receiving help from extramural institutions (mainly RIAGGs and outpatient departments). We can assume that few schizophrenics present to psychiatrists in private practice.

Table 6.2 **Utilization of services by patients diagnosed as schizophrenic (ICD 9) in psychiatric hospitals: in absolute numbers and as a proportion of all new patients and the standing patient population in each type of institution**

	New patients	Proportion of total	Standing population	Proportion of total
General psychiatric hospitals**	3967	15.4%	6376	29.6%
University psychiatric clinics***	325	11.6%	62	11.8%
Psychiatric units in general hospitals****	664	5.3%	90*	5.3%*
Psychiatric day treatment**	427	11.2%	318	12.4%
Total	**5383**		**6846**	

* Estimate. ** PIGG 1987.
*** PIGG 1986. **** LMR 1987.

It is not known how many schizophrenic patients receive care in the primary sector. A survey has shown that social workers and family doctors often see follow-up support for psychiatric patients as part of their function (De Ridder & Visser 1987); in some cases this is also true of the home-help and community-nursing services. Some family doctors regard the treatment of delusions as part of their job. Specific information is however lacking on diagnostic categories.

Private boarding houses, many of which were formerly funded by the health ministry but which now fall outside the sheltered-living schemes, form a grey area overlapping with that of provision for the homeless (on which little is also known).

Numerous 'alternative' organizations operate at the interface between formal and informal psychiatric care. Such bodies, whose role often receives insufficient attention, include self-help groups, drop-in centres and support structures, sometimes organized by the bodies established to promote patients' interests. Then there are the volunteer workers involved in such areas as supervised living, day activities, information, legal assistance, occupational rehabilitation and hospital visiting (Centrum PS 1989).

Many schizophrenics live with or are supported by members of their family. Here again it is not known how many people are involved. Giel (1984) refers to the study by Dumont, who found relatives of mentally handicapped children to devote an average of seven hours a day to caring for them. In terms of hours the informal care provided for patients by their families may well be a multiple of the volume of formal mental health care.

6.4.4 *Developments in schizophrenia care*

Current trends in provision for schizophrenia patients are towards more extramural care and greater integration of extramural and intramural services. Continuity and meeting individual clients' needs ('tailor-made care') are major objectives, both in crisis intervention in cases of acute decompensation and in the support of long-term care-dependent patients.

Social psychiatry is placing greater stress on such acute-situation procedures as family therapy, extramural crisis intervention and strategies for avoiding hospitalization. Where long-term support is involved the overarching concern is rehabilitation.

At public-policy level these developments are reflected in the movement to substitute sheltered-accommodation and day-treatment places for psychiatric-hospital beds and in the greater stress placed on the social-psychiatry function of the Regional Institutes of Ambulatory Mental Health Care (RIAGGs). Cooperation and coordination are being improved through Multi-Functional Units and the formation of the Regional Institutes of Mental Health Care (RIGGs).

Many studies have shown extramural treatments for schizophrenia to be at least the equal of intramural treatment. Gmür (1988) gives a comprehensive overview of controlled studies in this area:

1. Alternatives to intramural treatment. Home-based treatment (e.g. Langsley & Kaplan 1968), treatment in sheltered accommodation (e.g. Mosher *et al.* 1975), day treatment (e.g. Herz *et al.* 1971), training in community living (e.g. Stein & Test 1980) and outpatient treatment (Levenson *et al.* 1977) have been compared with intramural treatment. Such studies have demonstrated the feasibility of these alternatives, while their effectiveness has in broad terms been equivalent to that of intramural care. In cost terms the alternatives appear to be somewhat more efficient.
2. Shorter stays. The effects of briefer hospitalization (with various forms of aftercare) have been investigated in a number of studies involving control groups. Some of these studies (e.g. Endicott *et al.* 1978) have included day treatment with aftercare while others (e.g. Glick 1976) have covered extramural aftercare. The experimental treatments have proved broadly equivalent to the traditional approach.
3. Aftercare programmes. Various studies have compared the effects of different types of aftercare with situations in which no aftercare was provided. The Fountain House project (Beard *et al.* 1978), the

Quarterway House project (Gudeman *et al.* 1981), a comprehensive support programme (Dincin *et al.* 1982) and a psychoactive-drugs programme under which those receiving drugs were compared with a placebo group (Leff & Wing 1971) have all demonstrated their effectiveness in terms of falling numbers of readmissions and improvements in clients' social functioning. The more comprehensive and carefully thought-out the programmes were, the greater were their effects.
4. Community care. This heading covers various replacements for the asylum function of the psychiatric hospital, among them small-scale residential provision (e.g. Linn *et al.* 1977), group residences (Burger *et al.* 1977) and apartments (Chien *et al.* 1973). In demonstrating that alternative forms of accommodation can be found in the community for many, though not all, long-stay patients, such trials have shown the need for permanent inpatient care to have been greatly overstated.

Experience in the Netherlands points in the same direction: part-time treatment can replace inpatient care under certain conditions, as the Assen substitution project showed (Van Veldhuizen *et al.* 1988); the Psychosis Prevention Project in Rotterdam demonstrated that the number of days of intramural care could be cut by 61% (Vlaminck 1989); and a chronic ward of Santpoort Psychiatric Hospital has been successfully accommodated in apartments in the Bijlmermeer district of Amsterdam (Bleeker *et al.* 1987). The first two of these projects involved control groups; in Rotterdam only patients diagnosed as schizophrenic were involved, while in Amsterdam schizophrenic patients made up 70% of the total. Asselbergs (1989) found some improvement in the social functioning of schizophrenia patients in the Rotterdam project.

Gmür (1986) concludes that, despite many studies' methodological deficiencies (such as the selection of more motivated or less 'difficult' patients), these various attempts at deinstitutionalization have produced equivalent or better results compared with traditional inpatient care. Sometimes there is also a perceptible improvement in patients' social functioning. The effectiveness of alternatives to the psychiatric hospital depends on the extent to which substitutes are provided for its various functions (accommodation, activities, protection, support, treatment). Gmür enters a reservation here: the achievement of results equivalent to those obtained by inpatient care, universally criticized though it is, does not in itself constitute grounds for rejoicing. The key issue is whether treatment outside hospital improves patients' quality of life, and research results give us little information on this more subjective point.

The quality-of-life question could be answered in two ways: by determining relevant criteria and considering the factors which best assist in meeting them and, more concretely, by considering whether those concerned are more satisfied. Ideally these factors would need to be assessed in the context of the triadic relation (Petry 1989) between client, social network and care-givers.

With regard to possible criteria it is reasonable to associate patients' quality of life with their ability to function in their own environment and to play a full part in social life, and the shift towards non-institutional care would appear to offer increased scope for promoting that ability. With regard to patient satisfaction Stein and Test (1980) found higher levels in their experimental group, as did Hoult and Reynolds (1984), Mattes *et al.* (1977) and Asselbergs (1989).

Gmür found the cost of the projects he described to be the same as, or indeed lower than, those of inpatient care. Weisbrot *et al.* (1980) and Vlaminck (1989) give detailed cost analyses, the latter finding savings on mental health care costs while the former finds increased mental health care costs to be compensated by reduced indirect costs and greater effectiveness.

A number of studies have found the burden on families to be no greater (Fenton *et al.* 1979) or even less (Washburn 1976; Stein & Test 1980).

With regard to the risk of suicide Vlaminck (1989, 36) notes that no increase was observable in the experimental group and that hospitalization did not guarantee an absence of suicide attempts. Langsley and Kaplan (1968, 171) and Endicott *et al.* (1978) also found no increased risk of suicide in their experimental groups.

While research may show deinstitutionalization to be feasible we must guard against naive and overoptimistic moves in this direction. Giel (1984) points to a number of dangers which should not be ignored[4].

Various studies have shown that extramural support and supervision for schizophrenics must be ongoing: where trials have been terminated the results have quickly evaporated (Stein & Test 1980). Rehabilitation can reduce the need for care, since individuals

---

[4] Giel (1984) lists the following dangers of 'naive' deinstitutionalization: families' ability to cope may be overestimated; the selection of 'better' patients may have harmful effects, such as the development of blacklists; the social limitations of schizophrenics may be underestimated; current facilities for extramural care may be overestimated; it is illusory to assume patients' motivation for extramural care; the organization of extramural care may run aground on the shoals of bureaucracy; and the result may be an increase in the numbers of psychotic vagrants. Giel also points out that successful programmes have a high ratio of staff to patients and are funded in a way that guarantees continuity, so that support for patients can be maintained long-term. All these factors could mean that extramural alternatives are not in fact cheaper.

are enabled to function ever more independently (Van der Veen 1983), but this is not necessarily true of the need for support and supervision.

6.5 *Concluding remarks*

A research field as vast as that concerned with schizophrenia cannot be summarized in so short a space as this. Almost nothing has been said, for example, about the extensive biological research carried out into schizophrenia: while its results is still highly contradictory, there is great optimism regarding future breakthroughs thanks partly to continuing technical advances (CT scanning, PET scanning, rCBF, gene studies, genetic manipulation and so on). Expectations in this direction are however somewhat tempered by the dashing of past hopes and the repeated failure of loudly trumpeted breakthroughs.

Schizophrenia must be recognized as a provisional, open-ended and evolving concept. Adjustments are likely in the future; indeed, the concept may be replaced by a whole new paradigm. Diagnostic variation and the arbitrary boundaries drawn around the condition notwithstanding, the problem must not be trivialized: its consequences for the individual are often severe and disabling.

The prevalence rate of schizophrenia in the Netherlands can be put at around 7.5 per 1000 population; for a variety of reasons the condition is considerably commoner in large cities.

It is important to see schizophrenia as a complex phenomenon: monolithic standpoints belong in the past. All aspects of the genesis, course and treatment of the condition involve a multiplicity of interacting biological, psychological and social factors, and it is thus highly improbable that some miracle drug or other treatment will ever be found.

Four questions are important as we look to the future: is the prevalence of schizophrenia increasing? Can we expect better treatment methods to be developed? Is improved prevention a possibility? And can the quality of life of those stricken with schizophrenia be improved?

The answer to the first of these questions must be that on current understanding the prevalence of schizophrenia will remain at its present level, neither rising nor falling. While therapies can certainly be further improved, the likelihood is very remote of any major breakthrough which would lower prevalence rates. Even were a breakthrough achieved in our biological or genetic knowledge it is doubtful that this would enable practical or ethically permissible interventions. This is equally true of preventive measures: while primary prevention must certainly be developed further, it is unlikely to bring any very significant benefits in the short term.

The last of the four questions can be answered affirmatively. There is scope in the areas of prevention (secondary and tertiary), therapy and support for further alleviating the mental suffering of those afflicted by schizophrenia. In the short term measures to influence the course of the condition are likely to be most important. Major shifts in care provision are possible, bringing with them improvements in the care of schizophrenics and their quality of life.

Schizophrenia remains a baffling phenomenon. More research is needed, particularly into its long-term manifestations and effects. Such research should tell us among other things whether the incidence and prevalence of schizophrenia can be influenced or must be accepted as immutable facts.

This baseline analysis was completed in December 1989.

Part II Schizophrenia scenarios, 1990-2010

6.6 *Exploratory scenarios*[1]

6.6.1 *Scenario 1: Reference scenario*

Outline: The reference scenario is marked by relatively adverse economic trends and a slightly increased fragmentation and hardening of society. These developments influence not so much the prevalence of schizophrenia as its expression and the extent to which it is seen as a problem. The adverse impact on schizophrenics of these developments will however be offset by improvements in the structure and practice of care. While some measure of deinstitutionalization will take place most care will still be provided by psychiatric hospitals.

Incidence and prevalence

No significant change is envisaged in the incidence and prevalence of schizophrenia over the period 1990-2010. Prevalence will remain at 7.5 per 1000 18-65s, so that with population growth the total number of persons diagnosable as schizophrenic will increase by about 7%. The course and outcome of the condition will change owing to environmental factors.

The living conditions of lower-status groups in society will worsen as income differentials widen and unemployment remains high; long-term unemployment will be concentrated among the unskilled and unfit while social provision will be at a lower level and less accessible. Society will be more complex: information flows will intensify and participation in society become increasingly demanding. It will also tend to fragment, with family ties growing less important and people less willing to offer one another support and informal care. There will be less tolerance and understanding of those who deviate from social norms. These trends, which must be seen as gradual shifts rather than sudden qualitative changes, have a number of implications for those who are vulnerable to schizophrenia: they will be exposed to greater stress, in part because of the higher demands made on individuals' capacity to process information; at the same time they will receive less support from family and friends, thereby becoming less able to cope with stress. The result will be that schizophrenia manifests itself in younger people, that schizophrenic episodes recur more frequently and that the course of the condition and its social side-effects are adversely influenced.

These developments, damaging from the viewpoint of the schizophrenic patient's interests, will however be offset by improvements in

---

[1] The basic assumptions of the exploratory scenarios are set out in Appendix 1.

formal care. First, the continuity of care will benefit from, among other things, the formation of Multi-Functional Units. Second, care provision will be improved and expanded: schizophrenia will be diagnosed and treated sooner, thanks partly to improvements in diagnostics; the Regional Institutes of Ambulatory Mental Health Care will be better able to treat acute patients in their own homes; better and more selective psychoactive drugs will be developed and their reduced side-effects enhance compliance with the medication; and rehabilitation techniques will be further developed and more widely applied.

Efforts in the area of rehabilitation will be hampered by the changes taking place in society, however, with the social reintegration of schizophrenics being impeded by the reduced acceptance of deviant behaviour, people's decreased willingness to offer informal care, cuts in social provision and the higher barriers facing those seeking to enter employment.

The net effect of these various factors will be a slight improvement in the course and outcome of schizophrenia: it will slightly more often be possible to prevent chronicity, the relapse rate will fall and the residual symptoms of schizophrenia will generally be a little less severe.

While the prevalence of schizophrenia in general will not alter the severe forms of the condition will be slightly less common. The average level of functioning of schizophrenia patients, as regards e.g. coping ability and social participation, will improve somewhat.

Increased efforts in the area of prevention will have yet to produce results in terms of reduced prevalence: given the long delay between the genesis of a vulnerability to schizophrenia and the expression of symptoms, the effects of genetic counselling and prevention programmes for children in high-risk groups will not begin to make themselves felt until some time after 2010.

Services and their utilization

While the prevalence of schizophrenia will remain constant and patients' care needs diminish slightly the number making use of care provision will rise, reflecting overall population growth. Of greater importance, however, is the fact that the extent to which help is sought in connection with schizophrenia and the extent to which the disease is recognized and treated will increase markedly thanks to measures in the area of education and early diagnosis; the reduced acceptance of deviant behaviour will also increase the pressure on individuals to seek treatment. There will also be greater social pressure, notably from the associations of sufferers' families, to ensure that such treatment is available.

Care intensity (i.e. the average time devoted to each client) will remain constant despite increased utilization both of the formal services provided by institutions and of the informal care provided by volunteers and social networks.

The informal care provided by families will increase slightly: relatives may be less willing to provide care, they will be in a better position to do so thanks to the increased support available from the formal-care sector. The consistent use of family approaches (including family therapy, the 'expressed emotion' approach and psycho-education) will be of help here. On balance a greater volume of informal care will be provided by a smaller number of relatives.

The utilization of intramural-care services by schizophrenics will decline, reflecting a continuing if fairly weak policy of deinstitutionalization; the number of beds in general psychiatric hospitals will be cut by 10% and the resources thereby released shifted into psychiatric day treatment and sheltered living. The annual growth in volume wil also expand the social-psychiatry function of the Regional Institutes of Ambulatory Mental Health Care. More staff will be taken on, especially in the extramural sector, but the pressure on services will remain considerable.

Most schizophrenia care will continue to be provided by general psychiatric hospitals, albeit some residential psychiatric care will be switched into sheltered-living facilities.

The quality of life of schizophrenics can only be assessed by those involved (in the triadic relationship between client, care-giver and social network). The conditions for improved quality of life will be better in some respects (with more patients remaining in their own environment and better means of relieving their suffering becoming available) and worse in others (with patients participating less in normal life). On balance, however, the conditions determining patients' quality of life will be slightly improved.

The number of people vulnerable to schizophrenia who are not reached by the care services will decline somewhat but remain high. The number of homeless among them will not fall and many people will drop out of care or try to cope on their own; their quality of life will decline.

6.6.2 *Scenario 2: Marginalization*

Outline: This scenario envisages more adverse economic, social and cultural trends than the reference scenario. Society will become highly complex and fragmented, with a strong emphasis on individual performance, and growing numbers will fall by the wayside. A social divide will open up, and for the increasing numbers not in work income levels and social provision will decline. The pressure on the mental health system will grow considerably as a result, but the effectiveness of the care provided will decline. There will be greater room for voluntary and private initiatives and new services will be set up to mitigate the worst distress.

Incidence and prevalence

Like the reference scenario, this scenario envisages no change in the prevalence of schizophrenia over the period 1990-2010, with the total number of people diagnosable as schizophrenic rising by about 7% as a result of population growth. The prevalence of severe and chronic forms of the condition, however, will rise sharply owing to social, economic and cultural trends: society will be more complex, making heavier demands on individuals; the spread of automation will mean there is little demand for unskilled labour; people will tend to be harder and more calculating, reflected in greater self-centredness, less tolerance of deviant behaviour and an ongoing marginalization of those who are different and/or cannot take part in the production process. Income differentials will widen and a social divide open up. Family bonds will weaken and people become less willing to provide care and support in informal networks. Views of what constitutes normal mental functioning will harden and higher levels of performance will be expected, with the result that more people will fall by the wayside.

These trends will be strongest in the cities. Many already marginalized groups will continue to migrate to cities, a phenomenon further promoted by the abolition of frontiers in Europe.

Together these factors will raise social stress levels, causing those vulnerable to schizophrenia to decompensate more strongly and more frequently. Schizophrenics will be ostracized more quickly and will find it more difficult to reenter society. Rehabilitation and resocialization will be hampered by the lower levels of tolerance, social provision and willingness to provide informal care and by the growing difficulty of entering the labour market.

The result is that schizophrenia will become even more disabling, chronicity commoner and the social limitations associated with the condition greater. The care needs of schizophrenics will grow and the formal care system will be unable fully to meet them.

Responsibility for care will increasingly lie with the citizen rather than the state. This will mean greater scope for private and voluntary initiative and, partly at the instance of organizations representing patients and their families, new types of provision will develop.

Services and their utilization

Schizophrenic patients will make greater demands on the formal care system and the greater number of sufferers and, especially, the increased propensity to ostracize and reduced willingness to provide informal care will mean that the system is faced with more patients with severer problems. The pressure on services will increase considerably in consequence: while the volume of care will grow (mainly through the expansion of extramural provision) it will not keep pace with increasing demand and will therefore be less intensive.

Despite 10% cut in a intramural capacity and the conversion of beds into day-treatment and sheltered-living places there will be growing institutionalization: the number of admissions will increase as lengths of stay fall, while sheltered-living facilities will tend to develop into small institutions marked by isolation and the use of compulsion. In general care will be concerned more with control than with treatment. Continuity of care will deteriorate and provision for active resocialization and rehabilitation will be insufficient. The extramural sector will not be able to do much more than muddle through. More medication will be given, its effectiveness enhanced by the fact that it can be compulsorily prescribed for extramural patients. In some cases the payment of social benefits will be tied to medication to ensure that drugs are taken.

One result of these trends will be large groups of schizophrenia patients, inside and outside care facilities, who are permanently disabled and socially marginalized. Care facilities will be overloaded and increasing numbers of clients will receive little or no help. Another result will be growing homelessness and, owing partly to the decline in social tolerance, homeless people will increasingly find themselves caught up in the justice system.

The volume of care provided informally will decline, though many families, for lack of a better alternative, will continue to care for their relatives. This will produce stress, partly because no help will be available from an extramural sector which no longer has time to undertake home visits or family approaches.

These trends will necessitate new initiatives, in the form among other things of increased self-organization among patients (clubs and associations). Private clinics and commercial boarding-houses will be set up. More charitable refuges will be established aimed mainly at the homeless. A range of facilities will thus exist but in many cases they will provide only minimal care (bed, board and pills).

The conditions determining the quality of life of persons vulnerable to schizophrenia will deteriorate across the board: they will be less independent and more tied to care structures; they will be more likely to be forced out of their own environment and find it more difficult to reintegrate; little will be available by way of worthwhile activities and employment will be almost out of the question; mental suffering will not be adequately relieved but rather suppressed by medication.

The sight of patients wandering the streets and the nuisance they are perceived to cause, coupled with an anyway declining tolerance of inappropriate behaviour, will lead to new calls for the expansion of psychiatric hospitals.

6.6.3 *Scenario 3: Integration*

Outline: This scenario assumes economic, social and cultural trends to be more favourable than in the reference scenario, with a greater volume and a wider spread of employment, narrower social-status divisions and greater social cohesion. Society will be more inclined to accept deviant behaviour and ostracism less common. This will produce a decline in the severe and chronic forms of schizophrenia and will reduce pressure on services. A drawback associated with increased tolerance will be greater indifference, leading some groups of schizophrenia patients to be denied care.

Incidence and prevalence

Like the reference and marginalization scenarios this scenario envisages no change in the prevalence of schizophrenia over the period 1990-2010, with the total number of people diagnosable as schizophrenic rising by about 7% as a result of population growth. The prevalence of severe and chronic forms of the condition, however, will fall sharply as a result of social trends.

By 2010 the 'me age' will have made way for a new 'we age' as the values and norms associated with competition, self-centredness and performance are displaced by a desire for cooperation, community and involvement. Social cohesion will grow as family bonds strengthen and new forms of friendship network and communal life develope. There will be more contact between people, *inter alia* through modern communication systems (including computer networks). Deviant behaviour will be more tolerated and there will be greater willingness to offer mutual care and support.

Economic developments will strengthen these trends. Working hours will be further reduced, enabling employment to be spread more widely. The pressure to perform will weaken and new jobs will be created in many service occupations (janitors, handymen, nightwatchmen and so on). Income differentials will narrow and access to social provision be further democratized.

The rising average age of the population and the lowering of the pensionable age will produce a situation in which there are many elderly people with the time and ability to involve themselves actively in social life, giving a major impetus to the development of societies, cultural activities, voluntary work, action groups and the like.

At the same time a certain cultural complacency and lethargy will develop and the rate of social and economic progress slacken.

These social trends will lead to changes in the expression and course of schizophrenia. Lower levels of stress at work and in society and greater tolerance of deviant behaviour will make vulnerability to schizophrenia less likely to result in psychotic episodes and people will be better equipped to withstand stress thanks to higher levels of social support and cohesion. Schizophrenia will be less disabling, socially and otherwise, partly because the conditions for rehabilitation will have improved; long-term occupational incapacity as a result of schizophrenia will be the exception rather than the rule. Moreover schizophrenic symptoms will be less seen as problems necessitating professional care. Crises will more easily be dealt with in patients' social networks, reducing the need for intramural care.

Services and their utilization

Schizophrenics will put far less pressure on professional care: fewer patients will use services or enter institutions, despite population growth, because they are better able to cope independently and receive greater care and support within their social networks and because schizophrenic symptoms are less easily seen as psychiatric problems, while those patients who do make use of professional care will tend to have less serious problems. Schizophrenics will be better able to cope and will face fewer social handicaps across the board. In particular there will be a decline in the need for long-term nursing care.

Care intensity (i.e. the average time devoted to each client) will increase, with more time being devoted to 'non-motivated clients'. In the extramural sector there will be greater scope for labour-intensive approaches: home visits, rehabilitation activities and measures to prevent hospitalization will all be more common. Care-givers will need to have less resort to compulsion and there will be less pressure from society to apply it, with the result that patients are less mistrustful of care-givers and more easily reached and motivated. The number of homeless schizophrenics will fall.

The rate of deinstitutionalization will lag behind the growth in the options available; only 10% of the beds in general psychiatric hospitals will be replaced by additional extramural provision. The decline in psychiatric-hospital admissions will be accompanied by an intensification of care and an extension of the average stay (in part reflecting measures to prevent the development of overcapacity). In all sectors of mental health care there will be a tendency to relax admission criteria and reach out to new client groups.

Informal care will grow, with families, friends and neighbours more willing to provide care. Informal care will also benefit from the additional support available from the professional sector.

The conditions determining the quality of life of persons vulnerable to schizophrenia will improve: they will be better able to cope in their own environment, more involved in the life of society and more likely to obtain employment. Mental suffering will be less likely to engender such problems as prejudice and stigmatization and can more often be relieved.

The greater social tolerance of deviant behaviour will be accompanied by the drawback of greater indifference: to the extent that deviant behaviour is not recognized as a sign of mental suffering, the result may be that patients do not receive the care they need.

The greater numbers of schizophrenia patients remaining in the community will tend to constitute a social nuisance; where thresholds of tolerance are exceeded violent behaviour may result.

Professional care-givers will find their work more rewarding, with its increased stress on help and therapy and reduced need for supervision and control.

6.7 *Target-setting scenario: Continuity of tailor-made care*[2]

Outline: From 1990 to 2010 a consistent policy is pursued of improving the quality of life of persons vulnerable to schizophrenia, centred on deinstitutionalization and community care. The emphasis in mental health care is shifted toward extramural, community-focused care. Improvements are also made in intramural care; it will however lose its leading role, instead providing a back-up for extramural services. The conditions on which the achievement of these targets depends are: the restructuring of the organization and funding of care; the operation of consistent policies in other areas of society; the establishment of social support networks; improvement of the quality of care; and action against social prejudice.

[2] The basic assumptions of the target-setting scenario are set out in Appendix 1.

Objective: *To ensure that by 2010 the quality of life of those who are vulnerable to schizophrenia is considerably better than under the reference scenario (unchanged policy).*

Measures relating to the structure of care

The goal of 50%-lower consumption of intramural care by those vulnerable to schizophrenia by the year 2010 requires a systematic policy of deinstitutionalization. The number of psychiatric hospital beds must be cut by 50%, with an equivalent expansion of places in sheltered-living and, to a lesser extent, day-treatment facilities. This reform implies a reallocation, not a reduction, of resources.

Less should be invested in buildings and more in people. The RIAGGs' social-psychiatry services need to be expanded threefold, allowing both more outreach work and measures aimed at making hospitalization unnecessary and increasing the staff available to undertake rehabilitation (including the prevention of relapses), the support of informal networks (family, friends and neighbours) and case management (which should operate independently of the care service itself).

Intramural facilities must focus on crisis intervention and short-stay treatment in small-scale units and on the care and nursing of the most incapacitated patients.

Day treatment must replace full hospitalization, with day-treatment centres cooperating closely with the intramural and extramural services to ensure continuity of care (and where possible of the care-giver). Where necessary such centres should offer temporary accommodation.

Sheltered-living facilities of various types are needed, from residential communities and group and individual homes to temporary accommodation and refuges for the homeless. The supervision and support offered to residents must be flexible and in all cases independent living must be the aim. Day-activity centres must operate in all subregions; their services must include skill training, including cognitive training. They should also play a part in occupational rehabilitation and job placement.

In all regions the community support system has an important part to play, with case managers monitoring and maintaining the continuity and quality of care and ensuring that policy-makers are familiar with clients' needs.

The main emphasis in the services available to those with a vulnerability to schizophrenia needs to shift from 'cure' to 'care': support, protection, supervision and crisis relief are key concepts here, along with continuity and flexibility. The focus needs to be on the 'healthy' part of the client rather than the 'disease', implying among other things an attitude towards those vulnerable to schizophrenia which puts greater stress on their 'normality' and social role.

The 'cure' side must not be neglected, however. The scope offered by psychoactive drugs must be exploited. Greater therapeutic expertise needs to be developed by acute intervention teams, notably with regard to family- and system-focused approaches (e.g. in the treatment of adolescents in their first episode of decompensation). Greater stress is needed on supportive psychotherapy, with therapeutic insights being better incorporated into the day-to-day help given to clients.

Conditions

If the target scenario is to work a number of conditions need to be met in the organization and funding of care, in training and research, in housing and employment for clients, in social provision and in society's tolerance of deviant behaviour.

In all the measures taken priority must be given to the clients with the 'severest' problems, whether in the intramural or the extramural sector, to avoid the creation of new problem groups. Care provision also needs to be geared to and shaped by clients' needs as manifested in the various regions.

The scenario will not work unless the divisions between different services and levels are bridged. Policy must therefore be guided by the principles of *regionalism* and *client-centredness*: regionalism means that the full range of services is provided within each region, with the various facilities involved working together to ensure that this happens; client-centredness implies that care services are grouped into functions (accommodation, support, treatment, crisis intervention, day activities etc.) in such a way that an appropriate package of functions can be compiled for each individual client. The funding system will need to be restructured (see below) to achieve this situation and to ensure that the need for the various measures is recognized.

Collaboration among a region's institutions cannot be on a voluntary basis: it must be formalized, on the basis either of some form of merger or of contractual arrangements. In every region there needs to be central direction in which interest groups and clients' organizations are involved.

The obstacles to deinstitutionalization must be removed. Each region must have a budget from which initiatives can be funded without interference from central bodies. The funding legislation must incorporate incentives to encourage deinstitutionalization and discourage unnecessary bed occupancy.

Raising the standards of care must be made financially attractive, with a system of statutory quality criteria and perhaps rewards for high standards; it should also be possible to impose budget cuts where proven inefficiency is the result of conservatism. The process of deinstitutionalization must be separated from considerations relating to financial economies.

Carer-training needs to be improved. The particular need is for in-service training, since many professionals will be expected to exercise new skills. More practical and realistic approaches are needed in nurse education, which will need to include new subjects geared to the new functions (rehabilitation techniques, the supervision of day activities and of sheltered-living facilities, extramural crisis intervention, case management etc.). The status and pay of nurses (including community mental nurses) need to be raised.

Research has a part to play in achieving the target. Greater efforts are needed in the development and evaluation of rehabilitation techniques, and greater priority needs to be given to multidisciplinary (and specifically longitudinal) chronicity studies, from which more results can be expected in the medium term than from biological research. Experiments in new forms of care must be encouraged.

Appropriate action is also needed in other policy areas:
- occupational-rehabilitation schemes need to be developed, in the normal labour market, under the Sheltered Employment Act (WSW) and in new job projects;
- the housing market must be pushed into removing obstacles to the provision of accommodation for clients and ex-clients and to sheltered-living facilities;
- social provision must be made more accessible to those who are vulnerable to schizophrenia;
- public education is needed to promote the social acceptance of patients and ex-patients and to break down barriers across the board. In general attitudes must be fostered among both carers and clients which give greater scope to optimism and less to despair.

Specific measures

The role of central government will need to be more modest in some areas (notably the design of services at regional level) and more active in others (the creation of the right framework at national level).

Measures aimed at service coordination are needed at national level, e.g. accelerating the formation of Regional Institutes of Mental Health Care (RIGGs); the RIGGS' structure and management (including the involvement of clients and other groups) must be regulated by statute.

Funding measures must be geared to the various objectives: separate resource flows must give way to a system of regional budgets. The funding legislation must incorporate incentives for deinstitutionalization: newly created extramural-care places should attract the same funding as intramural places, limits are needed on the maximum number of days of nursing care in general psychiatric hospitals and the shortening of hospital stays must be rewarded. Hospital budgets need to be made fully independent of bed-occupancy levels. The conditions which an institution must meet to be recognized as eligible for public funding must be made more flexible and the regions must be given a greater say in the assessment of applications for recognition.

When budgets and funding arrangements are determined a long-term view is needed which allows temporary increases in spending to be offset at a later date.

Greater investment is needed in training, with supervision to ensure that new requirements are met. Resources need to be channelled into the development of expertise in various areas, notably rehabilitation in a broad sense, crisis intervention and case management. Greater emphasis is needed on therapeutic techniques (supportive psychotherapy, system-focused approaches) and their integration into the day-to-day support of clients. Medical education needs to focus more attention on the side-effects of psychoactive drugs and selectivity in their prescription. Different kinds of expertise need to be developed and deployed, geared e.g. to network development and the organization of social change.

At national level guidelines and funding procedures are needed for the coordination of care. The community support system has an important part to play here, in close cooperation with case managers. New initiatives must be undertaken as the need for them arises; voluntary work and alternative forms of care too should be supported through the community support system. In other policy areas both national measures (such as the full implementation of the Employment of Disabled Workers Act (WAGW)) and, particularly, regional measures are needed. The community support system will need to monitor the implementation of measures in other policy areas, and agreements will be needed at regional and local level on housing (municipal housing policy, housing associations) and employment (employment offices, sheltered employment, occupational rehabilitation). Public-information campaigns are needed, as is action against discrimination. Social provision must be made more accessible to clients and ex-clients, among other things by improving their income situation (paid employment, greater flexibility in charging arrangements).

Effects
While the target-setting scenario has no impact on the overall prevalence of schizophrenia it does affect the prevalence of its severer forms; social limitations, secondary handicaps and incapacity for regular employment could well be drastically reduced. Long-term care-dependence and chronicity will be less common (and less long-term). It must be borne in mind, however, that these are long-run effects and depend on ongoing and in some cases permanent support for clients.

The movement away from intramural care puts the focus on clients' integration and reintegration into society and makes it easier to avoid the development of dependence. This creates the conditions for a considerable improvement in the quality of life of people who are vulnerable to schizophrenia: they will be better able to cope in their own environment and have more opportunities and greater ability to participate in the life of society, and there will be greater scope for alleviating their suffering.

The cost of care in 2010 under the target-setting scenario is not much greater than under the reference scenario, though there are temporary cost increases as the process of restructuring gets underway.

Various side-effects are possible. The scenario could, for example, be misused as a vehicle for spending cuts: if the expectation is that deinstitutionalization will bring immediate savings, the result may be a dilution of care. A second danger is that the new care structure may be insufficiently underpinned by a consistent framework of policy in related fields. In both cases the result may be neglect, a growth in vagrancy and overconsumption of psychoactive drugs. The scenario could produce an excessive burden on families and the social environment, leading to protest and complaint. It is also possible that the inclination to ostracize could find an outlet in the justice system, with more patients finding themselves in prison.

Unless they are adequately prepared and carefully supervised the reforms could have damaging effects, in the shape e.g. of a higher suicide rate among patients, demotivation and reluctance among care staff, and intolerance and resistance in the population at large. The risk of such side-effects is greatest if the package of measures envisaged in the scenario is not seen and implemented as a whole.

Finally, there is a danger of new problem groups being created if the facilities created as part of the deinstitutionalization process are not adequate substitutes for the functions of their predecessors.

6.8 *Financial implications*

This section outlines a series of models with which an estimate can be made of the financial implications of the four scenarios, which vary various substitution processes within the overall field of mental health care. In this section we are concerned with costs relating to the care of schizophrenic patients. While the lack of data on the utilization of services specifically by schizophrenics makes exact calculations impossible, the models help bring out the order of magnitude of the costs involved and of the shifts taking place among them. The assumptions and estimates involved are indicated with numbers in the text and explained in the appendix at the end of the section.

The estimates allow for the phenomenon, noted by Häfner and An der Heiden (1989), that deinstitutionalization increases the average severity of problems in both the intramural and extramural sectors. This implies that care will need to be intensified if dilution is to be avoided. The tendency will grow as deinstitutionalization proceeds.

In what follows we outline first the cost factors involved in intramural and semi-intramural care and then those involved in extramural care. Overall costs, taking account of population growth, are covered in tables 6.7 and 6.8.

The main cost factor is the shift of capacity in intramural and semi-intramural care (see table 6.3). In the case of intramural and semi-intramural care cost can be related to capacity[5]; this is less true of extramural care, where the number of contacts or procedures is more significant. If more patients make use of extramural services this will be reflected in an increasing number of contacts or procedures involving the Regional Institutes of Ambulatory Mental Health Care and psychiatric outpatient departments (the role of psychiatrists in private practice is negligible).

Patient numbers are not the only factor affecting the form and cost of extramural provision: the severity of the problems concerned is also relevant.

Table 6.3 **Substition of semi-intramural for intramural places[1] for schizophrenia-patients**

	Today[2]	Reference scenario	Marginal-ization scenario	Integra-tion scenario	Target-setting scenario
Psychiatric hospitals	6380	5740	5740	5740	3190
Sheltered accommodation	1120[3]	1600	1600	1600	3510
Day treatment	190[4]	350	350	350	990
Total	**7690**	**7690**	**7690**	**7690**	**7690**

We look first at the changing pattern of the demand for services under the four scenarios, all of which assume constant prevalence. The baseline analysis included an estimate of the proportions of schizophrenics receiving and not receiving care; the ratio varies markedly between the scenarios, and these variations are shown in table 6.4. The exact figures are less important than the trends they indicate.

Table 6.4 **Shifts in the demand for care, 1990-2010**

	Today[6]	Reference scenario	Marginal-ization scenario	Integra-tion scenario	Target-setting scenario
Psychiatric hospitals	4000	-10%	-10%	-10%	-50%
Extramural care	20000	+20%	+25%	No change	+35%[7]
Not receiving care	17000	-10%	-20%	+10%	-10%
Homeless	9000	No change	+25%	-40%	-10%
Not recognized	17000	-10%	-20%	+10%	-10%
Prevalence	**67000**	**No change**	**No change**	**No change**	**No change**

Table 6.4 shows larger numbers using extramural services under all scenarios except the integration scenario. As well as patient numbers the kind of care needed is also an important factor, in that deinstitutionalization means that the extramural services will have to

deal with severer problems and will therefore need to provide more intensive care. The nature of the procedures involved can vary widely: a home visit is considerably more labour-intensive than a five-minute contact, and any shift in the pattern (towards more outreach work or less) has implications for extramural-care costs. In general the activities of outpatient departments are cheaper than RIAGG services, so that any shift between the two will affect overall costs. Finally, the cost of extramural care is related to its range of functions, and the case management and community support work included in the target-setting scenario are new functions with cost implications. The various factors are covered in table 6.5.

On the basis of the various cost determinants we can now make a reasonable assessment of trends in extramural-care costs under the four scenarios (table 6.6).

Table 6.5 **Factors affecting the cost of extramural care (outpatient departments and RIAGGs)**

	Reference scenario scenario	**Marginalization scenario**	**Integration scenario**	**Target-setting**
Patient numbers[8]	+ 20%	+ 25%	No change	+ 35%
Severer categories	Increase	Increase	Increase	Sharp increase
Care intensity	No change	Decrease	Increase	Sharp increase
Outreach work	Increase	Decrease	Increase	Sharp increase
Outpatient departments' share in extramural mental health care	No change	Increase	Decrease	Sharp decrease
Range of functions of extramural mental health care	No change	Decrease	No change	Sharp increase
Cost implication	Increase	Increase	Increase	Very sharp increase
Estimated cost increase[9]	**+ 40%**	**+ 30%**	**+ 30%**	**+150%**

Table 6.6 **Cost of extramural mental health services to schizophrenic patients (millions of guilders, 1988 prices)**

	Today[10]	Reference scenario	Marginalization scenario	Integration scenario	Target-setting scenario
Outpatient departments[11]	13	18	23	13	18
RIAGGs[12]	29	41	32	42	87
Total	**12**	**59**	**55**	**55**	**105**

We can now make an estimate of overall costs. Psychiatric-hospital costs are clearly an important element, but determining the resources released by the closure of a hospital bed is not straightforward. Three approaches are possible: (a) the saving could be equated with the average cost of a bed (e.g. Mootz 1985); (b) it could be equated with the average cost of a bed less overheads (which amount to around 40%) (NRV 1989); or (c) it could be equated with the average cost of a bed for certain patient categories (e.g. low-cost long-stay patients) less overheads (De Haen 1989). Table 6.7 uses approach (b), but with an assumption that overheads will fall as deinstitutionalization proceeds[13].

Finally, allowance must be made for population change. Under the Central Bureau of Statistics intermediate variant (1988) the population as a whole increases by 8% between 1990 and 2010. The number of 18-65s, who account for the vast majority of schizophrenia cases, rises by 7%, however, and the number of schizophrenic patients similarly is assumed also to rise by 7%. It is further assumed that the various institutions concerned are affected equally by the rise in the number of patients resulting from population growth and that costs rise in proportion.

In addition to direct mental health care costs the four scenarios have other cost implications which are harder to quantify. These are covered in table 6.8.

Table 6.7 **Cost of mental health care for schizophrenic patients (millions of guilders, 1988 prices)**

	Today[10]	Reference scenario	Marginalization scenario	Integration scenario	Target-setting scenario
General psychiatric hospitals	524	493	493	493	346[14]
Psychiatric units in general hospitals	8	8	8	8	8
Sheltered accommodation	38	55	55	5	132[14]
Day treatment	7	13	13	13	39[14]
Extramural care	42	59	55	55	105
Day activity centres	2[15]	3	3	3	6[16]
Occupational rehabilitation	1[17]	1	1	1	9[18]
Total	**622**	**632**	**628**	**628**	**645**
Total allowing for population growth		**676**	**672**	**672**	**690**

Table 6.8 **Indirect costs**

	Reference scenario	Marginalization scenario	Integration scenario	Target-setting scenario
Nursing pay[19]	No change	No change	No change	Increase
Other policy areas	No change	No change	No change	Increase
Social costs[20]	Increase	Sharp increase	Decrease	Decrease
Police, justice system etc.	No change	Increase	Decrease	Decrease
Provision for the homeless	No change	Increase	Decrease	Decrease

A final factor which is hard to quantify as a cost is the severity of the handicaps associated with schizophrenia. The integration and target-setting scenarios both envisage the severity of handicaps easing, and in the longer term this should produce savings in terms of the costs of care and general social costs.

Conclusion

Direct health-care costs under the three exploratory scenarios do not differ widely. The equal costs of the marginalization and integration scenarios reflect a constant volume of care; care functions vary differently under these two scenarios, however, and this is reflected in the indirect costs. Overall the integration scenario entails the lowest costs and the marginalization scenario the highest, the reference scenario falling between them.

Mental health-care costs are highest under the target-setting scenario, though they could be offset by lower indirect costs: given that schizophrenia's social cost in terms of benefit payments alone runs into hundreds of millions of guilders, there is evident scope for major cost shifts; these are difficult to quantify, however, not least because in some cases they will occur only in the long term.

The safest assumption is that the target-setting scenario entails a slight rise in costs as compared with the reference scenario.

Appendix: Calculations and assumptions in the cost assessment

1. The substitution of extramural places for hospital beds is assumed to take place on a one-for-one basis and to affect acute and long-stay beds equally. Acute beds are replaced with day-treatment places and long-stay beds with places in sheltered accommodation. Since service utilization is greater in the case of chronic patients than in that of acute/short-stay patients (according to PIGG figures, by a factor of three), three times more substitute places are created in sheltered accommodation than in day-treatment facilities. The figures in table 6.3 are rounded to the nearest ten. The capacities are not adjusted to take account of population growth.
2. See the data in the baseline analysis.
3. The estimate made in the baseline analysis is used in the case of sheltered accommodation, taking the average figure (37.5% of places are occupied by schizophrenic patients).
4. The capacity can be calculated from the number of patients receiving day treatment (see baseline analysis) by applying the conversion factor of 1.7 (Jacobs & Ketting 1989).
5. An intramural institution's costs are determined mainly by its capacity rather than its 'output', with the result that a sharp reduction in length of stay (i.e. a sharp increase in discharges or transfers to other forms of care) has little impact on costs (Endicott *et al.* 1978).
6. The figures relate to 18-65s.
7. The figure is rounded up to reflect the increased role of extramural care *vis a vis* sheltered accommodation. Under the other scenarios the role of sheltered accommodation is statistically negligible.
8. According to the indications in table 6.4.
9. The target-setting scenario's higher costs mainly reflect the tripling envisaged in the social-psychiatry function of the RIAGGs. The 150% rise in extramural-care costs appears realistic given the various mutually-reinforcing factors involved. This is less the case under the exploratory scenarios, where the different factors vary less widely and often offset one another. The cost increase thus reflects chiefly the increase in the number of patients (under the reference and marginalization scenarios) and increased care- and labour-intensity under the integration scenario.
10. According to the latest data from Jacobs and Ketting (1990) for 1988.
11. Schizophrenic patients are deemed to account for 20% of the

work of outpatient departments

12. Social psychiatry is deemed to account for 30% of RIAGG costs and schizophrenic patients are deemed to account for 20% of social-psychiatry costs.
13. The three exploratory scenarios assume 40% overheads for the replaced beds and the target-setting scenario assumes 20%. This is because major capacity cuts entail reorganizations and the reinvestment of capital and reserves. This general picture is confirmed by the experience of Trieste, where the replacement of at least 91% of beds was achieved without (in the end) any net cost increase (Dell'Acqua and Cogliati Dezza 1985).
14. A 10% cost increase is incorporated to cover the effect of deinstitutionalization, in accordance with Häfner and An der Heiden (1989).
15. A rough estimate, since no financial information is available on day activity centres as they currently exist. The three exploratory scenarios incorporate the recent (December 1989) grant scheme of the Health Insurance Funds Council.
16. Target-group size based on the NRV (1987) estimate; the figure also assumes 70 day-activity centres/Fountain Houses with a capacity of around 200 clients and is based on the average cost (300,000 guilders) of projects submitted for health-insurance funding (Hagen & Van Weeghel 1989). It is further assumed that 30% of clients can be diagnosed as schizophrenic.
17. A rough estimate, since no financial information is available on employment projects as they currently exist.
18. Based on the De Schalm model project, which costs 200,000 guilders a year and offers work to 35 people every year, of whom 34 move into mainstream employment (De Schalm 1988). It is assumed that half of those in the day-activity centres' target group are or wish to be eligible for occupational rehabilitation, so that around 140 projects are needed. It is estimated that 30% of their capacity is used for people diagnosed as schizophrenic.
19. Salary adjustments in line with general pay trends.
20. Production losses, benefit payments, etc.

7 Occupational incapacity due to mental disorders

Part I Baseline analysis

7.1 *Introduction*

This analysis focuses on people who are declared unfit for work owing to mental disorders. It is thus *not* primarily concerned with the psychological effects of occupational incapacity however caused (feelings of isolation, fatalism and so on); research in this field has been carried out by, among others, the Social and Cultural Planning Office (SCP 1986, pp. 81 ff.). Here in contrast we are concerned with what are known as Category V cases, people who are declared unfit for work with 'mental disorders' as their ICD-9 principal diagnosis and who therefore receive disability benefit under the relevant legislation.

The following diagram indicates how the occupational-incapacity process functions and what the main factors involved are.

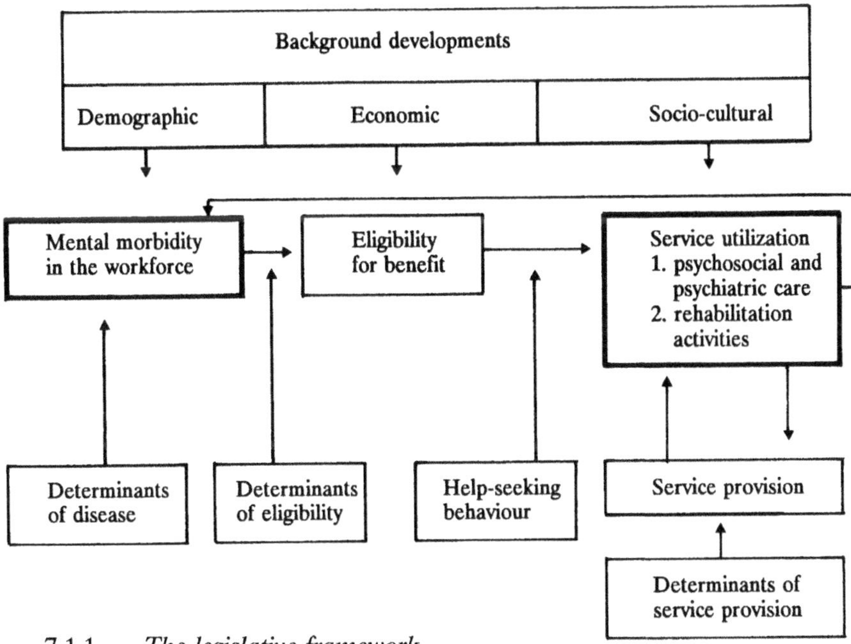

7.1.1 *The legislative framework*

Incapacity for work within the meaning of the Disability Insurance and General Disability Benefit Acts (WAO/AAW) is not a primarily medical matter and is not related solely to individuals' state of health; rather is it a legally sanctioned situation of long-term absence from work. When someone covered by the scheme reports sick a medical officer from an industrial insurance board determines whether sickness is present and whether there is entitlement to benefit (normally under the Sickness Benefit Act (Ziektewet)). After a year's payment of sickness benefit there follows a second assessment, this time to determine whether the individual concerned is entitled to benefit under disability legislation. The main focus in these assessments is not the individual's medical condition or functional disorder but rather the limitations on performance which result from that condition. What is a serious condition in medical terms (such as the loss of a limb) need not entail complete incapacity (not even for, say, a carpenter), where some other job (e.g. as a doorman) can reasonably be deemed possible given the individual's education and former employment. That job need not actually be available: what matters is the theoretical possibility of doing other work.

Another important point is that the disability legislation provides insurance cover not for unfitness for work as such but for *loss of income*. The link between an individual's medical condition or functional disorder and the formal degree of incapacity is a weak one; the direct link is between the degree of incapacity and the individual's former pay. The difference between what someone earned in their former work and what they could now earn in some other job which they are theoretically capable of doing determines the degree of incapacity, expressed as a percentage. The theoretically determined pay shortfall ('loss of earning capacity') decides the outcome, not the medical condition.

No benefit is payable under the Disability Insurance Act (WAO) where incapacity is less than 15%; in the case of the General Disability Benefit Act (AAW) the threshold is 25%. Setting these thresholds means that those whose position on the labour market is weakest - women and migrant workers in poorly paid jobs, often involving the greatest risk of sickness or disability - are ineligible for benefit (see also Den Heeten *et al.* 1987), since the gap between their former (low) wage and the theoretically determined new wage is often less than 15% or 25%. It is not known how many people there are who, though medically unfit for work, fall foul of this regulation and thus, being ineligible for benefit, do not appear in the statistics.

As will be evident from the above, any changes in social-security legislation can have a major impact on the number of those classed as unfit for work.

7.1.2 *Key data*

In 1988 over 893,000 people were in receipt of benefit at one time or another on account of long-term incapacity; these were people who, having been unable to work for more than a year, were entitled to full or partial benefit under the relevant disability legislation. (As well as the Disability Insurance Act, which covers employees, and the General Disability Benefit Act, which covers the self-employed and those who are handicapped from an early age, there are specific schemes for civil and public servants, railway employees and military personnel.) The total number receiving benefit at the end of 1988 stood at 794,000, i.e. just over 12% of the labour force. In 1987 the disability funds' outgoings totalled some 23 billion guilders.

Entitlement followed a 'mental disorders' diagnosis in the case of around a quarter of these benefit recipients and the cost of such 'Category V' benefits can thus be put at some 5.5 billion guilders a year; however, because this category tends to be found in the highest disability class the cost may will be greater. In addition there are those whose incapacity had lasted less than a year and who are thus still covered by the Sickness Benefit Act; at a rough estimate some 15% of these are diagnosable as having a mental disorder, giving a cost of 1.2 billion guilders in 1988. Total expenditure on benefits to persons declared occupationally incapacitated by mental problems in that year was thus over 6.5 billion guilders. This compares with total mental health care operating costs in the same year amounting to some five billion guilders.

Since the introduction of the Disability Insurance Act (WAO) in 1967 (the General Disability Benefit Act (AAW) followed in 1976) the total number of claimants has risen dramatically from 160,000 in 1968 to almost 800,000 in 1988; the 200,000 maximum expected when the 1967 legislation was introduced was in fact reached within three years. It is now expected that the total will rise to over a million in the year 2000, representing just over 13% of the labour force (as against 12.6% at present).

The rise in the number of Category V benefits has been, in proportional terms, faster still: where in 1968 11% of new claimants (4,100 people) had been diagnosed as suffering from mental disorders, by 1989 the proportion had risen to 32% (35,000 people). Of those receiving benefit at the end of 1988 26% - over 200,000 people - had been declared unfit on mental grounds.

It is generally accepted that other diagnoses than Category V also encompass mental health problems as part of the cause of incapacity, with estimates of their share ranging from 30% to 50%. If such estimates are correct, around a half of all those who are occupationally incapacitated are suffering from mental illness or problems. Social Insurance Council data indicate that among the recipients of disability benefit mental conditions are relatively frequent among civil and public servants (including teachers), health-care workers, printing workers and bank staff; also striking is the sharp increase within Category V in the 'adjustment reaction' diagnosis, which accounted for 23% of new entitlements in 1980 and 48% in 1988. While this is a weak indicator, it does appear to show that increasing numbers of people are unable to withstand the mental pressures of the work situation. A final point is that entitlement to benefit on mental grounds increasingly tends to arise at an early age: among the under-35s Category V is by far the commonest diagnosis where unfitness is found.

7.2 *Occupational incapacity in the Netherlands*

7.2.1 *Incidence and prevalence*

When the Disability Insurance Act (WAO) came into force in 1967 it was expected that the number of benefit recipients would not exceed 200,000. The total is now four times that number, and the forecast is that by the end of the century there will be over a million recipients of benefit under the Act. This growth is not due only to the growth of the labour force, since the number of people declared unfit is also increasing proportionally (see table 7.1); an important factor in this connection is the rising average age of the labour force. The sharpest rise in the absolute number of claimants is now behind us, however (see figure 7.1). The difference between the numbers of new and terminated entitlements has narrowed over the years, though according to the most recent data the annual increase in claimant numbers - currently a little over 20,000 per year - is again sharpening.

Table 7.1 **Labour force and benefit entitlement as at 1 January**

Year	**Labour force ('000) (1)**	**Incapacity ratio (2)(3)**	**WAO-Benefit recipients ('000) (3)**
1980	5493	12.0	660
1982	5752	12.2	700
1985	5967	12.6	751
1987	6149	12.6	771
1990	6471	12.6	815
2000	7100	13.3	944
2010	7197	14.0	1008

1. Central Bureau of Statistics, Statistical Yearbook. Central Planning Bureau (J. op de Beke), Revision of labour-supply trends 1985-2010 (1987).

2. The incapacity ratio is the ratio of the number of disability-benefit recipients to the total labour force.
3. Social Insurance Council (P. de Jong), Provisional projections to 2030 of the number of disability-benefit recipients, central variant (1984). Social Insurance Council (SVr) Annual Report 1986.

Figure 7.1 **New entitlements, terminated entitlements and the annual increase in claimant numbers**

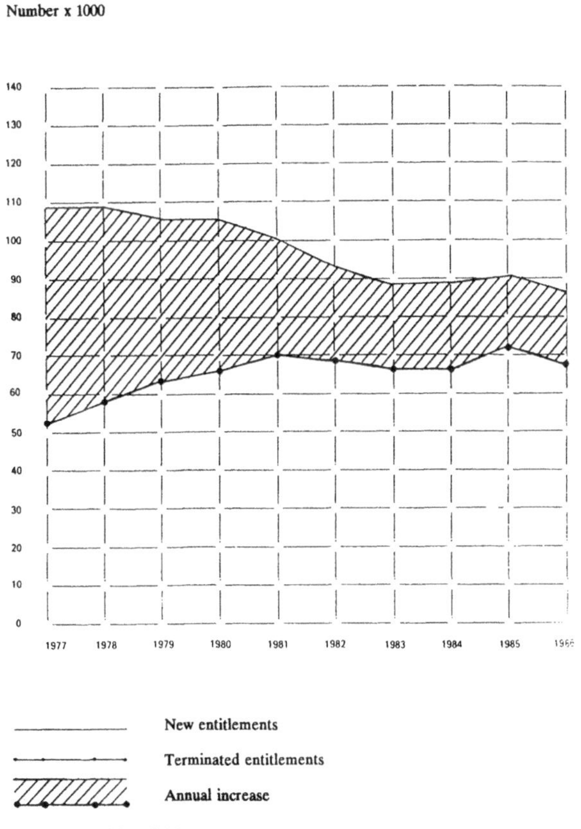

Source: SVr 1988.

82% of claimants are classed as fully (i.e. more than 80%) incapacitated, with a marked difference between the proportions of men (80%) and women (90%) so classed. It should be noted here that while the probability (expressed as a percentage of the population covered by the scheme) of women becoming entitled to benefit is smaller than that of men, where entitlement does arise the degree of incapacity tends to be greater among women.

Every year around 75,000 entitlements are terminated, half of them because the recipients have reached pensionable age. Recoveries - i.e. where claimants are found to be less than 15% (Disability Insurance Act (AOW)) or 25% disabled (General Disability Benefit Act (AAW)) and therefore lose entitlement - account for about 37% of the total, with marked disparities between different groups (see table 7.2). By no means all of the 37% can be regarded as having recovered in a medical sense, however, since a considerable proportion still have some degree of disorder or handicap, albeit not of such a nature as to render them unfit for work. This occurs notably in the case of those who, while they can no longer do their old job, are capable of undertaking some other kind of employment. The self-employed stand out as disadvantaged as regards the likelihood of recovery or the resumption of work after a period of incapacity.

Table 7.2 **Terminations of entitlement, by reason for termination and category, in percentages (1987)**

Reason for termination	**Category** Disability Insurance Act (WAO)	**Civil-service and related schemes**	**Self-employed**	**Disabled from childhood**	**Other**	**Total**
(Number)	(56005)	(12905)	(4882)	(1350)	(688)	(75830)
Recovery (less than 15 or 25% disabled)	37	45	10	24	8	37
Attainment of pensionable age	47	39	69	36	66	48
Death	14	10	18	38	20	14
Other	2	6	3	3	7	2
Total	**100**	**100**	**100**	**100**	**100**	**100**

Source: SVr 1989.

7.2.2 *Sex, age, diagnosis*

More men than women are occupationally incapacitated. Since there are more men than women in the labour force there are of course in absolute terms more men than women in receipt of disability benefit; however, there are also more male than female claimants relative to the total numbers of each sex in the labour force (see table 7.3).

Table 7.3 **Percentages of men and women in the labour force and among disability-benefit recipients**

Year	**Labour force**		**Benefit recipients**	
	% m	**% f**	**% m**	**% f**
1980	68.6	31.4	73.9	26.1
1985	65.1	34.9	72.6	27.4
1986	64.8	35.2	71.9	28.1
1987	64.3	35.7	70.5	29.5

Source: CBS 1988, SVr 1988.

The older age groups are strongly overrepresented among claimants. Table 7.4, which compares the age makeup of the labour force as a whole with that of the population of benefit recipients, brings out the sharp increase in the risk of incapacity from the age of 55 onwards.

Table 7.4 **Age makeup of the labour force and of the population of benefit recipients (end 1985)**

Age group	**Percentage of workforce**	**Percentage of benefit recipients**
15-39	65.3	23.0
40-54	27.2	36.0
55-59	5.1	19.0
60-64	2.3	22.0

Source: CBS Statistical Yearbook 1988.
CPB (J. op de Beke) 1987

Two diagnostic categories are particularly frequent as grounds for entitlement: musculoskeletal disorders and, almost as common, mental disorders. Table 7.5 shows the distribution of claimants among the ICD-9 principal categories in 1986 and 1987. The proportion of 'mental disorder' diagnoses is continuing to rise, accounting currently for just over a quarter of all principal diagnoses.

Table 7.5 **Entitlements to disability benefit in 1986 and 1987, by principal diagnostic category, totals and percentages**

		1986		**1987**	
		Number ('000)	**%**	**Number ('000)**	**%**
I	Infectious and parasitic diseases	7.6	0.9	6.0	0.7
II	Neoplasms	16.4	2.0	17.0	2.0
III	Endocrine, nutritional and metabolic diseases	8.3	1.0	9.2	1.1
IV	Diseases of the blood and blood-forming organs	1.4	0.2	1.4	0.1
V	Mental disorders	200.9	24.0	216.3	25.1
VI	Diseases of the nervous system and sense organs	41.3	4.9	42.5	4.9
VII	Disease of the circulatory system	89.7	10.7	89.9	10.4
VIII	Diseases of the respiratory system	32.3	3.9	31.8	3.7
IX	Diseases of the digestive system	21.1	2.5	21.3	2.5
X	Diseases of the genito-urinary system	9.3	1.1	9.1	1.0
XI	Complications of pregnancy, childbirth and the puerperium	1.0	0.1	1.1	0.1
XII	Diseases of the skin and subcutaneous tissue	6.4	0.8	6.5	0.7
XIII	Diseases of the musculoskeletal system	225.5	26.9	236.7	27.4
XIV XV	Congenital anomalies and Perinatal conditions	4.0	0.5	4.3	0.5
XVI	Symptoms	10.8	1.3	9.1	1.0
XVII	Injury and poisoning	43.8	5.2	48.3	5.6
	Unknown	118.5	14.1	113.9	13.1
Total 838.3		100	864.5	100	

Source: SVr Disability Funds Annual Reports 1986, 1987

7.3 *Incapacity due to mental disorders*

7.3.1 *Occurence and course*

7.3.1.1 *Incidence and prevalence*

Since 1982 the number of *new* entitlements arising annually under the various disability-benefit schemes has fluctuated around the 90-95,000 mark. The rapid increase in 1987 is due mainly to a different counting system, which raised the number of new cases by 6000. The share of Category V ('mental disorders') in the total (see table 7.6 and figure 7.2) has risen markedly, from 11% when the Disability Insurance Act took effect in 1968 to 28% in 1987; indeed, the most recent figures for entitlement to benefit under the Disability Insurance and General Disability Benefit Acts show the proportion to have risen to over 30% in 1988.

Table 7.6 **New entitlements to benefit under the main schemes, total and Category V)**

	1989*	**1988**	**1987**	**1986**	**1985**	**1984**	**1983**	**1982**	**1968**
New claimants ('000)	109.2	99.9	93.9	86.2	90.3	88.9	88.9	92.9	37.3
Of whom:									
Category V ('000)	35.1	31.9	27.7	22.3	24.7	23.0	22.4	22.2	4.1
Category V (%)	32.1	31.9	29.5	25.9	27.4	25.9	25.1	23.9	11.1

* 1989: provisional figures
Source: GMD (J.M. de Klerk *et al* 1986 - GMD Notes No. 7.
SVR.

The last line of table 7.6 is reproduced in graphic form in figure 7.2.

Figure 7.2 **New Category V entitlements to benefit under the main schemes, 1968-1987, as a percentage of all new entitlements**

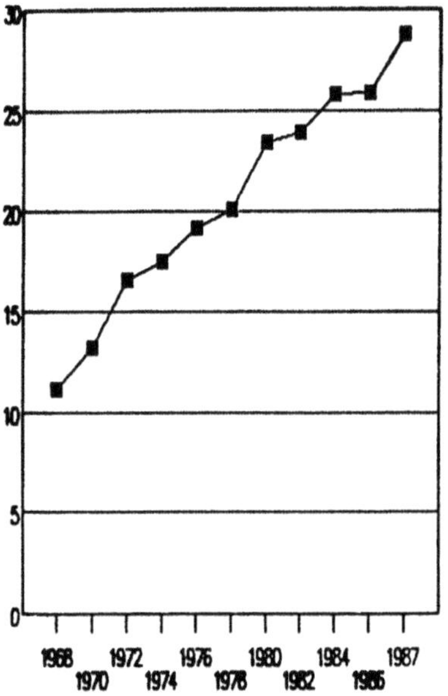

The numbers shown represent only 'recognized' cases of mental disorder: it is certain that a social and mental component is present in many other diagnoses, estimates of the number of cases with a non-somatic component ranging from 30% to 50% of the total. The main diagnostic areas involved are the digestive system, the musculoskeletal system and unspecific symptoms (categories IX, XIII, XV and XVI). Table 7.7 shows that the share of these 'subjective' syndromes in the total number of entitlements arising each year has also increased sharply.

Table 7.7 **New entitlements under the Disability Insurance and General Disability Benefit Acts: percentages of 'mental disorder' diagnoses and of 'objective' and 'subjective' syndromes, 1968-1987**

	1988	**1987**	**1986**	**1985**	**1984**	**1983**	**1982**	**1968**
Mental disorders (Category V)	30.9	28.0	25.9	27.4	25.9	25.1	23.9	11.1
Subjective syndromes (Categories V, IX, XIII, XV and XVI)	67	67	68	66	65	64	63	43
Objective syndromes (Other categories)	33	33	32	34	35	36	37	57

Source: GMD Annual Reports.
GMD (J.M. de Klerk *et al.*) 1986 - GMD Notes No. 7.

The continuing growth in Category V diagnoses among those becoming entitled to benefit has meant an increase in Category V's share in the total entitled to benefit at any one time.

The number of *terminations* of entitlement has always been lower than the number of new entitlements (see table 7.8).

Table 7.8 **New entitlements and terminations of entitlement ('000 cases)**

	1982	**1983**	**1984**	**1985**	**1986**	**1987**	**1988**	**1989**
New entitlements	22.2	22.4	23.0	24.7	22.3	27.7	31.9	35.1
Terminations	12.1	12.6	14.3	15.7	14.9	16.6	18.6	19.2

Source: SVr (Social Insurance Council)

It is revealing that the ratio of new entitlements to terminations is less auspicious in the case of Category V (1:0.67) than in that of the aggregate of all diagnoses (1:0.83). This underlines the fact that many Category V claimants remain unfit for work long-term, only leaving the schemes when they reach the age of 65 or on death.

Table 7.9 **Labour force and Category V entitlement to benefit as at 1 January**

Year	Workforce ('000) (1)	Category V benefit recipients ('000)	Category V as % of all benefit recipients	Category V incapacity ratio (2)
1980	5493	139		2.53
1982	5752	148	21.2	2.57
1985	5967	173	23.4	2.90
1987	6149	186	25.0	3.02
1990	6471	212	26.0	3.27
2000	7100	255	27.0	3.59
2010	7197	282	28.0	3.92

1. Sources: see table 7.1.
2. The Category V incapacity ratio is the ratio of the number of claimants with 'mental disorders' as their principal diagnosis (Category V) to the workforce as a whole (column 2 divided by column 1 (x 100)).

The projections shown in table 7.9 for the years 1990, 2000 and 2010 assume no radical change in the social-security system; they also make the conservative assumption that the share of Category V claimants in the total will rise only slowly from 25% at present to 28% in 2010. With the population of benefit recipients increasing proportionately more rapidly than the workforce as a whole, the Category V incapacity ratio will rise from 2.90 in 1985 to 3.92 in 2010: for every 100 members of the workforce there will be just under four claimants with 'mental disorders' as their principal diagnosis in 2010, as against just under three in 1985. In absolute terms too an uninterrupted increase is expected from 173,000 Category V claimants in 1985 to 282,000 in 2010.

7.3.1.2 *Degree and duration of incapacity*

Of those entitled to benefit under the Disability Insurance and General Disability Benefit Acts on 31 December 1987 82% were deemed fully (i.e. 80%-100%) incapacitated, while of those who became entitled to benefit under these schemes in 1988 80% were classed as fully incapacitated (GMD 1989). Mental disorders, despite the often minimal diagnosis, is relatively frequently associated with the highest degree of incapacity.

Table 7.10 **New benefit entitlements in the commonest diagnostic categories and at different degrees of incapacity**

	Degree of incapacity						Total
	15-45%		45-80%		80-100%		
	1986	1987	1986	1987	1986	1987	
Diagnostic category							
V Mental disorders	3	3	6	7	91	90	100%
VI Diseases of the nervous system	4	8	10	9	87	84	100%
VII Diseases of the circulatory system	4	9	14	18	82	73	100%
XIII Diseases of the musculo-skeletal system	4	16	10	13	85	72	100%
XVII Injury and poisoning	5	14	11	14	85	72	100%
I-XVII (All diagnoses)	4	10	9	11	87	78	100%

Source: GMD (Joint Medical Service of the Industrial Insurance Boards).

The effects of the social-security changes introduced in January 1987 are visible in table 7.10. In the case of the Disability Insurance and General Disability Benefit Acts the changes meant among other things that new applicants for benefit were assessed using different criteria, mainly as a result of ending the practice of taking account of the state of labour supply and demand in the occupation concerned. This is visible in the figures for new entitlements: the proportion of persons becoming eligible for disability benefit (normally after a year on sickness benefit) who were classed as fully incapacitated fell by nine percentage points in 1987 to 78%. It is all the more striking, then, that the diagnosis of mental disorder is among the very few in which there was little if any shift towards the lower categories of incapacity.

The data are not entirely hard, however. The benefit funds' annual reports indicate that the effect of the 1987 changes was minimal: the average degree of deemed incapacity was only 1% lower among new than among old cases.

A cohort study by Besseling (1986) found that full and permanent incapacity was associated with mental disorders more often than with other diagnoses; this was true for both men and women and across the whole age range. The disparity with other diagnoses was particularly marked in the case of men aged 20-34 (see table 7.11).

Table 7.11 **Percentage of fully incapacitated persons in cohorts of new benefit recipients in 1977-79 after some 4.5 years, by age, sex and principal diagnostic category**

	20-24		30-34		40-44		50-54	
Diagnostic category	**m**	**f**	**m**	**f**	**m**	**f**	**m**	**f**
V Mental disorders	59	43	56	51	64	60	76	80
VI Diseases of the nervous system	34	40	46	48	59	55	77	75
VII Diseases of the circulatory system	32	30	43	43	57	67	70	78
XIII Diseases of the musculo-skeletal system	13	16	27	29	46	45	77	77
I-XVII (All diagnoses)	30	31	38	41	52	53	73	75

Source: Besseling 1986

The study, mentioned earlier, by De Klerk *et al.* (1986) looked at claimants' situation 34 months after becoming eligible for benefit under the Disability Insurance Act. The results are shown in table 7.12.

Table 7.12 **The situation of Category V and other claimants after 34 months, by sex (%)**

Situation after	**All**		**Men**		**Women**	
34 months	**Cat. V**	**Others**	**Cat. V**	**Others**	**Cat. V**	**Others**
Full incapacity	38	29	46	33	24	23
Full/partial recovery, work resumed	26	35	23	28	35	57
Work resumed, fully/partially	17	25	19	33	14	8
GMD assessment not completed	16	7	12	6	27	12

Source: J.M. de Klerk, GMD Notes No. 4 1986

More people become fully incapacitated in Category V than in the other diagnostic categories, though the difference is found only among men. The number of recoveries is significantly lower among those

those found to be incapacitated by mental disorders, whether we look at those who have not (yet) resumed work or at those now in employment.

7.3.1.3 *Sex, age and occupation*

Mental disorder is more often diagnosed in women than in men: while women account for 28% of the whole population of benefit recipients, in the case of Category V recipients the proportion is 35% (Social Insurance Council). This disparity is of long standing and shows little if any sign of changing.

Mental disorders are proportionately more common among the young: 22.6% of all 'mental disorder' diagnoses relate to the 15-34 age group, even though this group accounts for only 14.1% of all entitlements (see table 7.13).

Table 7.13 **Benefit recipients (Disability Insurance and General Disability Benefit Acts) as at 31 December 1987, by age and diagnosis, in percentages**

Diagnosis	Age group 15-24	25-34	35-44	45-54	55-64	Total
Mental disorders	7.3	15.3	21.7	25.5	30.3	100
Musculoskeletal diseases	1.0	6.6	17.7	31.6	43.1	100
All diagnoses	3.6	10.5	18.4	27.3	40.2	100

Source: GMD

An examination of the four commonest diagnoses in each age group of benefit recipients brings out even more clearly that mental disorders as a cause of incapacity are notably common in the lowest age range.

Table 7.14 **Benefit recipients (Disability Insurance and General Disability Benefit Acts) as at 31 December 1987, by age and diagnosis, in percentages**

Diagnosis	Age group 15-24	25-34	35-44	45-54	55-64	Total
Mental disorders	51.2	36.2	29.4	23.3	18.8	25.0
Nervous diseases	14.1	8.0	5.9	5.0	4.4	5.5
Circulatory diseases	1.0	1.5	3.7	9.7	17.0	10.3
Musculoskeletal diseases	7.5	17.0	26.1	31.5	29.2	27.2
Other diagnoses	26.2	37.3	34.9	30.5	30.7	32.0
	100.0	**100.0**	**100.0**	**100.0**	**100.0**	**100.0**

Source: GMD.

Mental disorder accounts for over half of all diagnoses in the youngest age group, and it is not until after the age of 45 that diseases of the musculoskeletal system displace mental disorders as the main cause of incapacity.

Statistics from the Industrial Insurance Boards' Joint Medical Service (GMD) on new claimants show that the proportion of young people is greater among those becoming entitled to benefit than in the standing claimant population. Table 7.13 shows, for example, that in 1987 the 15-24 age group accounted for 3.6% of current claimants; among those becoming eligible for benefit in that year 12.5% were in this age group. The result will be a gradual fall in the average age of recipients. The 15-34 age group accounts for 22.6% of new entitlements on grounds of mental disorder, as against 40.8% of the recipient population at the end of 1987. The proportion of young claimants with a 'mental disorder' diagnosis is thus set to increase over the coming years.

While information on correlations between 'mental disorder' diagnoses and particular occupations is scarce, Social Insurance Council data do indicate the branches of industry in which relatively many or relatively few people are declared unfit for work owing to mental disorders.

The Industrial Insurance Boards whose insured populations include relatively large numbers of Category V recipients are those covering the printing industry, health care, banking and the state sector (including teachers; see also Van der Putten 1985): in both 1982 and 1986 the numbers of Category V entitlements for which these Boards accounted were at least 20% above the national average. Over the period 1982-86 there was a considerable increase across the board in the percentage of claimants with a 'mental disorder' diagnosis. The lack of information on the numbers of workers covered by each Board unfortunately means that no conclusions can be drawn regarding inter-industry differences in the incapacity ratio (the number of benefit recipients per hundred workers).

Table 7.15 **'Mental disorder' diagnoses as a percentage of all diagnoses, by Industrial Insurance Board (1986 and 1982)**

Industrial Insurance Board	**1986**	**1982**
Agriculture	8.9	7.8
Dairy	20.1	17.5
Timber	21.0	18.7
Textiles	23.7	11.0
Leather	8.4	21.7
Printing	31.7	26.7
Building materials	18.1	16.3
Metal production	22.1	19.8
Metal processing	21.3	19.5
Mining	14.0	11.9
Chemicals	24.5	21.9
Tobacco	25.4	22.7
Bakers	22.4	19.9
Butchers	18.4	15.8
Food	23.5	21.1
Retailing and crafts	27.1	25.8
Ports, inland shipping, fisheries	17.4	15.4
Merchant navy	19.1	18.5
Transport	22.2	20.0
Hotel and catering	26.2	24.5
Health care	33.4	29.9
State sector (central and local)	19.4	16.7
Banking	33.1	28.7
NAB	22.5	17.5
Construction	13.0	12.8
Painting and decorating	19.3	18.0
Dredging	16.0	15.1
Military	5.6	11.4
State pension fund employees	40.2	34.6
Railways	22.2	7.4
Total	**24.0**	**20.6**

Source: Social Insurance Council

7.3.1.4 *Diagnostic categories*

Where we have so far been concerned with mental health problems in general, in what follows we focus on specific disorders using ICD-9 codes. The data cover the period from 1980 onwards, since it was in that year that the benefit agencies switched from ICD-8 to ICD-9.

Table 7.16 relates to new entitlements, i.e. the incidence of benefit entitlement under the Disability Insurance and General Disability Benefit Acts.

Table 7.16 **Diagnoses (new entitlements) in Category V (mental disorders), by year (%)**

ICD 9 code and diagnosis	**1980**	**1982**	**1984**	**1986**	**1988**
290-299 Psychotic conditions	11	11	9	7	7
Of which: 296 Affective psychoses	5	5	4	3	3
300 Neurotic disorders	33	26	20	18	16
309 Adjustment reaction	23	30	38	44	48
311 Depressive disorders	10	10	11	11	13
Other diagnoses	23	24	22	20	16
	100	**100**	**100**	**100**	**100**

Source: Joint Medical Service (GMD) and Joint Administrative Centre (GAK) of the Industrial Insurance Boards.

Between 1980 and 1988 there was a sharp rise in the proportion of 'adjustment reaction' diagnoses, from 23% to 48% of new Category V entitlements. While the possibility of changing diagnostic practices cannot be excluded (note the sharp decline in 'neurotic disorder' diagnoses), this would appear to indicate that we are increasingly faced here with people who cannot cope with the mental stress of the work situation. Categories 300 (neurotic disorders) and 309 (adjustment reaction) are in a psychiatric sense a sort of non-diagnosis, and the large number of these vague diagnoses clearly indicates the difficulty facing the assessment agencies, in the many cases where people's health is adversely affected by their work situation, of finding an appropriate medical label (necessary if benefit is to be payable). There has been a relative decline in the severer psychiatric problems (codes 290-299) over the past eight years, while less easily classified (but not for that reason less serious) problems of a psychosocial or neurotic nature have shown a sharp increase.

7.4 *Determinants of incapacity and of the increase in entitlements on mental grounds*

7.4.1 *Introduction*

As the introduction to this baseline analysis indicated, we are here concerned with incapacity as defined by the Disability Insurance and General Disability Benefit Acts, i.e. with an entitlement to benefit assessed in accordance with statutory norms rather than with some objectively determined or exclusively health-related inability to undertake employment. Incapacity and benefit entitlement should be seen as the outcome of a decision process involving three parties, namely the individual employee, the employer and the assessment agency (specifically the medical officer acting for the insurance boards) (Bax 1984).

Against this background an account of the macro-level determinants of incapacity, those affecting the workforce as a whole, must encompass more than a description of factors adversely affecting employees' health in the immediate work situation. The chart in section 7.1 makes this clear. While such health-threatening and pathogenic influences are clearly of great importance in relation to incapacity, they can offer only a very partial explanation of the sharp growth over the last twenty years in the number of benefit recipients with a 'mental disorder' diagnosis. The main determinants are to be found in all the factors, not directly associated with the individual's health status, which play a part in the decision of the three parties mentioned that the individual is entitled to sickness or disability benefit.

The obvious explanation for the growth in the absolute number of claimants is the increasing size of the workforce, but there has also been a proportional increase: there are now more claimantsas a percentage of the labour force. Different authors have suggested very different explanations for this phenomenon.

De Klerk *et al.* (1983) offer the following summary (not intended as exhaustive) of the explanations found in the literature:

- There has been a real increase in problems and illnesses, mainly as a result of developments in society.
- The increase in the number of Category V diagnoses is related not to any change in the incidence of disease but to political and moral judgements.
- The increase reflects changing responses to illness rather than any increased incidence of mental disorders.
- The increase is due to expansion of the notions of what constitutes illness.

- The increase reflects attempts to protect the social system from change by focusing on individuals rather than the community.
- The increase is the result of redefinition on the basis of the frameworks set by professionals ('protoprofessionalization').

We would supplement the picture with the following explanations:
- Over the years working conditions in many industries have altered to such an extent that many employees cannot meet new skill requirements (mainly of a social and psychological nature). The relevant legislation - the Working Conditions Act (ARBO) - appears inadequate in this respect, focusing little if at all on the psychological and social aspects of working conditions and placing virtually exclusive stress on physically stressful factors (noise, toxic substances etc.).
- It is increasingly recognized that mental problems, like physical disorders, can restrict individuals' performance. The assessment agencies - employers' and insurance boards' medical officers - are diagnosing mental disorder with increasing frequency, and it may well be that in the past somatic diagnoses would have been made in similar cases.
- Changes in society in a number of important areas have raised levels of mental stress and rendered individuals more vulnerable while at the same time eroding the support available from the social environment. Significant factors include growing individualization, greater stress on performance and competition with colleagues.
- Employers have sometimes engineered entitlement to disability benefit for older employees who can no longer adequately cope, often with the latter's approval, as a way of bridging the gap until they reach pensionable age. The 'mental disorder' diagnosis offers a way of giving economic necessities a statutory medical legitimation.

This wide range of possible explanations for the growth in benefit entitlement on mental grounds can be reduced to four broad determinants, often acting simultaneously: *pathogenic* factors in the work situation, *social and cultural change* (e.g. in the work ethic and attitudes to illness), *economic change* (in the areas of employment and labour supply and demand) and *institutional change* (relating to the structure and operation of the social-security system).

It should be noted that most of the papers published on the determinants of disability deal in very general terms rather than particular diagnostic categories: little specific attention is devoted to the reasons for long-term 'mental incapacity'. Only occasionally have publications focused on industries or employee groups particular at risk for mental problems, and then generally from the viewpoint of a specific occupational group.

Much of what is adduced in the literature as background to and explanations of incapacity and of the trends within it is based on vague indications. Surprisingly little empirical research has been carried out in this field, given the extent of the problem, and this is particularly true of research specifically focusing on the determinants of mental incapacity. Subsequent sections will therefore comprise, to a greater extent than their predecessors, considerations of a mainly qualitative nature.

7.4.2 *Pathogenic factors in the work situation*

In this country and elsewhere much has been published on the links between work and health. Working conditions and the nature of work are known to have a major impact, positively and negatively, on workers' health. The qualitative aspects of work which affect individuals' physical and mental health are (WRR 1981):

- Job content. Relevant factors here include the nature and level of the work, responsibilities, autonomy and scope for self-development. Problems can arise if either too much or too little is expected of the employee in the light of his or her capacities.
- Working conditions, i.e. ergonomic conditions, noise, dirt/ cleanliness, safety/danger etc. The government policy statement 'Nota 2000' (1986) notes a shift from more physical to more psychosocial forms of stress; feelings of powerlessness and depression are often the result (Van 't Hullenaar & Van Koningsveld 1986).
- Labour relations in a broad sense: contacts, social relations, supervision and control, consultation and negotiation.
- Terms of employment: pay, training opportunities, job security, duration of work, working hours, prospects.

The qualitative aspects of work thus cover a wide range of factors. Not all are relevant to all industries or jobs, however, and not all weigh equally heavily in all circumstances, making it difficult to determine whether recent decades have seen a net improvement or deterioration in the overall nature of work in this country, or indeed whether progress has been made in some areas (e.g. workplace safety) but not others (e.g. job security and prospects). In any event it would be difficult to identify objective measures, since individuals' perceptions, strength and resilience are a major factor in deciding both what weight to accord to particular factors and whether a given change is an improvement or not. Those perceptions and that strength and resilience are in turn partly determined by such background factors as personal circumstances (whether and to what extent individuals receive emotional support in their private life, what positive or negative events they are experiencing, and so on), the nature of the individual personality (sensitivity, ambition, sociability, introversion/extraversion, rigidity etc.) and individuals' social status (as reflected e.g. in their educational level).

Views diverge on the question whether worsening (or at least changing) working conditions have contributed over the years to a deterioration in the health of the workforce and hence to an increase in the number of people classed as unfit to work (Den Heeten *et al.* 1987; Hilverink 1981; Schmitz 1988; Emanuel 1981).

Those who consider that work has become less 'worker-friendly', more incapacitating, in recent years (Hilverink 1981) point to such pathogenic developments as continuing and often rapid changes in job content and organization, growing labour mobility, sharpening requirements in terms of education, training, experience, flexibility and work rates, and the increase in the number of jobs involving predominantly mental stress. Any links between such general developments in the working situation and workers' mental health are still largely hypothetical and have yet to be extensively researched. It has however been shown (see e.g. Buys 1985 p. 473; Grosfeld 1988; Aarts *et al.* 1982) that there are vulnerable groups on the labour market who, partly on account of their working conditions, run an increased risk of sickness, whether physical or mental, and longer-term incapacity. The health of the lower social classes - people with a low educational level and, as a result, generally a low income and poor working conditions - is on average worse than that of higher socio-economic groups; this is due on the one hand to the greater burden that they experience and on the other to their relatively lower level of resilience (Bax 1984 p. 42). Focusing more specifically on mental problems and stress at the workplace it is known that these conditions are relatively common in certain jobs and industries: teachers, nurses, bus drivers. For these groups, which include relatively large numbers of women, the risk of long-term sickness absence and incapacity is particularly great.

7.4.3 *Social and cultural changes*

Since World War II there have been large-scale changes in social attitudes and values relating on the one hand to the role of work in people's lives and on the other to health and illness (Hagendoorn *et al.* 1981; SCP 1986; Bax 1984). The relevance of these changes to the rapid growth in the numbers classed as unfit for work (Category V diagnoses in particular) is often assumed but difficult to determine.

A Social and Cultural Planning Office report (SCP 1986) has dealt with Dutch people's changing attitudes to work since 1945. Contrary to what it usually believed (e.g Wiersma 1980), the report concludes that since the 1970s there has been little change in the beliefs and attitudes relating to work of those in full-time employment: there has for example been no increase in the value attached to leisure or the willingness to accept shorter working hours, and work continues to play a central part in people's lives. Changes among the unemployed have in some respects been more marked: their willingness to work has increased. The fluctuations observed in sickness-absence rates and the growth in the numbers classed as incapacitated cannot to any significant extent be ascribed to changing attitudes to work within the labour force.

Another area in which explanations for the growth in the numbers classed as incapacitated are often sought is that of changes in social attitudes to health and in the responses to illness that they engender. There can be no doubt that the notion of what constitutes illness has expanded in recent decades, implying a widening definition of disease encompassing mental and social malaise as well as physical complaints (Wiersma 1980). One effect of this expanded notion of illness has been to blur the distinction between being well and being ill, which can no longer be determined by doctors alone. A second trend has been the increasing 'medicalization' and 'protoprofessionalization' of society as the influence, both practical and normative, of medical and paramedical disciplines on society has grown (Bax 1984). Day-to-day happenings and problems in such diverse areas as environmental pollution, housing and physical exercise are increasingly discussed in medical terms; daily activities are marked with a medical endorsement or health warning derived from the conceptual framework of professional medicine. The question (and hence the uncertainty) as to whether one is well or ill has come to occupy an important place in many people's lives and the threshold for regarding oneself as ill and behaving accordingly has been lowered. This could help explain the rise in sickness absence and occupational incapacity.

Alongside attitudes to work and responses to illness attention is frequently drawn in the literature to other, more general, developments in Dutch society which are seen as not conducive to mental health and which could offer some explanation for the rise in sickness absence and occupational incapacity: increasing individualization, greater focus on consumption, 'privatism', the desintegration of social networks, secularization and the decline of traditional religious and other loyalties, increased social and geographical mobility and so on (Den Heeten *et al.* 1987; Bax 1984; Van 't Hullenaar & Van Koningsveld 1986). While such trends are no doubt relevant to individual cases of sickness absence and occupational incapacity, it is not yet clear whether and to what extent they also explain the national growth in the number of disability-benefit claimants in recent years.

The possibility must be borne in mind that these presumed adverse socio-cultural developments may be offset by other factors tending to promote physical and mental health, such as people's increased opportunities and ability to speak up for themselves and the greater personal freedom which now exists in areas like education, work and relationships: it could be that increased stress is compensated by an increased ability to withstand stress.

7.4.4 *Socio-economic changes*

The possible link between changing (and perhaps deteriorating) working conditions and incapacity was considered in section 7.4.2. Here we focus on the link between certain macro-economic developments relating to the labour market and the numbers of benefit claimants. Two major themes are covered, namely the mismatch between labour supply and demand and the obstacles facing the incapacitated on the road to re-employment.

A cause of the growth in occupational incapacity often mentioned in the literature is the qualitative mismatch which for some time exists between labour supply and demand (Hilverink 1981; Van den Bosch & Petersen 1981; Emanuel 1981). The rationalization of production, involving as it does ongoing reorganizations, redundant and rapid changes in working methods, job requirements and the division of functions, has left many workers with training, knowledge, skills and experience which are no longer relevant: the problem is worst in the case of older and less skilled employees, who find it difficult to adjust to changing circumstances, and it are these vulnerable groups, with their weak position on the labour market, who have accounted for much of the growth in occupational incapacity in recent years. Many publications note rising numbers of WAO-benefit claimants in industries marked by falling employment (Kuné 1982; Wiersma 1980; Douben & Herweyer 1979). The WAO has offered an alternative to unemployment benefit which has proved attractive to employers and employees alike: to employers because redundancy arrangements for unproductive workers under the Disability Benefit Act (WAO) are relatively straightforward, and to employees because until recently disability benefit was higher than unemployment benefit and because receipt of the former is socially more acceptable than receipt of the latter (Van den Bosch & Petersen 1981; SCP 1988).

The growing numbers of disability-benefit claimants reflect not just the high rate of new entitlements but also the relatively low rate of terminations of entitlement. The great majority of recipients are very unlikely to be able to resume work, and the likelihood of re-employment is least among Category V claimants (see section 7.3). The position on the labour market of workers with any degree of occupational incapacity is very weak. Den Heeten *et al.* (1987) mention three factors in this connection:

- Very few suitable jobs are available and the incapacitated face heavy competition from able-bodied job-seekers, school-leavers etc.
- More and more is now demanded of job-applicants; an incapacitated person for whom only a particular, clearly defined, job is suitable cannot show e.g. the adaptability now expected of employees.
- Firms believe that taking on incapacitated employees will have an adverse effect on the production process, not just because they may drop out frequently but also because the privileged position of such employees could lead to tension in relations with other members of the workforce. Incapacitated employees are also felt to underperform.

In the case of those with a Category V incapacity a fourth factor comes into play. Firms which do offer jobs to the disabled generally prefer a physically handicapped person to someone with a mental disorder; employers' ignorance and prejudices in respect of people with mental disorders and their work skills are an extra obstacle to the re-employment of the mentally incapacitated.

The Employment of Disabled Persons Act (WAGW) of July 1986 seeks to promote the employment of people with disabilities by the use of such instruments as subsidies covering pay and other employer outgoings, help from the industrial insurance boards' Joint Medical Service (GMD) while employees are covered by the Sickness Benefit Act, GMD job-placement services and financial penalties where quotas are not achieved. The aim is that disabled employees should eventually make up 3-7% of firms' workforces. In July 1989, following a three-year trial period, the Act was found to have borne only limited fruit and to have benefited mainly the physically incapacitated.

7.4.5 *Structure and operation of the social security system*

Since it is social-security legislation that determines who is classed as incapacitated and on what grounds, any amendments to such legislation and the operational practices based upon it inevitably affect the numbers of benefit entitlements: incapacity can be 'created', and just as easily 'cured', by legislative change.

The past decade has seen many changes: disability benefit has been cut, the notion of 'suitable work' has been expanded, the practice of taking account of the labour demand/supply position in claimants' occupations has been ended (in the most recent reform, dating from 1987), and legislation has been introduced to promote the employment and re-employment of people with disabilities. The number of disabled people is thus determined, quite independently of any changes in individuals' health and employment situation, by political and financial considerations and choices relating to the scale and structure of the social-security system.

There are many aspects of the existing system that are 'pathogenic', or at least tend to impede recovery: alongside factors making for unclarity and uncertainty - such as the institutional division (favouring chronicity and irreversibility) between the operation of sickness benefit by the industrial insurance boards and of disability benefit mainly by the Joint Medical Service and the different incapacity criteria under the two sets of legislation - the literature also refers extensively to the many elements in the assessment procedure that can have this effect.

The main points to emerge are: the virtual absence of objective criteria for determining the (remaining) work skills of those classed as mentally incapacitated; the highly individual focus of those involved in making assessments (the insurance boards' medical officers, occupational specialists, psychiatrists and tribunals); and the strict division of functions between agencies and persons with supervisory and therapeutic roles.

Much of the literature suggests that the validity of diagnoses, and the limitations on the work skills of the mentally incapacitated which they imply, constitutes a considerable problem (Kabela 1988; Knepper 1987; Schipper & Hoencamp 1984; Houben 1988; Schnitzler 1977). This applies not only to medical assessors working for the industrial insurance boards or the Joint Medical Service but also to the expert psychiatrists and psychologists brought in as consultants to give advice or help settle disputes. The psychiatric determination of occupational incapacity is often difficult, since the problems of the individuals concerned are generally located on the boundary between psychosocial suffering and psychopathology; psychiatrists must therefore cover many factors in their examination, taking account among other things of the physical and mental health and character structure of the person before them, the kind of work to which the examination relates and the social and cultural background (Kabela 1988).

We still know very little about the links between psychiatric diagnoses and the remaining work skills (or prognoses thereof) of the individuals concerned, so that psychiatrists' judgements on this central question are very debatable. Psychiatrists are also expected to make judgements in the other social, occupational and legal fields mentioned, even though these are outside their competence. Assessors' medical judgements in individual cases are thus based on many non-medical considerations and personal value-judgements. Kabela (1988) concludes that assessing psychiatrists can be classed as 'harsh' or 'mild', depending on whether they are more or less likely to confirm incapacity, while Ruijzendaal (1985) considers that no less than 85% of psychiatric reports on incapacity are based in some degree on prejudice or defective reasoning. Every year between 15,000 and 25,000 psychiatric reports are drawn up under the Sickness Benefit (ZW), Disability Insurance and General Disability Benefit Acts (WAO/AWW) (Kabela 1988; Knepper 1987), so that the problem is far from being marginal.

Recent publications have begun paving the way to greater objectivity in both diagnosis and the determination of limitations on work skills in cases of mental incapacity (Hoenkamp & Rijnhart 1988; Koele *et al.* 1989).

7.5 *Utilization of care by the occupational incapacitated*

Little is known regarding the utilization of medical and other services by disability-benefit claimants: only two studies focusing on this point (Slot & Steinbuch 1988; De Klerk *et al.* 1986) have been carried out among recipients of benefit under the WAO by the insurance boards' Joint Medical Service.

Table 7.17 lists the services used by benefit recipients over the past twelve months, comparing those with a Category V diagnosis with the remainder.

Table 7.17 **Services utilized in the previous twelve months (%) (NB one person may use more than one type of care)**

Service	**Persons with mental incapacity**	**Others**
Family doctors	83	70
Physiotherapists	16	34
Neurologists	23	31
Internal medicine	14	17
Orthopedics	6	21
Surgery	5	20
Cardiology	13	13
Psychiatrists (including Regional Institutes of Ambulatory Mental Health Care)	48	4
Ear, nose and throat	8	6
Other	11	12

Source: GMD Notes No. 14, Slot & Steinbuch 1988.

Less than half of the Category V claimants consulted a psychiatrist or presented to one of the Regional Institutes of Ambulatory Mental Health Care; moreover many in this group sought other forms of care, reflecting the fact that their mental disorders are generally accompanied by physical complaints or conditions.

An earlier Joint Medical Service (GMD) study of case dossiers (De Klerk 1986) found that 27% of Category V claimants had had no contact with any treating agency whatever since becoming entitled to disability benefit or during the preceding period of entitlement to sickness benefit; among other claimants the proportion was only 15%.

7.6 *Re-employment*

The introduction of the Employment of Disabled Persons Act (WAGW) in 1986 gave a new impetus to occupational rehabilitation and job-placement services for the incapacitated. The legislation places additional obligations on both claimants and employers with regard to the search for ways of promoting re-employment, assigning a major role to the Joint Medical Service (GMD). In such a short time it has of course not been possible to complete the process of developing the necessary instruments and reaching agreements on tasks and their distribution with the many bodies involved (local employment offices, industrial insurance boards, organizations for the handicapped, the sheltered-employment service, the factory inspectorate, employers). As conditions for getting re-employment activities underway nationally provision has been now made for (GMD 1989):

- Guarantees covering the benefit entitlement of incapacitated persons undertaking training.
- Trial placements. Incapacitated persons whose ability to resume employment is still uncertain are permitted, for a period not exceeding two months, to undertake productive work for an employer without pay but without losing their disability and/or unemployment benefit.
- Occupational therapy. Incapacitated persons may undertake a period of training in an occupational therapy/rehabilitation department.

The rehabilitation and job-placement services set up at regional level cover a wide range of activities. They include: canvassing employers for vacancies; promoting training, e.g. with the help of training budgets; establishing teams within the Joint Medical Service with the job of improving information and services to employers in the framework of the Employment of Disabled Persons Act (WAGW); and building up regional labour-market information.

Unfortunately the most recent Joint Medical Service data on the effects of the Employment of Disabled Persons Act conflate all the diagnostic categories and can thus give us no definite information about Category V claimants. Moreover they do not cover all benefit claimants, and since those receiving benefit under the civil-service scheme (ABP) are excluded there may be some distortion, in that Category V incapacity is relatively common within this group and Category V claimants have more limited scope as regards re-employment than other benefit recipients. This is evident from table 7.18.

Table 7.18 **Joint Medical Service employment activities for the incapacitated (%)**

Activity	**Persons with mental incapacity**	**Others**
Registration at local employment office	25	36
Contact with former employer	42	38
Attempt at placement with former employer	16	19
Attempt at placement with new employer	16	16
Vocational guidance sought	4	6
Suitable work identified	22	47

Source: GMD Notes No. 4, De Klerk *et al.* 1986.

The poorer prospects of those incapacitated by mental disorder are reflected in the significantly smaller number of cases in which suitable work is identified, the smaller number of contacts with former employers and the smaller number of registrations with local employment offices.

With this context in mind we turn now to re-employment outcomes.

In the vast majority of cases - 81% in both 1985 and 1987 - individuals resuming work returned to their former employer. There is a growing tendency for people to move to a new job with their old employer, working the same hours; the proportion of cases in which this occurs rose from 6% om 1985 to 13% in 1987. While these are very recent developments, these figures could indicate that firms are making greater efforts than in the past to find alternative work for incapacitated employees.

Table 7.19 **Re-employment of benefit recipients (Disability Insurance Act) an average of six months after inception of entitlement, 1987 and 1985 (%)**

	Men		Women		Total	
	1987	1985	1987	1985	1987	1985
Former job, in full	17	24	17	24	17	24
Former job, fewer hours	34	37	57	50	41	41
New job, same hours	16	8	6	1	13	6
New job, fewer hours	12	11	7	8	10	10
New employer, same hours	8	9	6	6	7	8
New employer, fewer hours	7	7	8	11	7	8
Self-employed, sheltered employment	7	3	-	-	5	3
Total	100	100	100	100	100	100

Source: GMD Annual Report 1988.

Turning to the total number of incapacitated workers whom the Joint Medical Services has sought to place, this has grown sharply from just over 60,000 in 1987 to 70,000 in 1988. In 1988 about 72% of the total had no job at the start of the process, falling to 55% on its completion (see table 7.20). The results of the process are thus such that only a minority of those concerned are able to resume work.

Table 7.20 **Job situation before and after activities geared to re-employment, 1987 and 1988**

Job situation	Before		After		Change	
	1987	1985	1987	1985	1987	1985
No job	50170	45100	38871	32400	-11299	-12700
Old job	10000	9800	15760	14500	+5760	+4700
New job	3237	1900	7878	8300	+4641	+6400
Self-employment	6220	3300	6599	3700	+379	+400
Sheltered employment	511	400	1030	1600	+519	+1200
Total	**70138**	**60500**	**70138**	**60500**		

Source: GMD Annual Report 1988.

The number of persons returning to their old employer rose from 4,700 in 1987 to 5,760 in 1988, an increase of just over 20%; in contrast, placements with new employers declined. Overall the number of placements fell from 12,700 in 1987 to 11,299 in 1988.

This baseline analysis was completed in November 1989.

Part II Scenarios for occupational incapacity due to mental disorders, 1990-2010

7.7 *Exploratory scenarios*[1]

7.7.1 *Scenario 1: Reference scenario*

Mental health problems in the workforce

Over the last twenty years changes at work and a weakening of the supports in individuals' personal lives have led to an increase in the number of people with mental health problems in the Dutch labour force; the next twenty years will bring a further rise, with stress-related problems, neurotic (adjustment) disorders and depressive states in particular becoming more common, generally manifested in the form of psychosomatic complaints. This represents a real increase in mental malaise rather than simply a greater willingness to apply the 'mental' label.

The increase is due mainly to a combination of general trends in Dutch society which threaten mental health and specific developments in many people's jobs and working conditions. An important general trend is the growing 'protoprofessionalization' and 'medicalization' of society, which leads the kinds of malaise that may be felt in many areas of life (including work) to be labelled a medical problem and individuals to seek help from health professionals. An important factor of a very different kind will be the continuing high level of unemployment and the associated job insecurity. For many people this situation will result in mental problems, not least because society will remain work-oriented, attaching great value to the possession of a job. The growing emphasis on individual satisfactions and the erosion of support from social and family networks will also give rise to more problems.

Health-threatening developments will also take place at work. The content and nature of many people's jobs will be a cause for concern, giving rise to mental problems because the work is either too demanding or not demanding enough. More and more work situations will be marked by monotony, isolation, pressure to work fast and so, while on the qualitative side - management styles, provision for consultation, delegation of responsibilities, etc. - the next twenty years will bring little improvement. The demands made on workers will continue to grow, changing moreover at an accelerating rate as a result among other things of ongoing automation, the growing numbers of jobs in which mental and social functioning is of prime importance, greater pressure of work and greater emphasis on performance. As change becomes the norm many workers will fall by

[1] The basic assumptions of the exploratory scenarios are set out in Appendix 1.

the wayside, despite efforts in the area of training and retraining: the mental stress will be too great. In particular there will be many more problems in service occupations such as teaching, nursing, the police and the care of the elderly and infirm; in part the increased problems will reflect the service sector's growth, in part they will result from the continuing (excessive) pressure of the work.

Women and first- and second-generation migrants will be among the most vulnerable. A growing proportion of women will enter the workforce over the next twenty years; the psychological risks they face will be aggravated by the double or even triple burden they will continue to bear as (often unskilled) workers, as partners and as mothers. Migrants will also become more vulnerable; their deficient education and society's declining tolerance will mean their employment prospects are poor and will condemn them, often, to jobs where health risks are relatively high.

Mental ill-health will also increase among employees aged 50 and over, many of whom will find it hard to adapt to the rapid changes taking place at work. Among younger workers too mental problems will grow, mainly owing to the discrepancy between their high expectations in connection with work on the one hand and the limited job and career opportunities actually available on the other.

While scope exists in many firms for modifying the work situation in such a way that mental problems can be prevented or influenced little systematic attempt will be made to exploit it; only individual cases will be tackled, in an *ad hoc* approach which will do nothing to counter the growth in mental ill-health mentioned above. Employees' mental well-being will not receive adequate attention in legislation on working conditions and the quality of work. The early detection of problem situations and the support of workers by firms' medical services will remain rarities, partly because of the low priority given to the prevention of mental disorders. The specialized mental health services will continue to play only a marginal role in the area of work-related problems and their prevention.

Benefit entitlement

Entitlement to disability benefit will remain a largely non-medical matter. Major factors affecting entitlement rates will continue to include the employment situation (job availability), financial and other constraints on the social-insurance system and the attitudes and activities of the agencies and individuals involved in determining entitlement.

The number of WAO/AAW-benefit claimants with mental disorders as their principal diagnosis will rise from 3% of the workforce in 1990 to 4.5% in 2010, an increase in absolute terms from 186,000 to 320,000 in twenty years. The causes are clear: the workforce will have grown and with it the number of workers with mental problems. Among women there will be a 'catching-up' process in terms of claimant numbers in all diagnostic groups, including mental disorder. Entitlement on mental grounds will be relatively common among migrants and older employee.

Changing diagnostic views and practices will also play a major part in the growth in the number of entitlements on grounds of mental disorder. The medical services of the larger firms in particular will be more alert to mental problems and this will have some preventive effect. Medical officers working for the industrial insurance boards and the Joint Medical Service will be more likely to recognize the mental component of many physical complaints, notably in conditions of the musculoskeletal system (back and neck problems) and cardiovascular disease. Mental problems will be diagnosed more commonly in cases where formerly a non-mental diagnosis would have been made, representing a shift in the labelling. The proportion of benefit claimants with mental disorders as their principal diagnosis will rise from 25% to 32%.

In twenty years there will be no significant progress towards greater competence, uniformity and objectivity in the diagnosis of individuals' condition and the determination of limitations on their work skills due to mental problems. Assessment procedures under the Disability Insurance and General Disability Benefit Acts (WAO/AWW) will continue to focus on individuals and their problems, even though these often result from 'supra-individual' causes in such areas as working conditions. No legislative moves are expected to set different or stricter standards for assessment.

A major problem will persist in the form of the often long qualifying periods (i.e. the first year of incapacity, when claimants receive sickness rather than disability benefit), which tend to promote incapacity and chronicity. The problem of rigidly divided tasks and responsibilities and inadequate information flows between those who operate the social security system and assess entitlement (the insurance agencies) and those who provide care and treatment (company medical officers, family doctors, the Regional Institutes of Ambulatory Mental Health Care (RIAGG), social workers, psychologists and psychiatrists in private practice, etc.) will not be overcome and will remain an obstacle to preventive measures.

Care and rehabilitation

Around half of all disability-benefit claimants with a 'mental disorder' diagnosis currently receive some form of care from mental health institutions. The proportion will rise slightly over the next few years as the taboo relating to mental problems weakens somewhat and family doctors and insurance-agency medical officers come increasingly to appreciate what mental health care-institutions have to offer and hence refer benefit claimants to specialists more often. The primary sector - family doctors and the community mental health services in particular - will gradually focus more attention on problems relating to work and the work situation and will develop greater expertise in this area. However, the emphasis will tend to remain on the psychological *consequences* rather than *causes* of incapacity, while the practical scope for care-provision and problem-solving will remain extremely limited owing to the close ties between the employment situation and occupational incapacity.

Individual psychosocial help and support for benefit recipients will continue to be provided in the first instance by family doctors. Organizations set up to represent claimants' interests will acquire somewhat greater significance. Company welfare officers, psychologists and medical officers will take on a much greater role, as will the medical officers of industrial insurance boards and the Joint Medical Service, albeit mainly in the initial period of entitlement to sickness rather than disability benefit when the employee has still not been lost from view. The community mental health care services (mainly the RIAGGs) will be involved more quickly and more often in the case of the more severe problems.

There will be little if any improvement in the re-employment prospects of claimants with a 'mental disorders' diagnosis and the numbers resuming work will remain small. Scientific knowledge regarding residual or alternative occupational capacity in the case of specific mental disorders will remain inadequate and little statutory provision will be made for compelling firms to employ ex-claimants. Considerations of efficiency and profitability mean that industry will show little enthusiasm for tailoring jobs to this particular group's needs. Where tighter legislation does enable more ex-claimants to resume work these will mainly be the physically incapacitated. Here again individuals' health is not the only factor determining the scope for their re-employment: the state of the economy also plays a major part.

Mental health and social-welfare services will continue to play only a marginal role in promoting and initiating the re-employment of the mentally incapacitated. Consultation and coordination between employers' and insurance agencies' medical officers on the one hand and the mainstream health services on the other will spread only very gradually, as will the view that re-employment is a joint responsibility.

7.7.2 *Scenario 2: Prevention*

Outline: Out of enlightened self-interest industry will undertake initiatives aimed at promoting employees' mental health and preventing long-term incapacity. The state will concern itself actively with these developments.

Mental health problems in the workforce

The social trends associated with the development of mental problems in the workforce parallel those in the reference scenario. In brief this means that the next twenty years will see a real increase in mental morbidity as a result of shifts in public attitudes and reactions to illness, developments in the economy and the trend towards greater mental stress in many people's work situation. While legislation covering social and psychological aspects of working conditions will be greatly expanded compared with the reference scenario its implementation and enforcement will prove extremely difficult. The immediate preventive impact of the legislation will thus be limited, being restricted mainly to a gradually increasing focus on and interest in questions of work and mental disorders.

Owing partly to the aging of the population many industries will find it difficult to recruit sufficient labour, leading employers to accord greater weight to human capital and to their own interest in preventing mental problems and minimizing employees' recourse to sickness and disability benefit. The number of people receiving advice and help from firms' medical services will increase sharply thanks partly to statutory requirements. Firms' medical and welfare officers will play a more active role, in both curative and preventive terms, putting greater emphasis on the early detection of mentally stressful work situations and on modifying them where necessary. They will also see it as part of their job to bring to management's attention any structural factors in working conditions and labour relations which are mentally unhealthy.

The more active approach adopted by firms' medical services will be manifested not only in growing preventive work but also in more and above all better advice and assistance for sick employees and in greater efforts to educate managers at all levels e.g. through courses on stress prevention and modern management. To ensure that the necessary expertise is available medical officers will frequently consult mental health professionals, who will concern themselves explicitly with the prevention of mental incapacity and will remedy current shortcomings in their knowledge of the links between work and mental problems. This scenario, unlike the reference scenario, envisages a general acceptance that the whole working situation should regularly be examined for its impact on both the physical and the mental well-being of the workforce and not just to the problems of individuals.

Benefit entitlement

The percentage of WAO/AWW-disability-benefit claimants with mental disorders as their principal diagnosis will rise only slightly, from 3% of the workforce at present to 3.5% in 2010. In absolute terms this represents an increase from 186,000 in 1987 to 252,000 in 2010. The increase will be due mainly to the growth in the labour force and the associated 'catching-up' increase in occupational incapacity among women.

Compared with the reference scenario, this scenario envisages a marked change in company medical services' attitudes to stress and mental problems at work: much time and money will be invested in the early identification of signs of excessive (or insufficient) mental pressure and checks on prospective employees' mental resilience will become a standard part of appointment procedures. The number of psychologically and psychiatrically trained company medical officers will slowly but surely increase over the next twenty years as appreciation grows across the board of the value to firm and individual employee alike of early and, where necessary, long-term psychosocial support. Efforts will be made during the period of entitlement to sickness benefit to prevent workers with mental problems moving more-or-less automatically onto disability benefit after twelve months, and contacts with the primary sector - notably family doctors, who generally knows the workers concerned best - will be intensified to that end. Larger employers will intervene quickly where there is a risk of mental problems in the workforce, though problems will remain in the small-business sector. The advice of external experts (such as mental health professionals) will be of great value in such circumstances, since firms' own medical services will be unable over the next twenty years fully to remedy their knowledge and skill deficiencies in the prevention of and response to mental problems.

Owing to these developments the industrial insurance boards' medical officers will increasingly be confronted with the 'severer' psychosocial and psychiatric problems. Thanks to their steadily growing knowledge and experience regarding the links between mental incapacities and work skills they will be able to offer advice within firms and thus to have a preventive impact. This more active role will be underpinned by new legislation clearly different in two respects from that envisaged in the reference scenario: first, the quality of the work done by the bodies involved in incapacity assessment (industrial insurance boards, Joint Medical Service, administrative appeals tribunals) will be monitored with a view to ensuring that decision-making is uniform and claimants' rights are clear; and second, entitlement will be further tightened, notably by requiring that it must be more clearly demonstrated that work is the main cause or occasion of the functional disorder or medical condition in question.

The effect of these developments is that the numbers classed as unfit on mental grounds will not rise above the present level of 25% of all disability-benefit claimants.

Care and rehabilitation

Theoretical and practical knowledge of the relations between mental problems and both short- and long-term limitations on individuals' working capacity will increase, albeit not in any spectacular fashion. In the mental health care sector the greatest progress in this area will result from experiments in the occupational rehabilitation of former psychiatric patients. In this non-ideal situation re-employment services for those classed as unfit on mental grounds will remain largely limited to special sheltered-employment projects; commercial objections will continue to prevent any major influx of Category V claimants into mainstream industry. The greatest re-employment efforts will be made in the public sector, partly thanks to tougher legislation (Employment of Disabled Persons Act, WAGW) on sanctions against employers who fail to meet quotas for physically and mentally incapacitated staff. Despite the example set by the state as an employer, many firms will prefer to pay up rather than implement statutory quotas.

As in the reference scenario, the mental health services will find themselves dealing with somewhat greater numbers of Category V disability-benefit recipients, thanks mainly to increased referrals by family doctors and company medical officers. The help available will, again as under the reference scenario, be equivocal: while the immediate alleviation of specific problems will be possible, in structural terms the services will have little to offer. Other types of help will be beyond their scope.

The preventive mental health services will become active in the area of assistance and advice to industry and in a number of cases will achieve improvements, in consultation with employers, in mentally stressful working conditions. Worryingly, it will be virtually only the large employers that are reached in this way; preventive work will not get under way in sectors with many small and medium-sized businesses.

7.7.3 *Scenario 3: Laisser faire*

Outline: This scenario envisages great reluctance on the part of both government and industry to take any preventive measures in relation to mental problems at work. The re-employment of the mentally incapacitated is also given low priority.

Mental health problems in the workforce

The social trends associated with the development of mental problems in the workforce parallel those in the reference and prevention scenarios. The virtual absence of legislation on the mental and social aspects of working conditions (reflecting the view that activities aimed at reducing occupational capacity are primarily the responsibility of industry), will result in a large increase in mental problems mainly of a psychosomatic and neurotic nature. The tendency will be reinforced by society's tendency to see problems in psychological terms. The health services, including company medical services, will not keep pace with these developments, not least because medical education will still include insufficient psychological and psychiatric training. Industry's understanding of and provision for prevention will thus remain extremely limited and strongly oriented towards the individual. There will be little contact between the primary and mental health sectors and firms' medical and welfare services.

Benefit entitlement

The number of WAO/AWW-benefit claimants with mental disorders as their principal diagnosis will rise sharply, from 3% of the workforce at present to 5.5% in 2010. In absolute terms this represents a more-than-doubling from 186,000 in 1987 to 396,000 in 2010. In other words, of the million or more entitlements over a twenty-year period, 40% will have a mental background. This rise reflects not just the overall growth in the workforce but also the deterioration, outlined above, in the mental health situation at work. Firms' awareness of and expertise in mental aspects of the work situation, pathogenic factors, stress prevention, at-risk groups and the like will not grow significantly. While more people will be entitled to sickness benefit as a result of mental problems, the lack of trained staff will mean they do not receive the help they need from employers' medical services. The relatively early 'abandonment' of sick workers to the disability-benefit scheme will become even more customary. People with mental disorders will still commonly be seen as an inconvenience: unproductive, inconvenient and a threat to the atmosphere at work. Attitudes thus remain markedly negative.

Over the years disability benefit will remain for many employers an attractive alternative pension provision for their less productive workers. The state's reluctance to impose regulations and restrictions will allow this situation to persist.

Despite the sharp increase in cases of mental incapacity, the psychiatric expertise possessed by the insurance organizations' medical officers will remain inadequate and assessment by external psychologists and psychiatrists will increasingly be used. The rights of sick workers (the potential claimants of disability benefit) will remain insecure, since little if anything will be done to develop instruments to check the quality such assessments.

Care and rehabilitation

Scientific knowledge of residual or alternative work skills in cases of mental incapacity will remain limited; with little call for such knowledge few initiatives will be undertaken to expand research in this area. Research will remain of marginal significance and its resourcing accordingly limited. This lack of knowledge and interest will be paralleled by a lack of commitment to the re-employment of those who are mentally incapacitated. Resistance will not only come from firms (see above): many claimants will prefer the certainty of benefit payments and an ordered and predictable existence to the risks of resuming work in an organization where working conditions have changed little if at all since they became incapacitated.

The health services, mental and somatic, will mainly serve to pick up the pieces. Lacking any influence with firms' medical services, insurance organizations' medical officers or occupational experts, the mental health services will concentrate on treating the incapacitated; their mainly individualistic focus will offer little scope for tackling the work situation of the incapacitated in a more structural fashion. Symptomatic treatment in the form of psychotherapy for disability-benefit recipients will be all that is feasible; prevention will be impossible. Growing claimant numbers will lead to a considerably greater demand for such care from the extramural mental health services. With health-care funding still output-related, preventive work in relation to employment will not be an attractive prospect for the primary sector or the mental health services.

The organizations set up to represent the interests of the occupationally incapacitated themselves will gain greatly in importance, and such non-professional bodies will supply a major part of the direct support, both psychosocial and material, available to the incapacitated.

7.7.4 *The three scenarios in brief*

The combinations of autonomous developments and government measures over the period 1990-2010 on which the exploratory scenarios are based

	Reference scenario	*Prevention scenario*	*Laisser faire scenario*
Context variables			
• Demography	CBS intermediate variant	Idem	Idem
• Economic trends	CPB intermediate variant (low growth, more women in workforce)	Idem	Idem
A. Determinants of mental problems in the labour force			
• Working conditions			
- at the workplace	Increased mental stress	Idem	Idem
- legislation and regulation	Limited	Extensive, binding	Very limited
• Socio-cultural developments			
- social tolerance of mental problems/deviant behaviour	No change (low)	Idem	Idem
- protoprofessionalization/ medicalization in society	Greater	Idem	Greater tendency to view cal problems in mental te
- work ethic	No change (strong)	Idem	Idem
- support form social network where mental problems arise	No change	Idem	Idem
- impact of lifestyles on mental health; high-risk behaviour	No change (little general concern)	Increase in preventive behaviour	Idem (little general concern)
• Developments in prevention and care			
- approach and activities of firms' medical and welfare services	Mainly individually oriented approach to problems	Recognition of broader commercial and social interests	Mainly individually oreint approach to problems
- approach and activities of other health and welfare services	Little role if any	Important role/collaboration with firms' medical/welfare services	Little role if any
B. Determinants of entitlement to WAO/AAW-benefit			
• Mental problems in the work-force (for determinants see above)	Marked increase	Increase	Sharp increase
• Activities and attitudes of firms' medical services	More early diagnosis, greater awareness of mental aspects of sickness	Major expansion of measures aimed at preventing long-term sickness absence, less ready referral to Joint Medical Service	Predominantly somatic o tion; relatively ready tran disability benefit
• Activities and attitudes of assessment agencies (insurance-board medical officers)	More early diagnosis in first year of incapacity, greater awareness of mental disorders	More active role vis a vis industry	Predominantly somatic o tion
• Legislation governing:			
- the social-security system, benefit rights and requirements	No fundamental changes	Reduced benefit entitlements	No fundamental changes
- role of assessment agencies	No fundamental changes	Insurance boards' medical officers are given curative functions	No fundamental changes
- quality of assessment agencies (insurance boards, Joint Medical Service, Admin. Appeals Tribunal)	General monitoring	Stricter standards	Monitoring only at margi
C. Determinants of service utilization and reemployment			
• Scientific and practical knowledge of relations between mental disorders and work skills	Very slight	Slight	Very slight
• Facilities for support and reemployment within firms	Very limited support; little effort at reemployment despite recognition of commercial value	Active policy, but only marginal provision for support and reemployment activities	No support; little desire o provision for reemployme
• Role of mental-health services	Help provided only after onset of incapacity; only a minority of benefit claimants helped	Active mainly in the area of prevention, not in that of reemployment	Marginal rol ('picking up pieces')
• Legislation (Employment of Disabled People Act, etc.)	No fundamental changes	Tighter rules, tougher sanctions	Dilution of Employment c Disabled People Act

7.8 *Target-setting scenario*[2]

Objective: * A structural decline in mental health problems in the workforce between 1990 and 2010, particularly in the categories of employee, employer and occupation currently seen as high-risk.
* A fall in the number of disability-benefit claimants with a 'mental disorders' diagnosis to 2% of the workforce (a decline in absolute terms from 185,000 in 1990 to 145,000 in 2010).
* The gradual creation, over twenty years, of a situation in which 90% of disability-benefit claimants (i.e. over 20,000 people every year) can return to some appropriate form of employment within two years of becoming entitled to benefit.

Necessary measures

1. General measures

Achieving the objective will necessitate a number of radical measures over the coming years aimed at improving working conditions, preventing the development of incapacity, helping claimants and promoting re-employment. Before detailing the measures required under these headings we first consider some more general areas in which action will be needed over the next twenty years.

- Public education: greater public education by government and the mental health services with the aim of removing mental problems (notably in relation to work) from the sphere of taboo, prejudice and discrimination. A similar campaign needs to be focused specifically on industry and the primary-care sector.
- Identification and recording: procedures for identifying and recording, within firms and at national level, mental problems associated with working conditions need to be expanded and greatly improved. In particular more specific information is urgently needed on high-risk groups, businesses and occupations.
- Radical improvements are needed in the (currently defective) procedures for information-exchange and the coordination of functions and activities between the various medical and non-medical services. A multidisciplinary approach is needed to prevention, social and medical care and support and the re-

[2] The basic assumptions of the target-setting scenario are set out in Appendix 1.

employment of the incapacitated; if necessary it should be made a statutory requirement.

- Mentally unhealthy work situations must be improved as a matter of urgency through a statutory requirement for preventive measures of a structural nature in the area of working conditions and labour relations. The government should guide developments and itself set an example as an employer. In the somewhat longer term an international approach is desirable.
- Scientific knowledge of the relations between work and mental disorders and between mental disorders and limitations on work skills is still in its infancy. Research needs to be promoted; both government and industry have an interest in progress in these areas.
- There is considerable room for improvement in the assessment procedures under disability-benefit legislation. A positive side-effect would be enhanced certainty regarding the rights of potential and current benefit claimants.

2. *Measures to reduce mental problems in the workforce*

Two (partially overlapping) sets of measures may be distinguished here: those aimed directly at improving 'shopfloor' working conditions and those whose purpose is more to set the right framework.

The measures needed are as follows.

- *Urgent preventive measures*
    - Enhanced knowledge and understanding within industry of sickness absence and incapacity on mental grounds and of the effects of possible preventive measures. Measures: the establishment of a uniform national system for recording absences and statutory provision for their publication.
    - Direct preventive measures in industry: better career planning and medical and welfare support for employees, greater willingness to adjust mental stress levels to employees' age. The need for action of this type is greatest among those in lower-grade jobs. Greater attention also needs to be focused on small and medium-sized businesses. Possibilities include adjustments to individuals' work or workload where the need emerges from appraisal interviews. Measures: an entitlement to six-monthly training sessions (including e.g. assertiveness training for clerical workers and conflict-management for middle managers) and/or provision for new career directions, job rotation, external assessment of mental pressures (excessive/inadequate) in the work situation.

- National structural measures aimed at improving mental and social working conditions: the introduction and strict enforcement of welfare provisions in the framework of the Working Conditions Act (ARBO). Concrete possibilities include the regular examination of employing organizations for situations which may threaten mental health. This should involve not only the Factory Inspectorate but also (given their special expertise) the mental health services and company medical services in an advisory role. The financial penalties for non-compliance with the Working Conditions Act need to be made considerably tougher.
- Ongoing information and training for managers, personnel departments and company medical services aimed at facilitating recognition of the signs of excessive (or insufficient) mental pressure on employees, more effective ways of dealing with sickness absence, and adjustments and improvements in management styles at middle and senior level. Greater knowledge and new attitudes are urgent necessities in this area. Possibilities include an information campaign on television aimed at the general public, together with specific information campaigns aimed at management-training institutions, at the professional associations of company medical officers and occupational-medicine specialists and at employers' associations and trade unions.
- Company medical teams should be multidisciplinary in makeup. A greater input of psychological and psychiatric expertise in insurance boards employees.
- Greater education at all levels of industry regarding the position of first- and second-generation migrants and the associated risks of occupational incapacity on mental grounds.
- Prevention and support programmes should be established as speedily as possible aimed at those occupations, industries and firms in which mental problems are known to be relatively common; these include teachers, welfare workers (home helps, nurses etc.), urban bus drivers and bank staff. It is the task of the trade unions in particular to draw attention to such problems; prime responsibility for treatment and support rests with the extramural mental health services.

- *Longer-term measures*
  - Work needs to be organized in ways which enable a faster and more flexible response to be made to changing requirements, including provision for 'sabbatical leave', training in advance of radical changes in such areas as automation and more flexible

working hours. Such measures are particularly necessary in the case of women, who will account for an increasing proportion of the workforce and often have to carry a double or triple burden. To help prevent mental problems developing there should be no raising of the age at which early retirement is possible. In addition to the extensive educational activities already mentioned firms, Works Councils need to be given stronger statutory powers in respect of initiatives to improve the work situation.

- Welfare provisions should be incorporated into individual and collective employment contracts. Employee welfare should be a regular topic of collective bargaining.
- Physicians in general and occupational-medicine specialists in particular need greater knowledge and expertise regarding the mental aspects of work and working conditions. Family doctors are particularly deficient in this area. The current curriculum should be checked for obsolete or redundant elements and for an excessively somatic emphasis.
- More research is needed in the areas of the relations between working conditions in particular industries and mental problems, stress as a causal factor in mental problems, prejudice and discrimination against those with mental problems, and prevention and support strategies in the work situation. The government should provide more resources for university and non-university research institutions and should commission more research. Industry should establish a research fund into which a fixed percentage of profits is paid.
- Occupational incapacity due to mental disorders is an issue which lies on the boundary between the responsibilities of the health and employment ministries. Greater coordination and cooperation is needed between the two ministries on such health-promoting measures as action against unemployment (notably youth unemployment), the more efficient application of the mental health services' existing knowledge and expertise regarding mental problems, action to help at-risk groups, enforcement of the Working Conditions Act and monitoring of the operation of company medical services. Ongoing consultations are needed at senior civil-service level, with inputs from experts, employers and trade unions, with a view to identifying problems in these areas and coordinating the formulation and implementation by the various ministries concerned of policy on working conditions and social security. The consultative body established for this purpose should be able to make proposals to parliament, at the latter's request and

on its own initiative. The National Health Council should focus explicitly on the theme of work and health.

3. *Measures aimed at reducing the number of disability-benefit claimants with a 'mental disorder' diagnosis to 2% of the workforce*

In addition to the various measures taken to improve working conditions, supplementary measures are needed to reduce the numbers of people needing disability benefit, thus allowing the number classed as unfit on mental grounds to be cut from 185,000 in 1990 to 145,000. In particular, changes are urgently needed in the assessment procedures under the Sickness Benefit (Ziekteweg) and Disability Insurance Acts (WAO).

The measures necessary to achieve this objective are as follows.

- *Urgent measures*
  - In industry: systematic measures are needed to ensure that contact is maintained between workers on sickness benefit and their employers and colleagues. In this way the numbers proceeding to disability benefit can be reduced and the resumption of work facilitated.
  - A consultative structure involving all the agencies concerned with occupational incapacity - company medical services, monitoring agencies, support agencies (primary and mental health care) and both sides of industry - should be established at the earliest opportunity with the job of detecting undesirable situations at regional or employer level and of deploying the available support services in effective and coordinated fashion.
  - In conjunction with the preceding point: provision is needed for case management, i.e. a procedure whereby a single coordinating medical or welfare officer remains in charge of the case of an employee who falls ill, if necessary until he or she becomes entitled to disability benefit. This approach will help ensure that individuals do not get lost between different agencies.
  - The legislation on entitlement to sickness and disability benefit should be evaluated and if necessary amended. Attention needs to be focused on: the pathogenic and incapacity-promoting effects of thc procedures, such as excessively long qualifying times, the uncertainty and arbitrariness resulting from repeated assessments by different agencies, the different incapacity criteria applying under the Sickness Benefit and Disability Insurance Acts, the shortcomings in the exchange of information between assessment and treatment agencies and the implications of the structural changes pending in the industrial

insurance boards and Joint Medical Service for the quality of assessment and of the medical and welfare support available for the incapacitated.
  - Legislative change is also needed to bring about a considerable improvement in the procedure for determining occupational incapacity. Priority should go to: compulsory in-service training for insurance-board medical officers and advising psychologists and psychiatrists and the development of instruments aimed at a more objective assessment of capacity and incapacity (primarily a task for science).

- *Longer-term measures*
  - Establishment of a system of financial rewards and penalties,among them differentiated contribution levels under the sickness- and disability-benefit schemes which reflect firms' rates of sickness absence on mental grounds and a requirement that firms replace any employee becoming entitled to disability benefit with another incapacitated employee.
  - Reform of the social-security system: integration of the unemployment- and disability-benefit schemes into a single scheme under which the reason why claimants cannot work is irrelevant to their rights and obligations.
  - Promotion of research into the relations between psychiatric conditions and residual work skills with a view to developing more uniform criteria of assessment, *inter alia* through the establishment of a university chair in insurance-related medicine and mental problems.
  - Extension of compulsory industrial health care to the entire workforce, facilitating the early identification of problems.
  - Provided that more valid assessment criteria can be developed: more regular psychological or psychiatric assessment of persons classed as incapacitated on mental grounds with a view to responding more rapidly to any changes, for better or worse, in individuals' situation.

4. *Measures aimed at ensuring that 90% of those classed as incapacitated on mental grounds return to work within two years*

Measures under this heading may relate to the help provided to those classed as occupationally incapacitated on mental grounds and to follow-up activities aimed at enabling them to return to mainstream employment. This aspect of the overall objective requires strong measures, since it involves creating jobs, if necessary suitably adapted, for over 20,000 people every year.

The measures necessary to achieve this objective are as follows.

- *Urgent measures*
  - Strengthening the state's power to guide and compel: the Employment of Disabled People Act (WAGW) should be amended in such a way as to promote the re-employment in particular of the mentally incapacitated. Discrimination in favour of the physically incapacitated at the expense of the mentally incapacitated should be prevented by the imposition of quotas for the numbers of mentally incapacitated workers on firms' payrolls, and such quotas should be complemented both by considerably tougher financial sanctions on employers not complying or making insufficient efforts to create suitable jobs and by a stricter requirement on the incapacitated to accept the work available.
  - Trial projects should be carried out in mainstream industry, with financial support from the state and the Disability Funds, involving the partial re-employment of the mentally incapacitated.

- *Longer-term measures*
  - Trial projects aimed at the occupational rehabilitation and re-employment of psychiatric patients need to be extended, partly with a view to building up knowledge and experience regarding the residual work skills of the mentally incapacitated. Mainstream industry, and in particular those sectors in which mental incapacity is currently relatively common, should be involved in such projects, e.g. through regular participation in consultations through the Regional Institutes of Mental Health (RIGGs).
  - The extramural mental health services must make help for people classed as occupationally incapacitated on mental ground a focus of their work. This requirement should be included in the criteria which institutions must meet to be eligible for public funding, and additional funding should be provided to enable them to comply with it. In the short term this will require new provision for in-service training and and a greater orientation towards industry and the labour market on the part of the Regional Institutes of Ambulatory Mental Health Care (RIAGGs). The existing training agencies (RINOs) will need to modify their courses accordingly.
  - The mental health services need to be involved as standing advisers on rehabilitation and re-employment. Consultations with the Joint Medical Service and the industrial insurance boards should be institutionalized.

- Research is needed into ways of exploiting the knowledge and experience which psychologists and psychiatrists in private practice have built up over the years in their role as experts in the assessment of occupational incapacity.
- Company medical services and industrial insurance boards must come to regard investigations into the scope for creating jobs for the mentally incapacitated as a central concern. The various educational and training activities aimed at changing attitudes and raising knowledge and skill levels are of great importance here.

7.9 *Staffing and financial implications*

The costs and benefits associated with the scenarios cannot be determined in detail: as is commonly the case in health economics, many of the data needed are unavailable and in some cases it is not possible, at least as yet, adequately to operationalize certain key concepts. Only a limited number of directly attributable costs and benefits can be calculated, while the more indirect costs and benefits can often be only roughly estimated if at all. This applies for example to the cost of production losses due to occupational incapacity: if this could be determined it would be an interesting and relevant element in comparisons between the scenarios, but unfortunately we lack both the time and the information needed to quantify this factor.

This section sets out the cost and, where relevant, staffing implications over the period 1990-2010 of the three reference scenarios and the target-setting scenario under the following headings:

- benefit entitlements under the Disability Insurance and General Disability Benefit Acts (WAO/AAW) and the civil-service scheme (ABP),
- company medical services,
- preventive activities undertaken by the Regional Institutes of Ambulatory Mental Health Care (RIAGGs),
- psychiatric assessments,
- activities relating to the re-employment of the mentally incapacitated,
- other costs and benefits.

The methods of calculation and assumptions involved are set out in the appendix at the end of this chapter.

Table 7.21 **Annual cost of benefit payments to persons classed as occupationally incapacitated on mental grounds, billions of guilders, 1987 prices (index 1987=100)**

	Reference Scenario	Prevention Scenario	Laisser Faire Scenario	Target-setting Scenario
1987	6.4 (100)	6.4 (100)	6.4 (100)	6.4 (100)
2000	8.9 (139)	7.8 (122)	9.9 (155)	5.9 (92)
2010	10.6 (166)	8.3 (130)	12.9 (202)	4.7 (73)

As this table shows, heavy investment in prevention and re-employment (see subsequent tables) can pay for itself through billion-guilder savings in benefit expenditure.

Table 7.22 **Capacity (fte) and annual cost of company medical services (millions of guilders, 1987 prices)**

	Reference Scenario		Prevention Scenario		Laisser Faire Scenario		Target-setting Scenario	
	Fte	Cost	Fte	Cost	Fte	Cost	Fte	Cost
1987	2632	322	2632	322	2632	322	2632	322
1990	2778	342	2872	353	2778	342	3159	389
2000	3161	389	3860	475	3161	389	4825	593
2010	3597	442	5187	638	3492	429	7781	957

Table 7.23 **Capacity (fte) and annual cost of preventive work undertaken by the Regional Institutes of Ambulatory Mental Health Care (RIAGG) specifically in connection with mental incapacity (millions of guilders, 1987 prices)**

	Reference Scenario		Prevention Scenario		Laisser Faire Scenario		Target-setting Scenario	
	Fte	Cost	Fte	Cost	Fte	Cost	Fte	Cost
1987	7	0.8	7	0.8	7	0.8	7	0.8
1990	8	0.9	8	0.9	7	0.8	13	1.3
2000	16	1.7	39	4.2	10	1.0	69	7.2
2010	21	2.2	83	8.8	13	1.3	167	17.5

Table 7.24 **Number and annual cost of psychiatric assessments carried out in connection with disability-benefit entitlement (millions of guilders, 1987 prices)**

	Reference Scenario		Prevention Scenario		Laisser Faire Scenario		Target-setting Scenario	
	No.	Cost	No.	Cost	No.	Cost	No.	Cost
1987	15500	16	15500	16	15500	16	15500	16
2000	18000	18	15500	16	19700	20	11700	12
2010	20000	20	15500	16	24000	24	9300	9

Table 7.25 **Number of cases and annual cost of the re-employment of persons classed as occupationally incapacitated on mental grounds (millions of guilders, 1987 prices)**

	Reference Scenario		Prevention Scenario		Laisser Faire Scenario		Target-setting Scenario	
	No.	Cost	No.	Cost	No.	Cost	No.	Cost
1987	6300	315	6300	315	6300	315	6300	315
1990	7100	355	7500	375	6500	325	10000	500
2000	9600	480	11500	575	7300	365	22500	1125
2010	12200	610	15600	780	8000	400	11300	565

Other costs and benefits

There are a number of costs and benefits which, though difficult or impossible to quantify, ought nevertheless to play a part in the assessment of the various scenarios. They include:

- the costs/benefits of in-service training for insurance-board medical officers, prevention officers, company medical and welfare officers, forensic psychiatrists, primary-care workers etc.;
- the costs/benefits of training new/more professionals in these categories;
- the costs/benefits of the use by the mentally incapacitated of drugs in general and psychoactive drugs in particular;
- production losses through incapacity and production gains through the re-employment of the mentally incapacitated;
- the costs/benefits of treatment in the mental and somatic health care for the mentally incapacitated;
- the cost (arising as a side-effect) of support, therapy etc. for the families of the mentally incapacitated;
- the costs/benefits of research and education relating to work and mental health.

Appendix Calculations and assumptions in the cost assessment

1. *Cost of disability-benefit payments to persons classed as occupationally incapacitated on mental grounds (Category V cases)*

Tables 7.10 and 7.11 in the background analysis show Category V cases to include a relatively large proportion of persons classed as fully incapacitated; it is therefore reasonable to suppose that such cases also account for a relative large proportion of total annual expenditure on disability benefit. In what follows we indicate how benefit spending can be corrected to reflect this.

Claimant numbers and benefit expenditure under the Disability Insurance and General Disability Benefit Acts and the civil-service scheme (WAO, AAW, ABP)

	No. as at 1 January	Index	Cost (billions of guilders, 1987 prices)
1987	771,000	100	21.9
2000	944,000	122	26.8
2010	1,008,000	131	28.6

Reference scenario, benefit expenditure, Category V cases

	No. as at 1 January	Index	Cost (billions)	Corrected cost (billions)
1987	186,000 (3% of workforce)	100	5.5 (25% of total)	6.4 (29% of total)
2000	270,000 (3.8% of workforce)	145	7.6 (29% of total)	8.9 (33% of total)
2010	320,000 (4.5% of workforce)	172	9.2 (32% of total)	10.6 (37% of total)

Calculation:
32% of claimants as at 1 January are in Category V, leaving 68% in the remaining categories. 90% of Category V claimants are fully incapacitated. Assuming that for all categories together the proportion is constant at 78% (see baseline analysis), it follows that just over 72% of non-Category-V claimants are fully incapacitated. The share of Category V entitlements in total benefit expenditure can then be determined with the help of the following equations:

Category V claimants as % of all claimants x fully incapacitated Category V claimants as % of all Category V claimants) = fully incapacitated Category V claimants as % of all claimants

Non-Category-V claimants as % of all claimants x fully incapacitated non-Category-V claimants as % of all non-Category-V claimants = fully incapacitated non-Category-V claimants as % of all claimants

Fully incapacitated Category-V claimants as % of all claimants + fully incapacitated non-Category-V claimants as % of all claimants = all fully incapacitated claimants as % of all claimants

Filling in the figures for 2010 from the reference scenario then gives us:

(32 x 90) + (68 x 72.4) = 100 x 78

2880 + 4920 = 7800

Since 2880/7800 = 37%, it follows that while Category V cases make up 32% of all entitlements, they account for an estimated 37% of total benefit expenditure (28.6 billion guilders in 2010).

The calculation can be performed in the same fashion for the remaining years and scenarios.

Prevention scenario, benefit expenditure, Category V cases

	No. as at 1 January	Index	Cost (billions)	Corrected cost (billions)
1987	186,000	100	5.5	6.4
	(3% of workforce)		(25% of total)	(29% of total)
2000	236,000	127	6.7	7.8
	(3.3% of workforce)		(25% of total)	(29% of total)
2010	252,000	135	7.2	8.3
	(3.5% of workforce)		(25% of total)	(29% of total)

Laisser faire scenario, benefit expenditure, Category V cases

	No. as at 1 January	Index	Cost (billions)	Corrected cost (billions)
1987	186,000 (3% of workforce)	100	5.5 (25% of total)	6.4 (29% of total)
2000	305,000 (4.3% of workforce)	164	8.7 (32% of total)	9.9 (37% of total)
2010	396,000 (5.5% of workforce)	213	11.2 (39% of total)	12.9 (45% of total)

Target-setting scenario, benefit expenditure, Category V cases

	No. as at 1 January	Index	Cost (billions)	Corrected cost (billions)
1987	186,000 (3% of workforce)	100	5.5 (25% of total)	6.4 (29% of total)
2000	178,000 (2.5% of workforce)	96	5.1 (19% of total)	5.9 (22% of total)
2010	145,000 (2% of workforce)	76	4.1 (14% of total)	4.7 (17% of total)

2. *Capacity and cost of company medical services*

The calculations start from the changes in capacity, expressed in terms of staff (full-time equivalent), envisaged under each of the scenarios. The Financial Overview of Care 1990 (Ministry of Welfare, Health and Cultural Affairs 1989) includes the following figures for capacity and operating costs since 1980.

	1980	1983	1984	1985	1986	1987	1988
Capacity (fte)	2430	2478	2527	2637	2645	2632	2707
Operating costs (millions of guilders)	263	293	305	315	318	322	331

Over the period 1980-88 capacity growth averaged 1.3% per year. The scenarios make different assumptions regarding future capacity changes. Fte capacity is converted into costs (1987 prices) on the basis of the unit operating cost in 1987 (123,000 guilders). The assumptions involved are as follows.

- Reference scenario: continued capacity growth of 1.3% per year.
- Prevention scenario: capacity growth of 3% per year.
- Laisser faire scenario: capacity growth of 1.3% per year to 2000 and 1% per year thereafter.
- Target scenario: growth rates as under the prevention scenario with additional increases, namely in 1990 prevention-scenario capacity + 10%, in 2000 prevention-scenario capacity + 25% and in 2010 prevention-scenario capacity + 50%.

3. *Capacity and cost of preventive activities undertaken by the Regional Institutes of Ambulatory Mental Health Care (RIAGGs)*

The calculations start from the changes in capacity, expressed in terms of staff (full-time equivalent) envisaged under each of the scenarios.

In Chapter 4 a calculation was made of the RIAGGs' total future capacity on the basis of past trends in their staffing. The figures obtained are also used here: 4741 fte in 1990, 6559 in 2000 and 8336 in 2010.

The scenarios make different assumptions regarding future changes in the capacity specifically devoted to the prevention of occupational incapacity due to mental disorders. Fte capacity is converted into costs (1987 prices) on the basis of the unit operating cost in 1987 (105,000 guilders). The assumptions involved are as follows.

In 1987 3% of the RIAGGs' fte capacity was devoted to preventive work (WAGG 1988); the target is 5%. It is assumed that in 1990 3.5% of RIAGG capacity is devoted to preventive work, rising to 5% in 2000 and 2010. The scenarios make the following assumptions regarding the share of available preventive capacity devoted specifically to the prevention of occupational incapacity due to mental disorders:
- reference scenario: 5% of total available preventive capacity throughout;
- prevention scenario: 5% in 1990, 12% in 2000 and 20% in 2010;
- laisser faire scenario: 3% throughout;
- target-setting scenario: growth rates as under the prevention scenario with additional increases, namely in 1990 prevention-scenario capacity + 50%, in 2000 prevention-scenario capacity + 75%, and in 2010 prevention-scenario capacity + 100%.

4. *Number and cost of psychiatric assessments*

The calculations start from the fact that around two thirds of new Category V cases involve a psychiatric assessment, whether when individuals become entitled to benefit or when cases go to appeal. The cost of an assessment, including the production of a report, is put at 1008 guilders, i.e. eight consultations at 126 guilders each (cost per psychiatric consultation based on Ketting & Jacobs 1989).

In 1987 new Category V cases totalled around 23,000, implying some 15,500 psychiatric assessments (Knepper 1987; Kabel 1988) at a cost of around 16 million guilders.

Each scenario envisages changes in the percentage of all entitlements for which

Category V cases account, and these changes are assumed to be reflected in and equal rise or fall in the number of new cases of entitlement on mental grounds. The assumptions made are as follows.

- Reference scenario: a rise in the proportion of Category V cases from 25% to 32% of the total, i.e. from 23,000 in 1987 to 32/25 x 23,000 = 29,500 in 2010. Two thirds of these involve a psychiatric assessment, giving a total of 20,000 per year. A similar calculation may be made for the year 2000.
- Prevention scenario: no rise in the proportion of Category V cases, which stay at 25%. The number of new cases of benefit entitlement on mental grounds remains at 23,000 per year, despite a growing workforce, and the number of assessments at 15,500 per year.
- Laisser faire scenario: a rise in the proportion of Category V cases from 25% to 39% of the total; further calculations as under the reference scenario.
- Target-setting scenario: a fall in the proportion of Category V cases from 25% to 15% of the total; further calculations as under the reference scenario.

5. *Number of cases and annual cost of re-employment*

Each scenario made assumptions as to the numbers of *new* entitlements to disability benefit; the actual figure in 1987 was 22,500. From the total numbers of entitlements in 2010 under each scenario we can calculate how many *terminations of benefit* are needed to arrive at that figure. Benefit is terminated on recovery/re-employment, reaching pensionable age or death. The number of terminations resulting from the reaching of pensionable age or death is assumed to stay constant at its 1987 level of 8,700 (SVr, GMD 1989). In 1987 there were 15,000 terminations of Category V benefit, of whom 15,000 - 8,700 = 6,300 were persons resuming employment. The calculations made were as follows.

- Reference scenario: a rise of 134,000 in the total number of Category V entitlements, from 186,000 in 1987 to 320,000 in 2010. The number of new entitlements is assumed to increase linearly from 22,500 per year to 25,000 in 2010. The total number of new entitlements over the 23-year period is thus 546,250, giving a total for terminations of entitlement of 546,250 - 134,000 = 412,250, an annual average of 17,924. Terminations also increase linearly, from 15,000 in 1987 to 20,850 in 2010. Subtracting 8,700 from both figures gives us the numbers of mentally incapacitated persons resuming work in 1987 and 2010.
- Prevention scenario: a rise of 66,000 in the total number of Category V entitlements, from 186,000 in 1987 to 252,000 in 2010. The number of new entitlements is assumed to be held at 22,500 per year. See above for the remainder of the calculation.
- Laisser faire scenario: a rise of 210,000 in the total number of Category V entitlements, from 186,000 in 1987 to 396,000 in 2010. The number of new entitlements is assumed to increase linearly from 22,500 per year to 27,500 in 2010. See above for the remainder of the calculation.
- Target-setting scenario: here a distinction is made between the periods

1987-2000 and 2000-2010. The target for the first period is a fall of 8000 in the number of entitlements, from 186,000 to 178,000; with the number of new entitlements assumed to remain constant at 22,500 per year, the current upward trend must therefore be reversed within thirteen years, implying a large number of returns to employment. A further fall of 33,000 (from 178,000 to 145,000) is targeted for the period 2000-2010, with the number of new entitlements assumed to decline linearly from 22,500 per year in 2000 to 20,000 in 2010. See above for the remainder of the calculation.

For the purpose of cost determination the cost of creating or adapting a job for a mentally incapacitated worker is assumed to average 50,000 guilders.

8 Emotional and behavioural problems in children and adolescents

Part I Baseline analysis

8.1 *Characterization*

The study was concerned with emotional and behavioural problems in children and adolescents (aged 0-17) which are severe enough to produce a breakdown of family relationships, failure at school or serious social problems. The definition excludes, mainly for practical reasons, the mentally handicapped, addicts and epileptics.

No attempt has been made to derive descriptions of children's mental health problems from a diagnostic and classification system such as ICD-9 or DSM-III. These systems lack clear descriptions for the main psychiatric disorders of children; indeed, aside from certain specific and rare syndromes such as infantile autism and Tourette's syndrome, there is little consensus within child psychiatry as to what is and what is not a disorder (and when). Several factors stand in the way of consensus (Verhulst 1985, Deboutte 1989):

- the role of maturation and development: what is normal behaviour in a two-year-old may be abnormal in a six-year-old and perhaps highly abnormal in an older child (thumb-sucking, fear of separation etc.);
- the situational dependence of children's behaviour: children often behave differently at home than at school or with friends;
- children's lack of awareness or understanding of illness: whether youngsters present to a medical or welfare agency is determined in the first instance by their parents, doctor or teachers, seldom by the children themselves; the need and demand for care is determined by persons other than the child;
- the uncertain boundary between the normal and the abnormal: most behaviours seen as symptomatic of a disorder are also found in normal children. Most disorders differ only quantitatively rather than qualitatively from normality.

Problem behaviour in adolescents always involves interactions with their environment: that is why the definition with which we began refers to problems in youngsters' three environments.

The definition is of course very broad and needs to be refined and made more specific. To produce a more differentiated overview of the field for the purposes of this baseline analysis we therefore distinguish between broad problem categories, such as emotional problems (manifesting themselves in anxieties, phobias, depression, inferiority feelings, social withdrawal, shyness, oversensitivity), behavioural problems (in the form of disobedience, destructiveness and aggression), hyperkinetic phenomena (hyperactivity, attention deficit, impulsiveness), developmental problems (learning problems, language problems, bedwetting), and psychoses.

Severe emotional and behavioural problems are estimated to affect

5-7% of youngsters, about twice as many of them boys as girls. The prevalence of such problems is slightly greater among adolescents than among younger children; often they extend over long periods of time. The background seems seldom to be strictly causal in nature: rather is it the case that mutually reinforcing adverse factors (such as family problems, low socio-economic status and biological factors) together exceed the capacity of the individual child and his or her environment.

8.2 *Occurrence, course and prognosis*

8.2.1 *Incidence and prevalence*

Most epidemiological studies concerned with emotional and behavioural problems in children and adolescents focus on prevalence; little research has been conducted into the incidence of such problems, given that it is very difficult to fix their precise onset.

The only large-scale epidemiological study that has so far been made of mental health problems in children in the Netherlands was carried out by Verhulst (1985) on a population of 8 and 11-year-olds, of Dutch nationality, living in the province of South Holland. The procedure used for determining prevalence was the two-stage method introduced by Rutter. This involves first the screening of the whole population by the use of a suitable instrument; Verhulst used the Child Behaviour Checklist (CBCL), a questionnaire completed by parents; the child's teacher completes a similar questionnaire. The checklist distinguishes between social competence and behavioural problems. The latter comprise two groups of items, namely externalizing and internalizing problem behaviours. Externalizing behaviours include aggression, hyperactivity, disobedience, destructiveness and stealing, i.e. conduct which disturbs those in the child's environment; internalizing behaviours include anxiety, withdrawal, dependence, shyness and crying.

The method's second stage involves a closer study of youngsters with high scores on the first stage (in the case of Verhulst's research this comprised a psychiatric interview with the child, a psychological test and a discussion with the parents), who are compared with a control group.

Table 8.1, which lists studies using this or a similar method (each one at least involved a psychiatric interview), shows that estimates of prevalence can vary widely even within the same country. The picture is however somewhat clearer if we limit ourselves to 'severe' disorders (albeit the designation is seldom defined). In addition to differences in the populations studied and in experimental designs, a major factor in the diversity of the results obtained is the subjectivity of clinical judgements. Verhulst himself notes that the percentages he found are slightly higher than in comparable research. In extrapolating Verhulst's results to the country as a whole account must be taken of the fact that South Holland is the Netherlands' most urban province, since the occurrence of problems is known to be related to urbanization levels (see section 8.3.3). A cautious estimate puts the prevalence of severe emotional and behavioural problems among children and adolescents in the Netherlands at 5-7% (SCP 1987), implying that between 166,000 and 233,000 youngsters are affected. Assuming that the percentage remains constant, we can expect the absolute numbers also to remain constant over the next twenty years (table 8.2).

Table 8.1 **Studies of the prevalence of mental health problems among children and adolescents**

Author, year of publication	Location	Sample size	Age range	Prevalence rate found
Connell et al. 1982	Queensland, Australia	779	10-11	10% with severe disorder
Earls 1980	Martha's Vinyard USA	100	3	11% with behavioural problems
Langner et al. 1974	Manhattan, New York, USA	1034	6-18	11.5% with disorder
Leslie, 1974	Blackburn, UK	1198	13-14	4.4% with severe disorder, 17.2% with disorder comparable with children in psychiatric clinic
Miller et al. 1974	Newcastle upon Tyne, UK	794	10	19.4% with maladjustment
Offord et al.	Ontario, Canada	2679	4-16	18.1% with one or more disorders (six-month prevalence)
Richman et al. 1975	London, UK	705	3	7.3% with moderate or severe disorder
Rutter et al 1970	Isle of Wight, UK	2199	10-11	6.8% with severe disorder, 12% with moderate or severe disorder
Graham and Rutter 1973	Isle of Wight, UK	2303	14-15	7.7% with severe disorder, 13% with moderate or severe disorder

Rutter et al. 1975	Isle of Wight, UK	1279	10	12% with severe disorder
	London, UK	1689	10	12.7% with severe disorder, 25.4% with moderate or severe disorder
Verhulst 1985	South Holland province, Netherlands	2076	8+11	7% with severe disorder, 26% with moderate or severe disorder
Vikan 1985	North Troendelag, Norway	1510	10	5.4% with a disorder

Source: Links 1983; Offord *et al.* 1987; Deboutte 1989.

Table 8.2 **Prevalence of severe emotional and behavioural problems in 0-17-year-olds in the Netherlands in 1990, 1995, 2000 and 2010 ('000 persons; total size of age group in parentheses)***

	0-12		**13-17**		**0-17**	
1989	140	(2334)	72	(1034)	212	(3368)
1995	146	(2429)	63	(905)	209	(3334)
2000	152	(2536)	56	(798)	208	(3427)
2010	141	(2351)	70	(1003)	211	(3354)

* The calculation starts from the Central Bureau of Statistics Population Forecast 1988 (intermediate variant) (CBS 1988). Constant percentages are assumed of 6% in the 0-12s and 7% in the 13-17s; see the next section for the reasoning behind the higher rate for the 13-17 age group.

Among the 5-7% of youngsters with severe problems, the psychiatric judgements suggest that emotional disorders form the largest group (45-55%), followed by behavioural disorders and hyperkinetic disorders (15-35% each) and developmental disorders. It should be borne in mind that one childe can involve several diagnoses.

8.2.2 *Sex and age*

Emotional and behavioural problems are generally more common in boys than in girls, albeit emotional disorders affect both sexes equally disorders to be 2.4 times commoner in boys; in the light of this and other research using comparable methodology the ratio of boys to girls among youngsters with severe psychiatric disorders can be put at 2:1 (Deboutte 1989). What is involved here is not so much the frequency of problems (which is only slightly greater among boys) but their nature: in general boys display more externalizing (socially undesirable) behaviour and girls slightly more internalizing behaviour (Verhulst 1985; see also table 8.3). Behaviour which is troublesome to the social environment is evidently more likely to be labelled disordered. A second point is that boys develop more slowly than girls, which may help to explain the greater frequency in boys of speech and toileting problems (Verhulst 1989).

Table 8.3 **Studies of sex-related differences and the nature of problem behaviour**

	No. of studies focusing on correlation	**No. of studies finding significant differences**
More problems in boys than in girls	15	10
More externalizing behavioural problems in boys	14	11
More internalizing behavioural problems in girls	14	10

Sources: Links 1983; Verhulst 1985; Vikan 1985; Offord *et al.* 1987.

Table 8.1 shows prevalence data for various age groups; they suggest that there are no great age-related differences in prevalence (the Isle of Wight studies in particular, which cover the same population, provide comparative material). Verhulst (1985), however, found a wide difference in the figures for severe disorders in 8- and 11-year-olds (13% and 4% respectively), but if moderate disorders are also included the gap narrows sharply (27% and 24%). We may provisionally assume that age-related prevalence differences are not great, albeit the prevalence of disorders appears to be slightly higher in 12-17s than in younger children (Graham & Rutter 1985; see also table 8.4).

An interaction is observable between age and sex, in that the relative frequency of mental health problems in girls *vis-à-vis* boys rises with age. This is visible in table 8.4, which shows the results of a prevalence study among 4-16-year-olds in Ontario, Canada (Offord *et al.* 1987); it should be noted that this study covered mild as well as severe disorders.

Table 8.4 **Six-month prevalence (per 100 children) of psychiatric disorders, by age and sex**

Age group (number)	Behavioural disorder	Hyper-activity	Emotional disorder	Somati-zation*	≥ 1 dis-order**
Boys					
4-11 (721)	6.5	10.1	10.2	-	19.5
12-16 (608)	10.4	7.3	4.9	4.5	18.8
4-16	8.1	8.9	7.9	-	19.2
Girls					
4-11 (721)	1.8	3.3	10.7	-	13.5
12-16 (624)	4.1	3.4	13.6	10.7	21.8
4-16 (1345)	2.7	3.3	11.9	-	16.9
Boys and girls					
4-11 (1442)	4.2	6.7	10.5	-	16.5
12-16 (1232)	7.3	5.4	9.3	7.6	20.3

Source: Offord *et al.* 1987.

* Somatization was so uncommon among the 4-11s that no reliable estimates were possible.

** ≥ 1 disorder: children in whom one or more of the disorders mentioned was diagnosed.

As table 8.4 shows, the nature of the problems differs from one age group to another, and in what follows we look briefly at a number of problems which affect (or whose onset occurs in) a particular age group.

In the first eighteen months of life the development of an emotional bond between children and parents (or parent figures) is of great importance, laying as it does the foundations for balanced social and emotional development. In infants of this age diagnosis is often limited to the identification of such phenomena as neglect and abuse, temperamental disorders and sleeping and eating disorders. Behavioural variations in this age group have little value as predictors of later individual differences.

During the next stage, from eighteen months to four years, children develop self-awareness, autonomy, language skills and social behaviour. Problems are often concerned with separation, the control of aggression, sleep, language, toileting and the development of a balance between dependence and independence. The commonest clinical picture is of a child who is restless, ungovernable and attention-seeking (Richman 1985); relatively few children are anxious or unhappy. It is generally in this age group that autism is diagnosed.

The next stage, from four to eleven years, sees a widening of the child's social environment; he or she becomes less egocentric and acquires increasing independence. The problems of children in this age group are more easily identified than those of younger children, since they are better able to put their problems into words; in principle, therefore, all the psychiatric disorders of children can be diagnosed at this stage. Since children start school during this stage, it is now that learning difficulties, attention disorders, school phobia and problems in contacts with contemporaries emerge.

The period of adolescence, from twelve to seventeen, is one of rapid growth, with changes in the skeleton and hormone system and the development of sexual differences. In general boys are more satisfied than girls with these physical changes; at this stage the proportion of girls who see themselves as fat and try dieting rises sharply to as much as 50% (Graham & Rutter 1985).

Social development accelerates during adolescence as youngsters begin to break away from their parents and develop their own identities; it is also a period of major choices in the areas of education and employment.

Adolescents' problems often differ considerably in nature from those of younger children, with bedwetting and hyperactivity becoming rarer and anorexia nervosa, bulimia, agoraphobia, depression and schizophrenia manifesting themselves for the first time. There is also a marked increase in alcohol and drug abuse and in delinquency. Feelings of depression, uncertainty and anxiety are common, affecting up to 50% of adolescents (more than any other age group). At the end of the spectrum of emotional satisfaction and dissatisfaction is suicide and attempted suicide. On the basis of her study of school and college students in the Netherlands Kienhorst (1988) estimates that 0.07% of boys and 0.16% of girls in the 14-20 age group attempt suicide at one time or another; of those covered by the study 3.5% overall (2.2% of boys and 5.2% of girls) had had suicidal thoughts in the recent past. In the 15-19 age group suicide is, after road accidents, the commonest cause of death (3.2 per 100,000, or around 40 cases a year; the corresponding figures for the 0-14 age group are 0.2 per 100,000 and ten a year; CBS 1988ab).

8.2.3 *Course*

Little research has been conducted into the course of emotional and behavioural problems in children and adolescents.

Richman *et al.* (1982) found that 63% of children with a problem in their third year of life still had a problem a year later; when the children were eight 62% of them had a problem (albeit not necessarily the same children or the same problems). The differences between boys (73% with problems) and girls (43%) were considerable.

Graham and Rutter (1973) found that of children on the Isle of Wight who showed psychiatric symptoms when they were ten or eleven years old 46% still had psychiatric problems when a follow-up study was carried out four years later. Here too relatively more boys than girls showed persistent problems.

When the various psychiatric disorders are considered separately, then according to Rutter and Gould (1985) the prognosis is best for emotional disorders (33% still affected after four years), less good for behavioural disorders, less good still for hyperkinetic disorders and worst of all for psychoses.

A recent Dutch study (Deboutte 1989) focused on youngsters who had presented to a Regional Institute of Ambulatory Mental Health Care (RIAGG) or been placed in a residential or semi-residential facility in 1983; interviews were conducted with their parents three or four years later and psychiatric diagnoses made on the basis of those interviews. The parents also completed the Child Behaviour Checklist (CBCL) to determine the current position: 54% of the children still had problems (52% in the case of those who had had contact with a RIAGG and 63% in that of those who had been placed in some form of institution; the difference is not significant). Among those with problems relatively many were diagnosed as having a behavioural disorder and relatively few as having an anxiety disorder (one of the emotional disorders): 32 of the 110 youngsters with an anxiety disorder still had problems three or four years later as against 66 out of the 68 with a behavioural disorder. This study thus confirms the picture sketched by Rutter and Gould (1985). The position should not be overstated, however: while children with problems tend to go on having them, there is significantly less stability in problem behaviour at the level of symptoms and syndromes (Richman *et al.* 1982, Verhulst & Althaus 1988).

The data presented in this chapter indicate fairly consistently that a large proportion (50-60%) of mental problems in youngsters are likely to be of a long-term nature.

While longitudinal studies following children into adulthood are very rare, there has been much retrospective research seeking to discover whether psychiatrically disordered adults had had problems in their childhood. In this connection Rutter (1985), reviewing research into four disorders, concludes that emotional and affective disorders do not appear to be preceded by any particular behaviour pattern in childhood, though there are indications that a lack of parental affection makes for vulnerability to affective disorders. Abnormal patterns are found in childhood in half of all schizophrenia cases, marked by such features as strange and unpredictable behaviour, social isolation, rejection by contemporaries and neurological and attention problems. Antisocial personality disorders, finally, are virtually always preceded by antisocial behaviour in childhood, though the reverse is certainly not the case: only a minority of children showing antisocial behaviour develop an antisocial personality disorder later in life.

8.3 *Background variables and risk factors*

This section focuses on factors relevant to child development and the genesis of emotional and behavioural problems. We look first at children's first and second environments (family and school), going on to consider socio-demographic factors and biological aspects of emotional and behavioural problems. Children's third environment (friends and leisure activity) is not discussed, since no systematic treatment of this topic was found in the literature.

8.3.1 *Family*

The family, here understood as the household or community in which children are cared for and brought up, determines in large measure the life that they will lead. Young children are entirely dependent on the family for the satisfaction of their emotional and material needs, and it is from the family that they derive the sense of basic trust. The upbringing, stimulation and opportunities which the family provides play a part in determining children's intelligence, school choice and occupational level.

Equally, many mental problems can be traced back to a deprived or disturbed family environment: problem youngsters often prove to have problem parents. Deboutte *et al.* (1987) found that 94.4% of 562 children registered with a RIAGG had problems in their home environment; among those who had been taken into care the proportion was 100%. The main problems in the home situation were: lack of guidance and instruction (29%), dysfunctional parenting (19%, including ambivalence, deprivation, exploitation and neglect), a mental disorder in another member of the family (14%) and an abnormal family structure (9%).

Van der Ploeg (1979) found illness, death or divorce/separation strongly overrepresented in the family backgrounds of children in children's homes.

Problems arise when burdens or stresses exceed the family's ability to bear them; this appears to be the situation of many one-parent families in which one adult has the double job of breadwinner and upbringer/housekeeper. Developments in family structure are considered in section 8.3.1.1. Children from 'abnormal' family structures are often regarded as at risk, i.e. as having a statistically greater likelihood of developing problems. The form of the household is not the only factor determining quality of upbringing, however; what matters is the context in which children are reared, i.e. the interactions which take place within the family (section 8.3.1.2). Family interactions which take the form of child abuse are considered separately (section 8.3.1.3).

8.3.1.1 *Changing patterns*

Family life has seen radical changes over the past thirty years. Reproductive patterns have altered, families have become smaller, divorce has become much commoner and the role of women has changed sharply. The availability of contraception has helped cut birth rates: where twenty years ago women had an average of three children, the current figure is 1.5 and stabilization at that level is expected. In addition the average age at which women have children has risen. Households have shrunk: the number of people in a household currently averages 2.6, and a further decline to 2.4 is expected by the end of the century (Raad voor het Jeugdbeleid (Council for Youth Policy) 1986a).

The number of divorces has risen sharply in recent decades: one in three marriages currently ends in divorce. One consequence of this is the growth in the number of one-parent families, a trend which is expected to continue (see table 8.5).

Table 8.5 **One-parent families**

	Number of one-parent families	Number of children in one-parent families
1985	203,500	325,000
2000	360,000	576,000

Source: SCP 1988.

The frequency of divorce has also led to an increase in the number of 'new stepfamilies' (Spruijt 1988). Children from one-parent families and stepfamilies constitute at-risk groups: according to the Social and Cultural Planning Office (SCP 1988a) children from one-parent families have more health problems, and this also appears to be true of children from stepfamilies (Spruijt 1989).

Divorce can have profound effects, particularly on younger chidren, which can go on making themselves felt for many years (Tusenius 1989). Adopted children, and especially foreign adopted children, are at risk (Hoksbergen *et al.* 1988); since 1976 the number of foreign adopted children has risen sharply, with some 60% of current adoptions (about 2,000) falling into this category.

8.3.1.2 *Family interactions*

Whether children are adopted or brought up in a traditional or one-parent family, their chances of healthy development will depend above all on the home climate, the affective relations within the family and the security provided.

Psychoanalysts and behaviourists have suggested that children's first experiences are of essential importance for their later well-being, with traumatic experiences such as separation from parents having an indelible effect. Research has shown, however, that children in their first two years of life are strikingly resilient: as long as a decent environment is provided thereafter the effect of negative experiences is often slight.

To give substance to the concept of 'quality of upbringing' Maccoby and Martin (1983) use two dimensions in their description of parenting styles, involvement and responsiveness on the one hand and setting requirements and exercising control on the other. A parenting style which scores moderately highly on both dimensions is considered best: a clear structure combined with attention to the child's wishes, with the child's independence encouraged. An authoritarian upbringing is associated with internalizing behavioural problems and a permissive upbringing with externalizing problems (Verhulst 1989). A vicious circle can develop in the interactions between parent and child where a lack of sensitivity on the former's part (perhaps determined in part by innate characteristics of the child) gives rise to behaviour patterns in the child (bad temper, stubbornness and poorly regulated emotions and impulses) which make it hard for the parent to support the child through new developmental challenges (Riksen-Walgraven & Geerts 1988, 52-53). "We should not however expect to find any simple interactions or transactions between characteristics of parent and child. Human beings are highly complex creatures who determine in good part their own developmental path" (Kalverboer 1988, 15).

Psychodynamic theories have contributed much to our understanding of developmental processes in growing children and how they can go wrong. Another line of thinking, which has taken hold particularly in child psychiatry (Stapert 1988) is the system-oriented approach in which the family is seen as a system in which the behaviour of each member links with that of all others. Within this approach some investigators stress the communicative system and others the power system. Within family interactions pathogenic patterns can emerge which lead to a member becoming an 'identified patient'. A familiar example is provided by the 'perverse triad' of father, mother and child in which one or other parent enters into unspoken coalitions with the child. Attention has also focused, notably in relation to the genesis of psychoses, on inconsistencies of communication. While research has required many claims to be moderated, some hypotheses have been empirically underpinned (Wynne *et al.* 1977; Goldstein 1985; Buurmeijer & Hermans 1988).

8.3.1.3 *Child abuse*

Child abuse is physical or emotional violence which children experience through the actions or omissions of their parents or others and which damages or can be expected to damage them (see also Baartman 1988). Five forms are distinguished: physical abuse and neglect, emotional abuse and neglect, and sexual abuse.

No reliable figures are available on the frequency of child abuse: research is hampered by methodological and practical problems and such data as exist probably represent only the tip of the iceberg. On the basis of American research the ratio of reported to unreported cases has been put at 1:5 (Dijkstra, Swets-Gronert 1989). In the light of figures from the Bureaus Vertrouwensartsen (BVA) (agencies to which child abuse may be notified in confidence) - 5856 confirmed cases in 1988 - it is conceivable that 1% or more of minors in this country are abused every year. Recent data on sexual abuse point however to a much higher figure.

Awareness of child abuse has grown in recent years. The clear increase in the number of notifications is attributable to the fact that the agencies concerned are now better known and people are more alert to the problem.

Abuse can result from heavy-handed child-rearing practices: an English study found that 62% of babies were hit before they were one year old (Freeman 1983).

The consequences of child abuse can be serious: in 1988 45 children died as a result of abuse in the Netherlands. As well as physical injuries there is also considerable psychological damage which can manifest itself in learning difficulties, emotional and behavioural problems, suicide attempts and delinquency (Dijkstra, Swets-Gronert 1989). Abuse is "an encroachment on children's right to exist, and for many of those who suffer it their right to exist remains in question throughout their lives" (Baartman 1988).

There is evidence that abused children become abusing parents: the 'intergenerational transmission of violence'. The links are complex, however, and child abuse is also associated with other factors: social and material stress (unemployment, financial and housing problems, social isolation), family size (abuse is commoner in large families), one-parent families and the 'ideology of parenting' (Baartman 1988; GHIGV 1986). Such associations must be interpreted with great caution. The reported link between low socio-economic status and child abuse (Kadushin & Martin 1981), for example, could have various causes: the likelihood of abuse being recognized may vary from one social group to another; in higher-status groups there may be more emotional abuse which is less often recognized.

The records indicate that abuse can occur at any age but is most frequent (24% of cases) in the 0-3 age group. Differences between boys and girls are minimal (GHIGV 1986).

Official agencies have in recent years been more cautious in the matter of taking children into care or involving the justice system. Reported child abuse does not generally lead to child-protection orders; BVA-records indicate that such orders are obtained in only 12% of cases, and these do not by any means always involve taking into care.

A specific form of child abuse on which more information is available is sexual abuse. In her study Draijer (1988) defines sexual contact as forced (and thus as abuse) where one or more of these criteria are met:

- the contact is perceived by the child as forced;
- authority, emotional pressure or obvious preponderance is applied in such a way that child is unable to refuse;
- the contact is between an adult and a child aged under 12.

On the basis of this definition Draijer found that 15.6% of a population of women in the 20-40 age group had experienced incest, 24% a forced sexual contact with an adult outside the immediate family and 34% had had forced sexual experiences with someone in and/or an adult outside the family.

Less is known about prevalence of abuse against boys. Draijer (1985) estimates that 1.5% of boys have had incest experiences; other forced sexual experiences with adults are perhaps four times commoner. Whether the objects of the abuse are boys or girls the abusers are generally men.

Many risk factors relating to sexual abuse have been identified, among them the long-term absence of one or both parents, upbringing by a stepfather or stepmother, an unhappy parental marriage (in which the parents show each other and the child little affection), long-term parental illness and sexual ignorance (Sandfort 1988). The parental situation thus appears to be the main determining factor in relation to forced sexual experiences both within and outside the family.

The long-term consequences of sexual abuse are often serious. In her study Draijer found that half of all women admitted to psychiatric hospital after the age of twenty had had an incest experience in their childhood.

In Sandfort's study of 66 adolescents (aged 18-23) who had had a very serious sexual experience in childood, 31 came into contact with the medical and welfare services (Goddijn & Sandfort 1988). Only in a few cases had the young people concerned told anyone else about the abuse while it was going on. The attention focused on the matter by the media and the welfare services is expected to make it easier to talk about and recognize sexual abuse, helping to shorten the period between the inception of abuse and its being brought to the welfare services' attention.

8.3.2 *School*

School plays a significant part in children's general upbringing. This is particularly true in cases of abnormal or difficult behaviour: the school is probably the main agency in relation to prevention, recognition, support and referral. For parents the school offers a meeting place and a source of social support.

Children often behave differently at school than at home and behaviour problems may manifest themselves in one of these environments but not the other. Verhulst (1985) found psychiatric judgements to approximate more closely to the judgement of parents than that of teachers (in each case on the basis of a behaviour checklist) and that the latter two tended to complement one another. Striking evidence is provided by the results of a study of the prevalence of behavioural disorders (Offord *et al.* 1986): of 62 children aged 4-11 48 were identified as having behavioural problems by teachers, eleven by parents and only three by both parents and teachers. Caution is needed in drawing conclusions from such material: not only is children's behaviour situationally determined, the conceptual framework of those making the assessment and the battery of instruments used may be of doubtful validity.

Regular schools are the main agencies referring children to special education, of which schools for children with learning and behavioural difficulties (LOM schools) and schools for the severely maladjusted (ZMOK schools) account for almost half. Most but not all mentally handicapped youngsters are to be found in schools for children with learning difficulties or schools for children with severe learning difficulties (MLK and ZMLK schools).

According to Van Weelden (1981) there is both appreciation and criticism of special education. The segregation of 'abnormal' children leads to isolation and stigmatization while little if any of the hoped-for remedial effect is obtained. Van Weelden therefore advocates an integrated form of education in which proper provision is made for children with special needs.

In the mid-1970s attention began to focus on the extension of care ('zorgverbreding') in regular schools for children with special needs:

> "We need to achieve a situation in which the educational process is better geared to pupils' wide-ranging circumstances and abilities, in which it is no longer the case that large numbers experience failure. The phenomena associated with educational failure - children having to repeat a school year, large numbers of transfers to special schools, the isolated nature of the extra help offered to children - should disappear" (Innovatiecommissie Basisschool 1979).

These views are reflected in the Primary Education Act (Wet op het Basisonderwijs) which came into force in 1985. Even so, the goal of care extension appears further away than ever: the numbers in LOM and ZMOK schools (for children with learning and behavioural difficulties and the severely maladjusted) have risen sharply in recent years, despite the overall drop in the number of school-age children (see section 8.4).

While special-school staffing has now been capped, such limits are under threat, as witness the legal actions instituted in the matter (Tweede Kamer (Lower House) 1989b). There are indications that foreign models will again be followed: in countries like Sweden, Denmark and Italy far-reaching forms of integration have been achieved between regular and special education.

School's role in relation to problem behaviour in children and adolescents can be summarized thus. School plays a major part in children's upbringing but can be a source of problems as well as of development. It is the school system's job to meet the needs of children who are 'different'; educational failure is often the result of inflexibility and narrowly focused approaches. The education service has many functions in relation to mental health; special schools also have a role in treatment.

8.3.3 *Socio-demographic factors*

Social class

The socio-economic status of families and children is often determined by reference to the parents' educational and occupational level. British and American investigators report a number of differences between social classes in the nature and quality of the methods of upbringing used (Gardner 1982; Wolkind & Rutter 1985), with the lowest-status groups making greater use of disciplinary measures, engaging in less discussion and showing less tolerance of deviant behaviour. Moreover birth complications are commonest in lower-class children, who also score lowest on intelligence tests (Verhulst 1989).

Given this combination of adverse social and physical factors a correlation between social class and emotional and behavioural problems is only to be expected, and research results do indeed point in this direction. Verhulst (1985) found that lower-status children scored more highly (parental judgement) in relation to 42 of the 112 types of behavioural problem; for the most part they were externalizing problems. Vikan's prevalence study (1985) found psychiatric disorders in the lowest social class to be 1.7 times commoner than in higher-status groups.

A study of the links between behavioural disorders and socio-demographic factors found such disorders to correlate with (in decreasing order of significance) dependence on welfare benefits, subsidized housing, crowded living conditions, low income, unemployment and a low level of education on the mother's part (Offord *et al.* 1986). The probability of behavioural disorders was 3.1 times greater than average in benefit-dependent families and 1.6 times greater in those where the mother's educational level was low.

Not every study has found correlations between behavioural disorders and socio-economic status, however. This is evident from table 8.6, which summarizes the results of prevalence studies up to 1983.

Table 8.6 **Studies of correlations between social class and behavioural problems**

	No. of studies focusing on correlation	No. of studies finding significant differences
Low social class	10	5
Family size	8	5
Low educational level of mother	4	2
Crowded living conditions	3	3

Source: Links (1983).

We may conclude that, while a clear correlation appears to exist between social class and behavioural problems, it is not confirmed in all studies and is contaminated by other factors such as intelligence and birth complications.

Urbanization

Rutter *et al.* studied children on the Isle of Wight and in inner London, finding twice the prevalence of problems in the latter case (see table 8.1). This greater frequency of psychiatric disorders was partly associated with family variables (marital conflict, missing parent, psychiatric disorders in the mother, criminal tendencies in the father), cramped and poor-quality housing, financial problems and a high turnover of teachers and pupils at school (Rutter 1973).

Offord *et al.* (1987) investigated the effects of environment - urban/rural - on the frequency of certain types of problem (see table 8.7). The differences were significant in the hyperactivity and one-or-more disorder categories and were in all cases of the type expected, i.e. with more disorders in urban areas. It thus seems reasonable to conclude that urban environments adversely affect mental health, albeit many intermediating factors may play a part.

Table 8.7 **Six-month prevalence (per 100 children) of mental health problems, by type of environment**

Environment (number of) children	Behavioural disorder	Hyper-activity	Emotional disorder	Somati-zation*	≥ 1 dis-order**
Urban (1648)	5.6	7.0	10.7	8.2	19.6
Rural (1031)	5.2	4.6	8.3	6.1	14.9

Source: Offord *et al.* 1987.

Ethnicity

Considerable attention is currently being focused on the position of young people from ethnic minorities. There is growing evidence that such youngsters' situation is a very difficult one, whether they belong to the intermediate generation (born elsewhere and brought up in the Netherlands), the second generation (born and brought up in the Netherlands) or the third and fourth generations (the second generation's children and grandchildren, e.g. in the Moluccan community). Their difficulties are reflected in overrepresentation among the clients of many welfare services:

- children from families originating from Surinam and the Netherlands Antilles in particular are overrepresented in special schools (SCP 1987);
- ethnic minorities (though not all categories) are overrepresented among the clients of the welfare services for drug users and the probation service and in State Treatment Institutions (see table 8.14) (Tweede Kamer (Lower House) 1989c);
- in the course of the 1980s Santpoort Psychiatric Hospital has noted a 400% increase in the number of patients, mainly young men, with Surinamese or Antillean origins; in many cases they were compulsorily admitted following involvement with the police (Werkgroep Etnopsychiatrie 1986);
- young people from ethnic minorities are more likely to come into contact with the police than those from the indigenous population, with young Moroccans (33%) heading the list (WODC 1989). This situation could reflect a higher crime rate, more energetic policing or both;
- ethnic minorities account for a disproportionate number of child-protection orders and their share is continuing to rise (see table 8.8)

Table 8.8 **Ethnic-minority children as a percentage of all children covered by child-protection orders**

	Guardianship	Supervision
1982	17.6	13.6
1983	19.7	15.4
1984	21.3	16.4
1985	23.0	18.9
1986	25.1	21.3
1987	25.4	21.6

Source: Tweede Kamer 1989c.

The picture which emerges is one of a growing overrepresentation of ethnic-minority youngsters particularly among the clients of the more control-oriented services.

There is also evidence that ethnic-minority youngsters are disadvantaged in many areas of life:

- youth unemployment among ethnic minorities runs at twice the already high level obtaining in the indigenous population (Tweede Kamer (Lower House) 1986c);
- the school drop-out rate is higher among ethnic-minority than among indigenous children, as is the percentage of youngsters leaving school without any qualifications (Tweede Kamer (Lower House) 1986a);
- even where ethnic-minority youngsters complete their education successfully their job prospects are worse than those of indigenous youngsters with similar (or even lower) levels of qualification (Raad voor het Jeugbeleid (Youth Policy Council) 1989, Tweede Kamer (Lower House) 1989a;
- ethnic minorities (with the exception of Turks) are overrepresented among young vagrants (Korf & Hoogenhout 1989).

The problems associated with young people from ethnic minorities are considerable and appear still to be growing, and in the light among other things of demographic trends (see table 8.9) there is a real possibility that they will take on explosive forms.

Table 8.9 **Forecast numbers of Turkish and Moroccan youngsters (0-19) in the Netherlands**

	Turks	Moroccans
1987	71,701	62,428
2000 (minimum)	84,222	96,630
2000 (maximum)	94,456	107,624

Source: NIDI 1987.

Current concerns at the position of ethnic minorities find expression in the report of the Scientific Advisory Council on Government Policy (WRR 1989) and in discussions in parliament and the media. As yet no vigorous policy has been adopted in this area.

8.3.4 *Biological and genetic factors*

Research into the extent to which behaviour is genetically determined makes extensive use of twin studies. Identical (monozygotic) twins share 100% of their genetic material and fraternal (dizygotic) twins 50%; environmental influences are assumed to be the same in either case. The differences in the incidence of a particular disorder found between the two groups then provide the basis, taking account of the prevalence of the disorder in the population at large, for a rough estimate of the genetic and environmental components of a particular characteristic.

Twin studies relating to behavioural problems point to a genetic component notably in schizophrenia, autism, reading difficulties and bedwetting (McGuffin & Gottesman 1985). The first two are rare and the second two, while relatively common, can hardly be considered severe behavioural problems; in the majority of problem behaviours a genetic component has yet to be confirmed (or excluded).

Studies of the links between brain damage and the development of emotional and behavioural problems are complicated by the fact that brain damage is often associated with low intelligence, learning difficulties and physical handicap, factors which themselves can lead to increased stress. To control for such factors Rutter, in his Isle of Wight study (Rutter, Graham, Yule 1970) compared a group of children with neurological diseases both with children from the general population and with children suffering from chronic diseases and/or handicaps of a non-neurological nature. Controlling for intelligence and social background Rutter found that psychiatric disorders were commonest in the group with neurological complications; the nature of the disorder was not significant. Most of the children in the neurological group did not have psychiatric disorders, however; it was children with an adverse social and family background that were most likely to develop disorders.

Children who receive prolonged treatment for perinatal complications in a neonatal intensive-care unit are also at risk. Van Engeland (1988) reports a study of 56 such children which found only 32% to function without problems, with 32% showing problem behaviour for which a child psychiatrist considered treatment to be indicated. Birth complications probably constitute a risk factor in their own right, but there is also evidence that intensive postnatal clinical care hampers the process of attachment between parent and child: on discharge from hospital parents of low-birth-weight babies have been found to be less actively involved with their child, to engage in less physical contact and to smile and to talk less to their child. (Verhulst 1989). The continuing growth of neonatological provision of care, enabling ever more babies with an ever lower birth weight to survive, thus entails a risk of increased problem behaviour in the future. Measures are needed to lessen the adverse effects of the hospitalization of young children (Kind en Ziekenhuis (Child and Hospital) 1989).

Brain damage and perinatal complications generally increase the risk of emotional and behavioural problems but are not a sufficient condition for their genesis (except perhaps in the case of autism). If children are brought up in a stable, secure and stimulating home environment the adverse effects can be greatly reduced (Shaffer 1985). The problem is that such children often need extra care, putting parents' coping ability to the test.

8.3.5 *Discussion*

It was noted earlier that emotional and behavioural problems can be seen as an aggregation of symptoms which also occur in 'normal' children. The same appears to be true of the background to such problems: it is rare that a strictly causal factor can be demonstrated, and in most cases problem behaviour arises through an adverse combination of biological, personality and environmental factors. The link between the adverse factors and the genesis of problems is non-specific, in that the *number* of adverse factors involved matters more than their *nature*. Where risk-increasing factors are accompanied by risk-reducing factors (for instance where family problems coexist with a good relationship with one of the parents) it is generally the case that no problem develops (Veerman 1988). Within the environment different correlations are hard to separate: low social class is associated with low income, poor housing, low intelligence in the child, perinatal complications and so on, *and* with behavioural problems, and our current knowledge is not sufficient to allow the weighting of these factors.

8.4 *Help-seeking*

There is a clear discrepancy between the number of youngsters with mental health problems and the smaller number coming into contact with welfare agencies. In part of the study by Verhulst which has already been cited on several occasions Verhulst and Van der Lee (1988) report that 2.0% of the parents questioned had sought help for their child, while 2.6% had needed help but had not approached any welfare or medical agency. Powerful filters would appear to be at work between the experience of a problem and its treatment.

A number of stages may be distinguished in the process of seeking and obtaining help: the recognition that a problem exists, its identification, contact with or referral to a welfare or medical agency and, where relevant, further referral. In the case of young children the actors in this process are virtually always the parents, the school, others in the child's environment and the welfare and medical agencies, but as children grow up they increasingly recognize and report problems for themselves.

This section describes how youngsters come into contact with welfare and medical agencies and what patterns are found in the agencies' referral and selection practices. The effect of care-agency involvement is sometimes to lock youngsters into a worsening problem situation or 'care career'.

8.4.1 *Initial admissions and referrals*

The child

Mental problems in young children can manifest themselves in a variety of ways in physical symptoms, troublesome behaviour or learning difficulties; whether or not the problems are recognized or identified as mental depends largely on adults. Often problems are not strictly individual in nature but arise in interactions with the environment. Slightly older children are better able to discuss their problems with parents, teachers or other adults; in cases of physical or sexual abuse, however, it is well known that many children are pressured into silence. A facility used by children from about the age of ten onwards is the child telephone helpline, and in 1983, for example, more children called helplines in connection with problems of sexual abuse than contacted the Bureaus Vertrouwensartsen (BVA) dealing in confidence with children's problems (SCP 1987); accessibility and anonymity play a part here. The majority (65%) of those calling children's helplines are girls; possible explanations include girls' greater propensity to express feelings and their earlier independence and greater verbal skills.

How problems are designated depends very much on the viewpoint of those who designate them. Every year around 30,000 youngsters in the 12-18 age range run away from home (Ministry of Welfare, Health and Cultural Affairs 1989); a further 2500-3000 run away from children's homes (Raad voor het Jeugdbeleid (Youth Policy Council) 1986). Running away attracts a wide range of designations (and reactions), from 'problem behaviour' (Van der Ploeg 1979), 'behavioural disorder' 'manifestation of mental illness' and 'relational problem' to 'normal behaviour' (Raad voor het Jeugdbeleid (Youth Policy Council) 1986). Help-givers who are psychoanalytically inclined may see a 'disturbed development of the ego' in running away, while Youth Advice Centre staff often regard it as a normal response to an undesirable home situation in the context of a healthy striving towards independence.

The parents

In many cases it is up to parents to seek out professional help, but even where such help is needed it does not always follow that it is sought. Table 8.10 summarizes the reasons parents give for not seeking help.

Table 8.10 **Reasons why parents needing help have not, or not yet, sought it**

Reason	**Number (N=53)**
Active involvement with problem (help may yet be sought) or: help sought, but not from a particular agency	16
"We'll wait and see", "It will pass"	10
"We'll deal with it ourselves"	7
Mistrust of welfare and medical agencies, despondency	6
Problems resolved	5
Don't know or unknown	9

Source: Verhulst & Van der Lee (1988).

The same authors also asked parents (N=1799) whom they would approach for help with mental health problems should the need arise: 12% said they would contact specialized youth-care services (Regional Institutes of Ambulatory Mental Health Care, Outpatient Child Psychiatry Clinics, psychologists and therapists for children with special needs; most (62%) would opt for the family doctor and a significant number (11%) would try the school (educational advisory service, school medical service, teachers); only 5% would not seek professional help but would try to deal with the problem on their own or with the help of family and friends. In most cases, therefore, help would be sought in the medical sphere.

How children's problems are designated and what help is sought in dealing with them depends in part on the parents' educational level and the extent of their 'protoprofessionalization'.

Garralda and Baily (1986) found concentrations of children with mental health problems in general practices in districts of high socio-economic status. Verhulst and Van der Lee (1988) found that the need for and receiving of help did not depend on social class, though problems proved to be more often reported in the lower socio-economic groups (see also section 8.3.3). An explanation for this discrepancy could be that people in this group are less familiar with the existence and working of (mental) health care agencies: knowing about agencies is of great importance in the decision whether or not to seek help (Goldberg & Huxley 1980).

In cases where parents are 'protoprofessionalized' difficulties tend to be more quickly designated as problems, problems to be regarded as treatable and professional help to be sought (Brinkgreve *et al* 1979), and protoprofessionalization is thought to occur most readily in networks of which professionals form part. While such networks are evidently most likely in higher-status groups, Oosterbaan and Zeldenrust (1985) found the extent of protoprofessionalization to depend on the nature rather than the level of parents' educational background and occupation. Protoprofessionalization was commonest in the case of those with 'modern interpersonal training and occupations'

Parents' ability to cope can affect the search for help, and both a lack of parenting and teaching skills and poor personal, material and social circumstances can lead to an inability to cope. Housing conditions, income, employment, health, childcare facilities, support from family and friends and the relationship with the partner can all determine when parents can manage and when they must seek help.

Forms of help which are voluntarily obtained differ in a number of respects from those which are imposed: the first are sought, the second avoided where possible. Referral patterns in the area of imposed help correlate for example with the policies operated by the police and the Child Protection Service.

School

After parents, school - particularly primary school - is the main detector of mental health problems in children. Cases of abuse are often noticed by teachers, though they may be reluctant to take any formal steps because of the risk that these may lead to greater harm (removal of the child from the parental home). Teachers will tend to note first of all those problems which lead to class disruption or poor performance at school.

The educational guidance service (Schooladviesdienst, SAD) is usually the first agency to be involved when problems arise at school. Where physical or mental difficulties are suspected a school doctor may be consulted; he or she then examines the child to determine the nature of the problem. The school doctor and the educational guidance service are involved in the special-education placement committees. When carrying out regular medical examinations (made three or four times while children are at primary school, perhaps twice during their secondary careers) school doctors devote little time and attention to youngsters' mental functioning; they do not provide treatment themselves, instead referring children mainly to other doctors or to the RIAGGs.

Referrals by schools are mainly to special education, family doctors and RIAGGs.

The number of children in special schools rose sharply between 1966 and 1986 (see table 8.11), almost all of the growth being concentrated in schools for children with learning and behavioural difficulties (LOM schools) and schools for the severely maladjusted (ZMOK schools). Suggested causes include: increased workloads and more intensive detection and tighter selection in mainstream schools, together with the increasing number and range of special-education facilities (Doornbos & Stevens 1987; SCP 1987).

According to Pijl (1989) the special-education referral system does not work satisfactorily: the tests made by the placement committees following registration with a special school seldom lead to any change in the choice of school; in practice IQ tests play the crucial role; placement criteria are vague, reflecting a lack of clarity as to both the kinds of problem for which special schools are expected to offer solutions and the kinds of solution that they can offer.

Table 8.11 **Pupils in mainstream and special primary (4-12) schools, 1966-87**

	Special primary schools				Mainstream primary schools		LOM+ZMOK/ mainstream
	All types		LOM+ZMOK				
	Number	Index	Number	Index	Number	Index	Index
1966	64,900	100	11,300	100	1,887,700	100	100
1970	74,061	114	18,313	162	1,953,881	104	157
1974	81,352	125	26,952	239	1,962,200	104	230
1978	87,135	134	32,480	287	1,851,255	98	293
1982	95,708	147	39,428	349	1,598,458	85	412
1986/1987	103,047	159	47,542	421	1,447,776	77	549

Note LOM schools: for children with learning and behavioural difficulties; ZMOK schools: for the severely maladjusted. The last column shows the ratio of children in LOM/ZMOK schools to children in mainstream primary education.

Source: Central Bureau of Statistics, Statistical Yearbooks for 1967-1988.

Twice as many boys as girls are placed in special schools; in the case of LOM and ZMOK schools the ratio is as high as three to one. This can be explained by the fact that boys display more externalizing, and girls more internalizing, problem behaviour (see section 8.2.2), combined with the observation that transfer to special education is often determined not so much by children's problems as by mainstream teachers' inability to cope with them (Wijnstra 1986). It seems therefore that it are mainly 'nuisance' children that are transferred to special schools.

Family doctors

Family doctors are mainly consulted in connection with physical symptoms: Garralda and Bailey (1986) found that in Manchester 22% of 7-12-year-olds attending general practice had physical problems; only in 1% of cases were mental problems the reason for consulting a doctor.

According to Deboutte (1989) general practitioners refer children with mental problems mainly to the RIAGGs, to a lesser extent to outpatient clinics and occasionally to intramural psychiatric services. There are indications that referrals to RIAGGs mainly concern children from higher-status groups (SCP 1987; Oosterbaan & Zeldenrust 1985).

Police

In 1985 there were 46,145 contacts between youngsters and the police (CBS 1985), a quarter of them in the Netherlands' three largest cities (Amsterdam, Rotterdam and The Hague). Contacts relating to criminal law (with theft as the largest category) formed 67% of the total and those relating to civil law (largest category: runaways) the remaining 33% (Scholte 1988). Criminal contacts mainly involve boys (around 87%); in the case of civil contacts the sexes are more or less equally represented. The main age group comprises 15-16-year-olds. The criminal statistics are distorted by selectivity: not all crimes are reported to the policy, and the police and the Department of Public Prosecutions operate selective arrest and prosecution policies. Van der Hoeven (1986) found the decision whether or not to prosecute to depend on the seriousness of the offence, the age of the suspect and the suspect's record; more subjective social factors also played a part, such as the suspect's 'development prospects' (corrective environment, likelihood of recidivism). The availability of some kind of formal help and support may also be grounds for not prosecuting (Junger-Tas 1986). The Department of Public Prosecutions can make non-prosecution conditional on compliance with alternative sanctions. In only 4.5% of cases do the police refer youngsters to welfare agencies; often these are social rather then medical in nature (refuges, Child Protection Board, social work).

Regional Institutes of Ambulatory Mental Health Care (RIAGG)

The services provided by the RIAGGs comprise direct help and support, preventive work focused on at-risk groups and back-up for other medical and welfare agencies. Their youth sections' target group comprises youngsters aged 0-17 with mental health problems. Ten Horn *et al.* (1985) found that family problems were mentioned as the reason (or part of the reason) for contacting a RIAGG in a quarter of cases.

In 1987 12,836 boys and 10,279 girls aged up to 17 were registered with RIAGGs: family doctors (29%) and school (18%) were the main referrers (NVAGG 1988). Significant numbers of contacts (21%) were made on individuals' own initiative or the advice of family or friends. Boys are overrepresented among clients aged under 17, the position being reversed among those aged 17 and over. The lower social classes are underrepresented among the RIAGGs' young clients; different filters are evidently in operation in their case (SCP 1987).

The Child Protection Boards, the guardianship agencies and the Youth and Family Guidance Bureaus provide help and support on both a compulsory (child protection orders) and a voluntary basis; in the order shown the emphasis moves from compulsory intervention to voluntary help, and over time there has been an across-the-board shift in the same direction. 'Voluntary' help is not always entirely voluntary, however, since there is often an implied threat of compulsion; in part compulsion has been replaced by pressure. The Youth and Family Guidance Bureaus provide help on a voluntary basis but refer 31% of their clients to the justice system (SCP 1987).

Child protection orders are issued by juvenile courts on the basis of reports by family guardians (persons appointed by the court to oversee 'problem' families in which the children have not (yet) been made wards of court) or Child Protection Board staff (generally social workers). Van Nijnatten (1986) found the substance of such reports to be extremely vague and concluded that report compilers had an interest in such vagueness, since it avoided conflict with their clients and helped them influence court decisions. Van Nijnatten describes the reports as a kind of 'social evidence' which contrasts with the criminal evidence required by criminal courts: where criminal evidence requires facts on the basis of which the suspect's guilt can be determined, in 'social evidence' suspicions, opinions and atmospheric descriptions form a context which can give rise to insinuations of guilt.

The criteria for taking children out of the parental home into care are in practice vague (Kooistra 1982), placement decisions being made by individual welfare workers who are allowed considerable autonomy; institutions' placement policies vary widely, with the youngsters themselves having little say (Bijker *et al.* 1981).

The reasons for taking children into care bear little relation to the form of care in which they eventually find themselves or to the involvement or otherwise of the police and courts. It appears to be in the more serious problem cases that placement orders are used, though 'for a substantial group it is relatively a chance matter whether children are taken into care voluntarily or as a result of judicial procedures' (SCP 1987).

8.4.2 *Patterns of referral to residential care*

Referrals to residential facilities appear to take place in a somewhat arbitrary and chance manner (Knorth 1989; Bol 1978). The quality of the decision-making process leaves something to be desired: no alternative is considered in almost half of all cases and cost/benefit analyses are uncommon (Knorth 1987). The referral process is influenced by many factors unrelated to the problems of the individual child or the requirements of rational decision-making. Knorth (1987) summarizes the literature on this subject from the Netherlands and elsewhere. The decision to take a child into care proves to relate less to the child's problems than to the attitudes, norms and values of the welfare or medical worker or agency concerned; the type of work done by the care provider and the institution in which he or she works also strongly influence the recommendations made. A study of four observation centres found that placement recommendations coincided in only 25% of cases (Brinkman & Kars 1974). In their assessment of problems referrers are influenced, consciously or otherwise, by the availability of suitable provision; in other words, how a problem is designated may shift, in the course of the referral process, in the direction of the kinds of provision available. Whether or not a referral actually takes place also depends on the selection made by the residential facility itself; in practice the main criteria proved to be whether the young person in question was seen as manageable and whether another (more specialized) form of provision might be more suitable (Knorth 1989). A third consideration, of an economic nature, may also come into play: admission is more likely where facilities are under capacity (Bol 1978, Van der Ploeg 1984).

So far we have been mainly concerned with residential care in children's homes, but there are indications that the picture is not very different in the case of the psychiatric hospitals for children and adolescents. Deboutte (1989) found that they belonged to different referral routes, namely the health route (school or family doctor, RIAGG, intramural psychiatric care) and the justice/welfare route (social workers, youth guidance centres, extramural child protection, temporary homes, children's homes, fostering), with the great majority of referrals taking place along one or other. Where a youngster's 'care career' begins seems to depend neither on the nature of his or her problem nor on the diagnosis reached; Deboutte found the route taken to correlate with the socio-economic status of the district from which the youngster comes, with those from higher-status areas predominantly following the medical route and those from lower-status areas the justice/welfare route. The fact that diagnoses do not discriminate between the two may also have another explanation: Deboutte himself suspects the diagnoses made by child psychiatrists to be of doubtful value.

Other data corroborate Deboutte's observation. The Interdepartmental Working Group on Residential and Semiresidential Provision for Young People (IWRV 1980) noted many similarities in terms of clientele and treatment methods between children's homes (particularly those which are more treatment-oriented) and intramural psychiatric facilities for young people. Van Nijnatten and Van Bavel (1984) found little difference between the two where very intensive treatment was concerned: "The type of client does not vary from the one to the other; the difference, such as it is, lies in the kind of language used." It thus seems that considerations relating to treatment do not play any dominant part in determining where young clients are accommodated.

8.4.3 *Escalating careers of care*

Many placements in children's homes are not first placements: Van der Ploeg (1979) found that around 50% of residents had been placed in a home on at least one previous occasion and 20% on two or more occasions. In part this reflects the fact that many youngsters - around 25-40% every year, according to the Youth Policy Council (Raad voor het Jeugdbeleid 1986b) - run away from children's homes. This may indicate ineffectiveness on the homes' part, perhaps partly reflecting the fact that they cannot do much about the essential problem, namely the youngster's disturbed relationship with the family (SCP 1987). "There are evidently some youngsters who make a largely unprofitable trek round the various child-protection homes" (SCP 1987).

Even so, where a youngster is placed in a home for a second time it is not so much the correctness of the earlier placement as its intensity that comes into question; an earlier placement tends to be seen as one which offered insufficient treatment. Junger-Tas (1983) found repeated placements to be associated with an increasingly unfavourable prognosis for the child. Deboutte (1989) found that the likelihood of placement in a treatment setting increased with repeated placements. Children's-home selection criteria, which in practice come down mainly to the two questions of the child's manageability and the availability of more specialized provision elsewhere (see section 4.2), could well bear some relation to this fact. The result may be that youngsters' 'care careers' go in an unfavourable direction.

8.5 *Sectors of care*

8.5.1 *The sectors*

This section gives a quantitatively detailed summary of the various care and support facilities with which youngsters with emotional and behavioural problems may come into contact. Thefacilities fall into three groups, namely those operated by the welfare services, the health services and the justice system; they are listed in table 8.12. The basic health services are excluded.

Table 8.12 **Care and support facilities for young people**

Residential and semi-residential facilities	
Health	- Psychiatric facilities for young people
	- Homes for the mentally handicapped
Justice	- State Treatment Institutions
	- Private residential homes offering very intensive treatment
	- Private centres at which preventive detention is implemented
	- Therapeutic family care
	- Fostering
	- Independent living
Welfare	- Boddaert centres (day centres for school-age children)
	- Residential facilities for special youth work
	- Long-term residential facilities providing care and support
	- Temporary residential-care facilities
	- Homes for single parents and their children
	- Private residential homes (child protection)
	- Family-style residential units
	- Residential and semi-residential projects
	- Foster care
	- Supervised independent living
	- Training centres for independent living
	- Medical children's homes
	- Medical day nurseries
Health	- Youth Sections of the Regional Institutes of Ambulatory Mental Health Care
	- Child-abuse notification offices (Bureaus Vertrouwensartsen, BVA)

(Note: 'private' here means that the facility is operated by a non-governmental organization but funded by the state.)

- *Table 8.12* -

Extramural and preventive provision

Justice	- Guardianship and family guardianship agencies
	- Foster-family organizations
	- Home training
Welfare	- Youth and Family Guidance Bureaus
	- Child telephone helplines
	- Youth guidance centres
	- Home training
	- Foster-family organizations
	- Training in parenthood
	- Refuges for runaways
	- Other projects

Source: Tweede Kamer (Lower House) 1988.

In 1987 a number of facilities were transferred from the justice to the welfare system, among them some private homes and the family-style hostels. In view of these changes, and given that the distinction between the justice and welfare categories is not always a sharp one, they are discussed together in what follows. Table 8.13 covers the facilities which come under the health heading and table 8.14 those which come under the welfare and justice heading. We then look in more detail at the residential and semi-residential facilities, going on finally to summarize statistical trends over the period 1983-87.

Table 8.13 **Nature, scale and cost of health-service facilities**

Facility	Nature of service	Target group	Users[1] 1983	Users[1] 1987	Places 1983	Places 1987	Cost (millions of guilders, nominal) 1983	Cost (millions of guilders, nominal) 1987
Extramural								
RIAGG Youth Sections	Treatment	Children aged 0-17 with mental/psychiatric problems	<	24295[2]	-	-	98	118
Child-abuse notification offices (BVA)	Notification, mediation, referral	Abused and at-risk children aged 0-18 and their parents	2619	5856	-	-	2.5	4.8
Psychiatric outpatient departments	Treatment	Children aged 0-17 with mental/psychiatric problems	<	1511[3]	-	-		6
Semiresidential								
Psychiatric day treatment	Daytime treatment on weekdays	Youngsters aged up to 18 with mental disorder	102[5]	172[4]	115	155		6
Residential								
Psychiatric hospitals for children and adolescents	Medical treatment, nursing, care	Youngsters aged up to 18 with mental disorder	420	550	423	535	51	69
Psychiatric wards for children and adolescents in psychiatric hospitals	Medical treatment, nursing, care	Youngsters aged up to 18 with mental disorder	<	384[4]		384[6]		86
Homes for the mentally handicapped	Nursing, care	Youngsters aged 6-18 with mild mental handicap	1690	1830	1889	1950	108	124

Notes

1. In the case of extramural facilities the total number of users per year is shown, except where otherwise indicated. In the case of residential and semiresidential facilities average use has been estimated by multiplying occupancy rates by capacity.
2. This is the total number of youngsters aged up to and including 17 registered with RIAGGs. The total number of persons registered with Regional Institute Youth Sections in 1987, including both young people and their parents/carers, was 44,955.
3. The total number of persons registered in the course of a year.
4. Total number as at 1 January 1988; occupancy rate estimated at 100%.
5. 1982.
6. 1986.

< Where no data were available an estimate was made of the likely trend in the use of facilities; '<' in the 1983 column indicates an upward trend from 1983 to 1987.

Sources: SCP 1987, NVAGG 1988, Tweede Kamer (Lower House) 1988, Jacobs & Ketting 1989, Deboutte 1989.

Table 8.14 **Nature, scale and cost of welfare-service and justice-system facilities**

Facility	Nature of service	Target group	Users[1]		Places		Cost (millions of guilders, nominal)	
			1983	1987	1983	1987	1983	1987
Extramural								
Youth and Family Guidance Centres	Treatment, support, advice, crisis intervention	Youngsters aged 14-20 and their parents/carers	9374[6]	>	-	-	4.4	6.8
Telephone helplines	Information, advice, help	Children aged 8-15	65000		-	-	0.4	1.1
Youth Guidance Centres	Information, advice, mediation, treatment, crisis intervention	Youngsters aged 12-25	c. 40000	>	-	-	6.6	9.8
Home training	Home treatment aimed at avoiding need to take children into care	Children with severe social development problems and their parents		>	-	-		1.6
Training in parenthood	Information and advice	Parents of young children		>	-	-	2.9	4.7
Child Protection Board	Legal functions, information, advice	Children and young people aged 0-21 and their parents/carers	9849[2,6,8]	<	-	-	77[9]	-
Guardianship agencies	Exercise of authority support	Children and adolescents aged 0-20 and their parents/carers	19166[8]	<	-	-	80	78
Fostering units	Recruitment and selection of foster families, mediation	Children and young people aged 0-21 and their parents/carers		>	-	-	4.7	7.5
Semi-residential								
Boddaert centres (day centres for school-age children)	Support and treatment during the day and outside school hours	School-age children and their parents with problems in their daily lives	880	1230	981	1322	35	52

- **Table 8.14** -

Crisis centres and refuges	Short-term accommodation and support	Youngsters in crisis situations, runaways, those thrown out by their parents		1284[6]		c.135		17
Medical day nurseries	Medical examination, treatment, care	Children from 18 months to 6 years with (potential) developmental disorder	1720	1900	1735	1935	79	97
Residential								
State Treatment Institutions	Upbringing, care, treatment	Mainly minors in need of discipline, generally admitted by court order	270	260	317	317	41	44
Residential centres for special youth work	Upbringing, care, education	Older youngsters, working or at school	890	780	943	859	59	54
TSJ residential centres[3]			2020	1260	2256	1346	98	85
Medical children's homes	Medical treatment, nursing, care	Under-15s whose physical or mental health is damaged or seriously at risk	700	620	781	671	46	48
Private residential homes[4] (child protection)			6450	5700	6618	6047	382	371
Family-style residential units	Upbringing and care in units based on family structures	Minors of all ages	220	240	238	280	6	6
Residential family support treatment	Treatment, support, upbringing, care	Families in which relationships are in danger of breaking down or have done so			21[5]	21[5]		

Fostercare								
Therapeutic family care	Housing, care, upbringing, intensive support and treatment	Youngsters whose problems are such that fostering is likely to fail	260	286		290	6.9	7.5
Fostering (judicial) and supervised independent living	Housing, care and upbringing	Youngsters removed from their families by judicial order	5677	5500[9]			60.4	61.5
Fostering (voluntary) and supervision	Housing, care and upbringing	Youngsters temporarily or permanently unable to live with their parents	2744	3623[8]	4300		19.5	37.9

1. In the case of extramural facilities the total number of users per year is given. In the case of residential and semiresidential facilities average use has been estimated by multiplying occupancy rates by capacity. Where no data were available an estimate was made of the likely trend in the use of facilities; '<' in the 1983 column indicates an upward trend and '>' a downward trend from 1983 to 1987.
2. This is the number of visitors; 19,651 investigations were made and 8,215 recommendations issued.
3. These are institutions funded under the TSJ temporary grant scheme for youth welfare. They include residential centres for the long-term care of young people, temporary hostels and homes for lone parents and their children.
4. These homes, run by non-governmental organizations but funded by the state, include treatment institutions (including centres for very intensive treatment), combined institutions, specialist residential centres and other private institutions.
5. This is the number of places for families.
6. Total number of registrations in one year.
7. Total as at 1 January 1988.
8. 1984.
9. 1985.

Sources: SCP 1987, NVAGG 1988, Tweede Kamer (Lower House) 1988, Jacobs & Ketting 1989, Deboutte 1989.

8.5.2 *Public health sector*

Semi-residential facilities

Medical day nurseries provide day treatment and are used mainly by children with severe long-term behavioural, developmental and emotional problems. A survey of day nurseries (Federation of Medical Day Nurseries, cited in SCP 1987) collected information on in- and outflows: 32% were referred to special schools and 13-15% were placed in residential care or a psychiatric hospital for children. Despite the fall in the total number of children, the number of day-nursery places rose from 1068 in 1975 to 1935 in 1987, while costs rose from 26 million guilders in 1976 to 97 million in 1987.

Psychiatric day treatment for children is still on a small scale: in 1987 there were 155 places in all, a significant proportion of them providing preparation for or follow-up after residential treatment (Deboutte 1989).

Residential facilities

Medical children's homes were originally concerned with somatic problems, but places are now provided both for children with chronic somatic disorders and, particularly, those with severe mental and psychosocial problems. Stays average around a year. The number of places has fallen sharply in recent years, from 1583 in 1975 to 671 in 1987. This contrasts with the growth experienced by other residential facilities, notably *psychiatric hospitals for children* and *children's wards of psychiatric hospitals*.

8.5.3 *Welfare and justice sector*

Semi-residential facilities

Day centres for school-age children - *Boddaert Centres* - offer treatment and support in cases of severe psychosocial problems affecting young people and their parents. The service is provided Monday-to-Friday, outside school hours. Capacity has grown from 981 places in 1983 to 1430 in 1988.

The ten *pedological institutes*, which are funded by the education ministry rather than the health or justice ministry, focus on a similar target group. They undertake testing as well as providing help and a school is linked to each of them. Diagnosis and treatment expressly encompass personality, family and school problems (SCP 1987). In 1983 the linked schools had 886 pupils; in 1988 there were eleven such schools, with 1086 pupils.

Residential facilities

In 1987 the residential facilities operated by the welfare services and the justice system had around 8,000 users (Timmermans 1989); the majority (5,700) were in private (i.e. non-governmental) child-protection homes. These fall into the following categories:
- reception homes, providing short-term care where a final placement has yet to be decided or is currently unavailable;
- observation homes, where comprehensive personality studies are carried out;
- 'institutions for upbringing', a collective term embracing institutions

for normal children, mentally handicapped children and unmarried mothers and institutions providing psychotherapeutic treatment and education and training;

- special-treatment institutions, accommodating severely maladjusted children unsuitable for treatment in an 'institution for upbringing';
- institutions for very intensive treatment, for which the admission criteria include the failure of earlier support and treatment, lack of alternative placements, behavioural and relational problems and insuperable difficulties in daily living.

As section 8.4.2 noted, all residential facilities, in whatever sector, provide broadly similar kinds of help and support, for all that the wide differences in terms of funding and target groups suggest otherwise. There are also many similarities in their clients' problems and backgrounds, with the residents of homes for 'normal' youngsters having fewest (SCP 1987). There are however differences between those whose placement is voluntary and those who have been placed in a home under a child-protection order, in that the latter have more adverse home circumstances and show more problem behaviour.

The last 25 years have seen a number of significant developments in children's homes. Total capacity has fallen markedly, the number of voluntary placements has shown a proportionately sharp increase, average stays are now shorter and the ratio of (highly trained) staff to children has risen. The decline in capacity is ascribed to the rapid expansion of foster care, itself linked to the growing realization that living in a home is harmful to children.

Of those placed in a home under a child-protection order 7% are aged under six and 77% twelve or over. A children's home is not now seen as a desirable environment for 0-5s and the Social and Cultural Planning Office (SCP 1987) has argued that no capacity should be provided for this group. The SCP also notes that children's homes focus excessively on the problems of the individual child, failing to devote due attention to problems and conflicts within the family, and that stays are still too long. Insufficient consideration is given to alternatives to the children's home and clear upbringing or treatment plans are lacking.

Fostering

Where parents cannot or will not look after a child he or she may be placed in a foster family. In the past permanent fostering was the norm, but recent decades have seen a growth in therapeutic and temporary (for a part of the week or short periods) foster placements. Around 10,200 youngsters were in foster care in 1987 (Timmermans 1989). The sharp rise witnessed in recent decades is due entirely to the growth in voluntary placements. A study covering three provinces found that in 1984 and 1985 12% of voluntary placements involved children aged under seven while 76% involved over-12s (Berben *et al.* 1986); among those fostered in pursuance of a child-protection order 17% were aged under six and 59% twelve or over (Timmermans 1989). Among those covered by child-protection orders younger children are more likely to be placed with a foster family and older children in a home, while those aged twelve or over are the majority in both foster care and children's homes. The risk that a foster placement will fail is relatively great in this last group (SCP 1987). No research has been done to discover whether in the long term fostering benefits or harms a child more or less than living in a children's home or with his or her own family (whether or not it is a problem family).

8.5.4 *Conclusion*

We concur with Deboutte (1989) that "The child-care system is made up of a complex and extensive network of institutions, functions, methodologies and funding streams." The figures for 1983 and 1987 set out in tables 8.13 and 8.14 show that even over this short period the number of youngsters in most forms of care has risen markedly. Table 8.15 outlines the changes between 1983 and 1987 (the picture is a general one, since data were not available for all types of facility).

Table 8.15 **Changes in youth care, 1983-87**

	Clients	**Places**	**Cost (nominal)**
Health services			
- extramural	>	-	+22%
- semi-residential	+14%	+13%	+23%
- residential	+ 7%	+ 2%	+18%
Total	>	+ 6%	+20%
Welfare/justice system			
- extramural	>	-	+ 9%
- semi-residential	>	+35%	+49%
- residential	-15%	-20%	- 4%
- foster care	>	+19%	+23%
Total	>	- 3%	+ 2.5%
Total	**>**	**- 1%**	**+ 8%**

> denotes rising trend.
Sources: see tables 8.13 and 8.14.

The number of clients increased in both the facilities operated by the health services and those operated by the welfare and justice systems, and this despite the 7% fall in the number of youngsters aged 0-17 in the Netherlands which took place over the same period. The scale and cost of provision rose, with the exception of the residential facilities in the welfare/justice group. The drop here appears to be offset by the growth in semi-residential and foster care: deinstitutionalization seems to be more successful in the welfare/justice category of provision than in the health-services category.

The table shows a striking increase in the cost of child-care provision in the health-services category: in 1983 such provision formed around a quarter of total child-care capacity but accounted for around a third of total costs, and the imbalance now is even greater. This can be put another way: the welfare/justice system is having to cope with an increasing number of youngsters with fewer places and shrinking resources, while health-services provision can offer help to only a small proportion of them.

This background analysis was completed in January 1990.

Part II Likely developments and desirable policies, 1990-2010

8.6 *Introduction: obstacles to scenario construction*

Departing from the pattern used for the other three themes, this section does not outline scenarios for the future but instead outlines likely developments and desirable policies in the area of the emotional and behavioural problems of children and adolescents. The method used was the same as that applied to the other themes, the decision to adopt a different pattern being made when the three rounds of the Delphi process failed to produce sufficient consistent material.

The factors preventing the construction of scenarios for this area were broadly as follows.

- A lack of basic data: few if any epidemiological data exist in the Netherlands covering all of the topic or the age range.
- Child-care provision is extremely complex, falling under different administrative headings and showing both extensive fragmentation and a large measure of overlap between apparently different facilities; moreover the territory is not yet fully mapped.
- The decision to look at an age-related field rather than a specific problem (such as dementia) means that we are faced with a wide range of problems and relevant topics which cannot easily be assembled into a coherent whole.
- Youngsters' problems are even more difficult to classify than adults', in part because they are more dependent on, and interwoven with, environmental factors. The lack of any diagnostic system or generally accepted classification of problems makes it difficult to build up a clear picture of the field as a whole.
- Many different disciplines, and different types of facility, can concern themselves with the same kind of problem behaviour; views can differ widely (cf. the interpretations of running away reported in the baseline analysis).
- The Delphi panel, encompassing as it did a diversity of disciplines and expertise, produced a great variety of opinions and attitudes which proved difficult to combine into a coherent whole. On the one hand individuals whose expertise was limited to specific fields were asked to give views in all; on the other there were so many fields that insufficient experts were available for consultation on any one (e.g. only one panel member was an expert on special education). On a number of points it proved impossible to achieve consensus within the panel.
- It proved difficult to limit the field, both for the reasons already mentioned and because the theme was chosen precisely in order to include a broad and above all socially and culturally relevant field in the study. This made it difficult to operationalize problem

behaviour in terms of a small number of clearly defined categories (such as autism or eating disorders).

Given the current situation and the deficiencies in our epidemiological knowledge of the emotional and behavioural problems of children and adolescents, the conclusion was that no consistent exploration of likely future developments was possible. A far more wide-ranging study would be required for that purpose, and indeed it is desirable that such a study be made. Preliminary studies would need to be carried out in order to chart the area more accurately and to add to our knowledge of the incidence of problems and their determinants.

Rather than set out a reference scenario, subsequent sections formulate a series of possibilities for the future based on the majority views of the Delphi panel and data from the baseline analysis. We then look at desirable policies as considered by the Delphi panel. In the Delphi process the definition of emotional and behavioural problems was limited to 'problem behaviour'; this covers the more serious problems which can give rise to a requirement for residential care.

8.7 *Likely developments 1990-2010*

Social trends

The majority of the panel take a pessimistic view of likely trends over the period 1990-2010, forecasting a widening social divide in the areas of income, employment and access to social provision. Further erosion of the welfare state, retrenchment in all sectors, continued high unemployment and a hardening of society will lead to a worsening of living conditions for the lower-status groups. Individualistic trends will continue, manifesting themselves in among other things a further erosion of traditional family life.

Prevalence of problem behaviour

A majority of the panel foresee a rise in the prevalence of problem behaviour in children and adolescents, generally of the order of 5-20%.

A number of in part related factors are suggested as causes of this increase. Worsening living conditions in the poorest sections of society, where problems anyway cumulate, will lead to a rise in problem behaviour. Where parents have less income and worse prospects, worse housing and less access to social provision, the result will be that less attention is devoted to children and fewer resources are available to look after them and bring them up.

A second factor suggested is the erosion of the traditional family as the divorce rate remains high and the number of single-parent families and new stepfamilies increases. While growing up in a single-parent family is not necessary problematic, problems become more likely where there is also a lack of money and prospects or of child-daynursery facilities and other forms of support.

In the panel's view child day-care facilities will remain inadequate, with access increasingly dependent on parents' ability to pay. The number of working mothers will increase, partly as a matter of economic necessity, while the help given by fathers will not be enough to ensure that children receive sufficient attention.

The panel is virtually unanimous in expecting the situation of ethnic minorities to worsen. Inadequate progress on racial integration, *inter alia* in the areas of housing, employment and education, will ensure that minorities retain their generally low socio-economic status. If the education system fails to break free of ethnocentrism and to raise the educational standards of children from ethnic minorities and the employment prospects of such children remain poor or even deteriorate, minority groups will increasingly be forced to turn in on themselves; the result will be a further rise in the number of child-protection orders issued, in homelessness among young people and in juvenile crime (including in youth gangs). This trend, already visible in the major cities among young people of Moroccan origin, could well be strengthened by the growth in the ethnic-minority population.

The panel sees youth unemployment remaining a problem, even though demographic trends point to a decline. Unemployment blocks youngsters' prospects, erodes their motivation at school and encourages early leaving.

Problem behaviour in young people will also be stimulated as retrenchment in the area of social and cultural welfare work leads to a further decline in the support available from the agencies set up to help teenagers and young drop-outs and to undertake multicultural activities.

The education system will be unable to cope with the increased problem workload. Any further retrenchment is likely to produce an increase in class sizes, thereby reducing the amount of individual attention given to pupils. The growing size of schools is also seen as contributing to feelings of anonymity in pupils and as hampering teachers' attempts to deal appropriately with problem behaviour. Heavier demands will be made on pupils, notably in cognitive terms, reducing the time available for personal and social education. Retrenchment in special education is also expected, without adequate compensating provision in mainstream schools.

Finally, the panel expects children's upbringing in the future to be marked by greater uncertainty on parents' part as to what is required. In a rapidly changing and ever more complex society parents will find it harder to know what goals to pursue in bringing up their children but will tend - partly out of uncertainty, partly in response to society's emphasis on achievement - to demand higher standards of them. It is expected in this connection that problem behaviour will increasingly be approached from an individualistic and medicalistic standpoint, making it more difficult to resolve problems of a social and relational nature. Children will display more problem behaviour because they will deviate more quickly from the expectations set for them and because such deviation will be viewed on a more individual basis and will be more likely to be designated problem behaviour. These trends will be strengthened by increasing efforts in the area of the early identification of problem behaviour and by information campaigns in the media.

Alongside these trends and developments which tend to generate and sustain problem behaviour the panel also identify a number of factors whose impact is more favourable. As preventive activities and treatment options are expanded and improved it will become possible to prevent or treat many forms of problem.

In the area of prevention the panel expects growing scientific knowledge to enable more effective measures to be developed. At-risk groups will be more clearly identified and more effective strategies developed and applied; in particular there will be improvements in the prevention of physical and sexual abuse. The increased provision for supporting parents in the area of child-rearing (*inter alia* through expansion of the 'home training' scheme) will also have a preventive effection.

Better ways will be found of helping children and adolescents develop their coping skills and the acquisition of coping strategies will be given greater emphasis e.g. in secondary education. Schools will focus greater attention on psychosocial health education. The adverse impact of educational retrenchment will in part be offset by expanded preventive activity; the larger schools will appoint prevention officers and initial teacher training will put greater stress on the early recognition of emotional and behavioural problems.

Treatments for behavioural problems will be better and more widely available. The expansion of facilities and the development of new methods will allow more problems to be treated successfully or at least alleviated. Improvements are expected first of all in the diagnostic field. As progress is made in the early identification of problems it will often be possible to intervene at an earlier stage, enabling the effects of physical abnormalities and traumas such as brain damage to be limited. Improved treatment methods are expected in the areas of pharmacotherapy, family therapy and, to a lesser extent, remedial education and psychotherapy. Psychoactive drugs will be prescribed more often and more systematically. Better ways will also be available of influencing parents and family relationships in a favourable direction. Finally, the availability of extramural and semi-intramural treatment and support will increase, partly because residential places will remain in relatively short supply (forcing the extramural services to provide substitutes for intramural care) and partly because more will be invested in extramural care. This will allow treatment to be directed less one-sidedly at the child and more at the home situation and social environment.

Utilization of services

The panel expects the prevalence of problem behaviour in children and adolescents to increase and greater use to be made of all services. The extent to which help is sought will not alter in total, albeit there is a difference here between the social classes. The volume of care provided will grow, more in the semi-residential and extramural sectors than in the intramural sector. Residential provision will be expanded in the area of child psychiatry and at the more control-oriented end of the justice system, namely juvenile prisons and other institutions.

The distinction between justice/welfare facilities on the one hand and medical provision on the other will sharpen and access to them will increasingly be determined by clients' socio-economic status. In the lower-status groups less use will be made of facilities, partly because of the increased cost, and where they are used it will increasingly be on a compulsory basis; the number of child-protection orders and other sanctions will increase, notably among minors from ethnic minorities. In the higher-status groups, in contrast, more help will be sought as early-detection programmes and information campaigns lead more parents to consult (mainly medical) experts and to do so at an earlier stage. As well as helping to improve prevention, information campaigns and prevention programmes also lead to an increase in the utilization of services, and this increase will made itself felt mainly on the medical side.

While cooperation between the various categories and levels of provision will increase, strong institutional barriers will remain in place. Justice-system facilities could well become a virtual 'dustbin', with advanced and expensive treatments being restricted to those who can afford, and can find their way around, the facilities provided by the health services.

8.8 *Desirable policies*

In the course of the Delphi process panel members were able to indicate what they saw as desirable future policies in provision for children and adolescents displaying problem behaviour. Two general objectives were virtually unanimously endorsed as 'desirable' or 'highly desirable', namely a considerable reduction in the prevalence of problem behaviour and the improved social integration of young people with problems. Although these objectives overlap to a large extent, partly owing to the definition of problem behaviour adopted, the first emphasizes the prevention and treatment of problems (thereby reducing the need to take children into care) while the second puts the stress on preventing the taking of children into care or, where this is inevitable, on providing a replacement home environment (implying that problems must be made 'manageable').

The policies suggested by the panel fall under six headings:
- prevention,
- the organization and coordination of care,
- foster care,
- extension of care by the educational system
- the quality of care,
- research.

Prevention

The great majority of panel members believe that the prevention of problem behaviour should be approached in the first instance through a general policy of improving the living conditions of the poorer sections of society through higher incomes, a better spread of employment and improved and more easily accessible social provision. High priority also needs to be given to ethnic integration, while more specific measures include the reduction of youth unemployment, the expansion of child-care facilities, action against sexual violence and the development of social and cultural welfare services.

Preventive measures are also needed in respect of high-risk situations (such as the admission of children to hospital) and groups (one-parent families on minimum incomes, young parents with a background of problems in their own childhood, and so on). Such measures need to be associated with the greater development and exploitation of scientific knowledge regarding both the identification of at-risk groups and risk determinants and the nature and evaluation of the effectiveness of interventions.

Both primary and secondary prevention need to be promoted through systematic measures in the areas of early identification, health education and back-up for parents.

In the area of early identification the panel recommends that more psychosocial experts be appointed to guidance clinics and early-diagnosis teams. The early detection of psychosocial problems should be covered in the training of family doctors, pediatricians, teachers, social workers and the police. Police sections dealing with youth affairs could be more involved in prevention projects where police contacts with minors indicate psychosocial problems. It is important that sufficient capacity be available to deal with the problems identified, including those of a structural nature. Expansion of the child-abuse notification offices is recommended.

Health education needs to focus more on psychosocial problems. Psychosocial health education should be covered by all schools, whether as a subject in its own right or incorporated into the teaching of others; it should be a permanent feature of the secondary curriculum, encompassing the acquisition of social skills and coping strategies and education for parenthood. The courses for prospective and new parents provided e.g. by the community-nursing service should focus greater attention on psychosocial questions.

Back-up for parents needs to be extended through the expansion of child-care provision and the development of social and cultural welfare services; the 'home training' scheme also needs to be expanded. Temporary foster parents in the child's own environment, for which the child may show a preference, also offer a way of strengthening back-up for parents.

In all these areas greater cooperation is needed among the various agencies concerned: schools, family doctors, pediatricians, the prevention services of the RIAGGs, the health-education service, early-diagnosis teams, social works, child-protection agencies and the police. Such cooperation could be organized at neighbourhood level.

Organization and coordination

The panel believes that systematic measures are needed to improve the organization and coordination of medical and welfare services for children and adolescents. Policy in this area should seek to:

- overcome the current compartmentalization as between levels, specialties and providers;
- prevent the shifting of responsibilities;

- achieve greater flexibility, with services being more client-centred and less institution-centred;
- promote continuity of care, with the different stages of the treatment process merging together more smoothly and linked more to persons than to institutions;
- transfer expertise (including diagnostic expertise) from specialized institutions to GP and social work;
- avoid overcapacity in residential provision;
- expand semi-residential and extramural provision which can genuinely substitute for residential facilities (crisis intervention, 'home training' schemes, specialist family care, part-time treatment, day care, foster care, therapeutic family care).

These objectives are best pursued at regional level, with a comprehensive range of provision in each region for which the various services take joint responsibility. Greater flexibility and continuity of care could be achieved by reorganizing provision into functions which can be combined at individual level ('client-centred care'); this would require restructuring of the funding system.

A number of conditions need to be met as this policy is implemented:

- the coordination of care and care functions. This must be ensured at the level of individual clients, e.g. by case managers;
- the periodic evaluation of placements (in homes, hospitals, special schools), with an active policy of returning youngsters to their own environment where possible;
- restrictions of residential care coupled with measures to improve its quality. More generalist approaches are needed to ensure that clients with multiple problems receive the kind of help they need;
- a client-centred approach which extends across all providers, but with a sharper division between the functions of the justice system and those of the health and welfare services. A shift of emphasis from control to care is desirable, with detention being replaced with alternative sanctions where possible.

A client-centred 'functional' approach can be associated with many forms of inter-institutional cooperation, which should be organized regionally rather than nationally. In the cities preference should be given to the establishment of neighbourhood-level information, support and treatment centres; such 'child protective' agencies should operate in close conjunction with the general preventive services.

Fostering

The panel sees the expansion and improvement of foster care as desirable. Host families could be involved more often in crisis situations; where there is no option but to remove children from their own families fostering is often preferable to placement in a children's home, and therapeutic family care could replace residential treatment in more cases.

The panel is unhappy at continued retrenchment in the anyway relatively inexpensive area of foster care; indeed, more resources are needed to ensure proper remuneration and adequate support for foster parents. On the organizational side steps are needed to minimize the bureaucracy involved in fostering; the unnecessarily complex funding structure also requires simplification. Finally, any prejudice which may exist in relation to the selection of foster families needs to be countered.

Education

Mainstream schools need to accept wider responsibility for both preventing and dealing with problems. Improving the primary pupil:teacher ratio and moving towards smaller secondary schools would make it easier to give pupils personal attention; there is also a need for more individual approaches in place of class teaching.

Greater extension of care in school is seen as requiring:

- a shift away from the one-sidedly cognitive emphasis of education towards more social and psychosocial aspects. Schools must focus on children's personal and social development, helping them learn to deal with their feelings and to acquire social skills: articulacy, coping, living in a multiracial society;
- improvements in educational methods, in particular with a view to helping disadvantaged children (including those disadvantaged as a result of cultural differences);
- improvements in teachers' pay structure;
- improvements in the support structure (school guidance services, back-up from the mental health services, the youth welfare service and special education);
- improvements in teacher-training, with a greater emphasis on individual approaches, health education, psychosocial prevention and the detection of problems.

Greater integration can also be promoted by expanding the education system's caring and support functions, for instance by:

- attaching to schools welfare workers who can help where problems arise in children's home environment;
- giving schools some responsibility for out-of-school care, if necessary helping to find temporary host families for children with problems.

The special schools' role should be gradually reduced. This must not be allowed to lead to any decline in standards and indeed should be accompanied by systematic measures to improve the quality of the service provided. Tighter criteria should be introduced for placement in a special school; their application should be supervised by multidisciplinary teams whose function should include an active policy of returning children to regular schools. Reducing the number of children placed in special schools will release teachers who can take on advisory and support functions in mainstream education.

The education system needs to develop more concrete projects and programmes concerned with equal opportunities and ethnic integration. How children are treated should depend on their developmental level, not on their sex. Where ethnocentrism - 'white dominance' - leads ethnic minorities to turn in on themselves and, for lack of training and job opportunities, to engage in group delinquency, there is little point in repressive measures; what is needed is a preventive approach which starts in primary school.

Quality of care

The panel believes that standards of care can be raised by means of more and better research, improved training in this area and structural measures.

Training courses should put more stress on practical experience (e.g. requiring more periods of teaching practice) and more people with practical experience should transfer to training posts. The training course for youth workers should be retained and improved and greater provision made for in-service training. A second phase of occupational training should be available for educationists and psychologists. The shortage of child psychiatrists must be remedied and priority needs to be given to training professional helpers from ethnic minorities.

In many cases smallness of scale is a precondition for quality. Case managers should be appointed to improve the coordination of care. Procedures need to be developed notably within the RIAGGs which are more appropriate for 'unmotivated' or 'troublesome' clients, with greater stress on outreach work especially with ethnic minorities and lower-status groups in society. More development is needed of multidisciplinary approaches to diagnosis and treatment. In many cases the treatment of emotional and behavioural problems focuses too much on the individual youngster him- or herself; what is needed is an approach which also encompasses the home situation. Home and family must be included in the treatment given, with more use being made of family therapy, 'home training' and other family-oriented approached.

Higher standards in the area of curative treatment should not be bought at the expense of ongoing care. Where problems are of a persistent nature more and earlier support needs to be offered with a view to avoiding or reversing separation from the three environments of home, school and friends.

Research

More evaluative research is needed on all fronts to determine the effects of care, prevention and policy. The effectiveness of traditional residential care and newer alternatives (day care, home training) needs to be investigated. Studies aimed at development of new methods of care must however come first.

We need to develop our understanding of the determinants of problem behaviour, notably anti-social behaviour and persisent conduct disorders. Research is needed of both a biological and a psychosocial nature. Developments in genetic science must be evaluated for their possible contribution to genetic counselling. Factors which tend to increase or reduce the risk of problems need to be investigated; in the process attention must be focused on young people's own experiences and perceptions and on their views as to the causes of problems and the kinds of help needed.

Research needs to be of greater practical relevance, devoting greater attention to the issues and problems facing youngsters and their carers. More intersectoral research is also needed.

9 Caring for mental health in the future

9.1 *Introduction*

This final chapter attempts to draw together the various strands of preceding sections, enabling the progress of a perspective regarding the developments in mental health and mental health care. We begin by focusing on a number of the report's key points.

Chapters 2 and 3 raised the question of the nature of mental ill-health problems and set about determining its prevalence. The picture that emerged was a differentiated one. Mental health problems vary widely as regards, for example, the background to their genesis, the extent to which they involve subjective suffering, their socially disabling consequences, their short- or long-term nature, the intensity of care required, the likelihood of cure, the nuisance they cause to others and finally the frequency with which they occur. The main classification criterion adopted was the extent to which mental health problems and the care relating to them were socially and culturally determined.

With regard to incidence and prevalence we concluded that, on internationally accepted definitions, mental health problems were very common: in any one year around one fifth of the population face such problems, though by no means all of them become the target of professional mental health care. What is meant here is not malaise of a transitory nature but psychiatrically diagnosable problems.

Chapter 4 went on to give a broad overview of quantitative trends in mental health care, showing that the number of people making use of such care is increasing. Statistics on the utilization of services must be treated with some caution, however, since they can easily give rise to misunderstandings. For example, while the numbers seeking care grew by almost 60% through the 1980s, a considerable proportion of that growth is apparent rather than real in that many of these 'new' clients had already received care on some previous occasion. The increasing number of 'repeat' clients is due in part to the policy of returning patients to independent life in the community as quickly as possible and of minimizing the risk of care-dependence. We must also presume that some clients present to more than one mental health agency. Such statistical difficulties can be only resolved with the help of nationally representative case registers.

These methodological problems do not alter the fact in all

probability there has been a real and substantial growth in the number of people receiving care. The increase is only in the extramural and semi-intramural sectors; in the intramural sector there has been a fall in the number of people receiving care at any one time, albeit by a considerably smaller margin than the increase in the other two sectors. Current best estimates put the number of people receiving mental health care at the end of 1980 at 13.2 per thousand population, rising to 18.4 per thousand in 1990 and, if current policies remain in place, at 25.8 per thousand by the end of the century. While this growth partly reflects the increasing numbers of elderly and very elderly people, other factors are also involved and it is these in particular that require further consideration.

Given that the population of the Netherlands is still growing, the absolute growth in the number of people receiving care is in fact slightly greater than indicated by the above ratios.

The last four chapters built up a picture of four very different mental health issues and of trends and possible and desirable developments within them. The four themes were dementia, schizophrenia, occupational incapacity due to mental problems and finally emotional and behavioural problems in children and adolescents.

A major consideration behind the choice of these themes was the need adequately to reflect the enormous diversity of the concept of mental health, notably with regard to its cultural dependence. A second consideration was that between them the four themes needed to cover a substantial proportion of the mental health care field.

These considerations were of importance particularly since the results of the study were to serve as a basis for formulating conclusions covering the entire field of mental health and mental health care.

The foregoing mean that this final and consolidating chapter needs to address four questions:

1. *What are the main results of the study in the four areas covered, and to what extent do they coincide or diverge?*
2. *How are the results to be interpreted?*
3. *Starting from that interpretative framework, to what extent is it possible to make generalizations covering the entire field of mental health and mental health care?*
4. *What general conclusions and policy options emerge?*

These questions provided the starting point for the subsequent discussion.

9.2 *The results in the four areas*

The central question addressed in the scenario project was formulated in Chapter 2:

> *"What developments are possible over the next two decades in the area of mental health and the associated need for care, what are their likely consequences, and to what extent can they be influenced?"*

The general expectation regarding the prevalence of problems is that it will continue to increase, and while a variety of causes are involved some are common to all four areas.

In the case of dementia the growth in the number of old people is the main explanation of increasing prevalence, but other factors also play an important part: the life expectancy of demented patients is being extended by improvements in medical care, leading to an increase in the total number at any one time; in addition it is likely that dementia will tend to be diagnosed earlier, producing an increase in the number of recorded cases.

The prevalence of schizophrenia is expected to remain roughly constant. This is not the main issue, however; what matters more is the extent to which the condition manifests itself and causes problems for patients and those around them. On this point the expectation is that the disease will manifest itself more strongly in the future, as a result of increasing social stress and eroding social support, but that this adverse tendency will partly be offset by considerable improvements in care. Finally, as in the case of dementia, it is likely that the condition will tend to be recognized earlier.

The prevalence of occupational incapacity due to mental problems is also expected to continue rising if current policies remain in place. The reasons are various, as one would expect in such a broad and diverse field. The rapid changes affecting working conditions and the increasingly demanding nature of many jobs play an important part here; other significant factos include the earlier recognition of problems and their more frequent designation as mental.

Finally, the outlook is also gloomy in the area of emotional and behavioural problems in children and adolescents. The relative deterioration in the social and economic position of certain groups, notably ethnic minorities, at the bottom of the social ladder is seen as one major factor in the increase in such problems; another is the further erosion of the family. In addition, the increasing demands made on young people and the ever more rigorous expectations held of their functioning could well produce a widening gap between what children can achieve and what adults regard as desirable or normal.

What are the implications of these various developments for the future demand for care services? The general trend would appear to be one of a general increase.

9.3 *Likely causes of the growing demand for services*

Setting aside a multitude of necessary qualifications and refinements, there would appear to be six general factors, closely interwoven one with another, tending to increase the demand for professional care in connection with mental problems.

First, mental problems in general are tending to be diagnosed as such both at an earlier stage and with greater accuracy. This tendency - visible in all four areas, whether we are concerned with early diagnosis in young children, the prevention of occupational incapacity or the growing need for screening for Alzheimer's disease - reflects above all the belief that early intervention improves the prospects of promoting recovery or at least preventing deterioration. Improvements in detection have a twofold effect: more problems are identified, inviting more interventions of one kind or another.

Second, people are increasingly inclined when faced with mental problems to want and actively to seek professional help. In this connection it is important to recall that, where at the beginning of the century all psychiatric admissions were compulsory committals, in recent decades the picture has changed radically: patients ('clients' is a better term in this context) have achieved emancipation and the doctor-patient relationship has become a much more equal one, with the result that the patient's authentic wish for treatment can now be taken as legitimate grounds for providing it (cf. Mol & Van Lieshout 1989, chapter 3).

Third, services have become available, in terms of both accessibility and affordability, to an ever increasing proportion of the population. Care has thus been democratized: it is no longer the preserve of a social elite and is decreasingly seen as such by potential clients.

Fourth, the range and effectiveness of professional treatments have increased considerably. Not only has our knowledge of the causes of mental disorders and of appropriate forms of treatment and their effectiveness grown more comprehensive, differentiated and accurate, the number of people who possess and can apply that knowledge and therapeutic expertise has also increased.

Fifth, there seems to be a trends towards a reduced acceptance of deviation, or perhaps rather a reduced ability to cope with it and to integrate it into the everyday world: such apparently unrelated phenomena as the pressure from families and the social environment to admit troublesome schizophrenics to hospital, the shunting of less efficient employees onto disability benefit or the transfer of pupils who have difficulty coping in mainstream schools into an ever expanding special-education sector may well have a common element, namely the belief that the deviant should be dealt with deviantly.

The sixth and final factor, closely tied up with the previous one, is an apparent decline in the social support available to 'people with problems'. This decline no doubt reflects not simply a diminishing willingness to help but a trend towards an atomized society of self-centred individuals marked by increasing insularity at the individual level and a growing emphasis on the individual interests at the expense of wider considerations.

Behind this outline of likely causes of the growing demand for professional care lies the more fundamental question of how society sees mental problems: what perceptions of mental problems predominate?

9.4 *The dominant perception of mental health problems*

As we have seen, mental problems are extremely diverse, to the point indeed that they cannot be comprehended in their totality from just one angle. This implies that the aggregate of 'mental problems', considered as a whole, exists only thanks to a particular viewpoint: some deviant behaviours or mental states which our culture defines as mental problems are seen in others as signs of divine intervention or possession by evil spirits or simply as antisocial or even criminal behaviour and a disgrace to the family. The angle from which mental health problems are lit determines not only how they are seen but also what is and what is not perceived as a problem, with every culture having its own range of meanings for the term.

In our culture the dominant picture has come to be one of mentalill-health as an undesirable condition which is to be prevented or remedied and for which medical science offers the most appropriate explanatory and interpretative framework and foundation for action. The dominant view of mental problems is as disease, and even where they are not seen as diseases in the somatic sense people's perceptions still involve analogies with somatic conditions.

A mental problem is seen primarily as a discrete phenomenon which can and should be described and classified on the grounds of a number of observable characteristics, whose genesis can in principle be explained, which can in principle be eliminated by means of certain interventions and which should where possible be so eliminated.

Mental health problems are regarded not so much as aspects, attributes or qualities of an individual or of life, rather as un-optional extras: an individual is said to 'have' a mourning problem rather than to be suffering intense grief at the loss of a loved one, for example, while a child that is not very bright is said to 'have' a learning difficulty. While it is not of course the case that every mourning process or learning problem is designated as a mental dysfunction by the health and welfare services, the intensive study of such phenomena and widespread professional involvement with them have led to a gradual narrowing of what is seen as normal and acceptable.

A mental problem is seen as a sort of tumor which results from some ascertainable cause, may deteriorate and needs to be removed by expert intervention. Mental problems are things which attach themselves to individuals, things which can be seen and counted, if sometimes with difficulty.

A key feature of this attitude is its strong focus on the individual: it is individuals who are seen as having something wrong with them, even if others play a significant part in their condition's genesis, persistence, deterioration or improvement. Seeing mental problems mainly as a particular kind of disease evokes two more or less opposing effects in that it renders the experience and designation of certain behaviours or mental states as mental problems both more and less appealing, a simultaneous attraction and repulsion which affects the individuals directly concerned, those around them and society as a whole.

The repulsion derives of course above all from the negative associations of the concept of disease: disease is an unwanted state of affairs, eliciting *inter alia* defensiveness and denial on the part of those affected: "there's nothing wrong with me", "I'll manage", "I'm not mad". Earlier chapters have repeatedly noted that epidemiological studies of a psychiatric nature always uncover far more 'mental problems' than ever present to the health and welfare services. In part this probably reflects the fact that the investigators are far less inclined than individual subjects to react with defensiveness and denial.

Underlying the attractive effect of defining mental problems as disease are two important factors. First, 'disease' is still very much a guilt-free notion (albeit this is now beginning to change): in our culture illness is something that happens to us, something that threatens us from outside and creeps up on us and against which we generally cannot defend ourselves; it is not a punishment for sin or the outcome of irresponsible actions. Prime responsibility for the genesis of illness does not lie with the individuals concerned; rather have they 'got' a disease. The disease definition allows people with 'mental problems' to explain their condition without becoming its moral victim, without having to take responsibility for it in an existential sense (though it must be said that in general people are seen as more responsible for the state of their mental than their physical health).

Second, the strong association with disease also has clearly positive aspects: it frees individuals from certain social obligations and confers an entitlement to care and attention; perhaps more important, it generally implies a prospect of recovery, and while that prospect cannot by any means always be realized the notion of disease nevertheless leads naturally on to that of treatment and cure. Medicine's function is seen primarily as one of repair, and where it cannot - yet - fulfil that function it is felt to have failed. Whether or not this perception is accurate or morally acceptable is unimportant here; what matters is that it is the dominant one and affects us accordingly. The fact that in recent years there has been pressure for a shift of emphasis from 'cure' to 'care' merely shows the predominantly curative view taken of medicine: were this not the case pressure for change would be redundant. Designating certain states of mind, experiences and behaviours as 'mental problems' and hence as disease not only gives them a name but also makes them in principle soluble (provided that the contrary has not, at least as yet, been found to be the case).

9.5 *A shifting balance*

We now turn to the important question of possible shifts in the balance of the attraction and repulsion associated with the definition of mental problems as treatable diseases.

The view defended here is that our society is undergoing a process of development in which the disease definition is more and more taken for granted as certain positive consequences become more significant and certain negative consequences less.

The forces tending to promote the disease definition of mental problems are as follows.

First, the taboo associated with mental problems is gradually dissipating as they emerge into the daylight from the enclosed world of individual experience. Television has played a major part here: talk shows and current-affairs programmes have dealt at one time or another with almost every mental condition. And while sexual abuse has received by far the greatest coverage topics as varied as schizophrenia, phobias, dementia and the effects on children of marital breakdown (to name only a few) have also been raised, often extensively, in the media. One result has been to promote the social acceptance of the disease definition, since problems are seldom presented as a fate: indeed, whenever the media cover a problem someone immediately appears telling us that something can (and should) be done about it. However, it is by no means always the case that the dissipation of taboo leads immediately to greater acceptance on the part of those directly concerned: the implications of the fact that certain problems can now be publicly discussed can be very different at the level of the individual and of society.

Second, as society places growing emphasis on individuals and their interests it becomes ever easier to be a 'patient' in a socially invisible fashion. While a considerable taboo still attaches to mental illness - it can involve individual shame and social disgrace, and public acknowledgements of mental conditions and their treatment can still shock - in an increasingly self-centred society such social factors lose their significance. Many psychiatric patients lack a social network; to put it in extreme terms, they have no-one to disgrace. More generally, the individual has greater scope for being a 'patient' without his or her immediate social environment becoming aware of that fact; the strong emphasis placed on the protection of mental patients' privacy can be seen partly in this light.

While this second trend may appear to be opposed to the first, this is not really the case. The fact that public awareness of the existence and significance of certain disorders is growing does not imply any diminution of individuals' fear of exposing themselves and their condition to the public gaze.

The attractions of defining mental problems as disease are also enhanced by society's growing tendency to reward - or at least decreasing tendency to punish - mental illness, in that for example the mentally ill are now entitled to a guaranteed income. (This point was covered in detail in the chapter on occupational incapacity.) They are also entitled to treatment, i.e. to socially legitimated attention and the confirmation of their role as sufferers.

A final important point to be made here is that in recent decades mental health care has, rightly or wrongly, taken on a much more curative character than ever before. This has happened in very different ways, but one of the effects has always been to strengthen the perception of mental problems as treatable conditions. As has already been emphasized, this is of course due primarily to the great increase in the range and effectiveness of available treatments, but other factors are also involved. The image of mental hospitals as asylums to which people with an irreversible condition are consigned for life has changed considerably, thanks in large part to the transfer elsewhere of the care of the mentally handicapped and of psychogeriatric patients. Also the process which has got under way in recent years of moving the chronic sick for whom no further treatment is indicated to forms of sheltered accommodation will no doubt further strengthen the perception of mental hospitals as therapeutic institutions. Not that the psychiatric hospital is now seen principally as a place where patients are 'cured': the shift has been only relative, with the asylum function remaining in practice very important (as witness the fact that in 1987 56% of patients in mental hospitals had been 'living' there for two years or more (PIGG 1987)). Nevertheless the dismantling of the asylum function is a consistent policy goal. Also of importance is the fact that treatment, with its implication of a possible cure, is accorded higher value than nursing and general care and therefore confers greater prestige upon the practitioners concerned and enhances their status.

The establishment of the Regional Institutes of Ambulatory Mental Health Care (RIAGG), partly on the foundations of institutions not formerly accounted part of the mental health care system, has also accentuated the therapeutic element of care.

In brief, all these developments both contribute to and are a manifestation of the changing picture of mental problems. That picture has been transformed into one of treatable conditions, with the result that the prospect of recovery now implicit in the 'mental illness' label has increasingly displaced its earlier implication of doom.

9.6 *Mental health problems as a policy issue*

The foregoing discussion renders the question whether and to what extent certain mental problems ought to be regarded as an illness (or, in stronger terms, whether they are an illness at all) somewhat meaningless. Whether mental conditions are viewed as diseases is up to a point a matter of social choice, even if in practice it is seldom perceived as such. The definition of mental problems as disease is the final outcome of a process of interaction between the culturally determined attitudes and perceptions of those who experience mental problems, their social environment and those who treat them and of the politicians, policy-makers and insurers who regulate access to services.

The question is thus whether science, in the shape of specialists in mental health and illness, can show to what extent mental problems should be regarded as forms of disease and hence as conditions requiring professional treatment. A problem arises here, however, in that the answer which science gives - that around 20% of the population, or around ten times more people than are currently receiving professional treatment, are mentally ill - is neither socially and politically acceptable nor practically useful: such an answer can offer no real basis for the conduct of policy. This is a core problem in mental health care.

The gradual extension of the view of mental problems as disease has brought with it a need for new demarcation criteria at policy level. If the total field of mental problems vastly exceeds the capacity of professional care some redefinition is needed within it. The question repeatedly raised is "Are certain problems *wrongly* labelled as illnesses requiring treatment or care?" (implying that there exists somewhere a more or less objective criterion).

Various answers to this question have been suggested; none has proved entirely satisfactory. Repeated attempts have been made to separate problems (or illnesses) which require professional care or treatment from those which do not, with distinctions being proposed e.g. between severe and mild problems, between mental conditions and mere malaise, and between psychiatric and psychosocial problems. In practice such distinctions are of little help, since they do not adequately differentiate in operationally relevant terms; the criteria which have to be applied in practice include the need for care, the extent of professional intervention required in consequence, the extent to which individuals are troubled by their problems and hence unable to function normally, and the extent to which patients are a nuisance to those around them. Attempts at nominal demarcation are thus not useful in practice, and the field of mental problems continues to expand.

9.7 *Culture-dependence as an approach*

The difficulties attaching to the search for demarcation criteria which are relevant and acceptable in policy terms do not alter the fact that within the overall field of mental problems there is considerable variation in the nature of those problems. One criterion of policy relevance (assuming policy to be concerned with more than just the size, nature and location of facilities) could be the extent to which disorders, conditions or problems are dependent as regards their genesis, duration and effects on social and cultural circumstances.

Problems such as loneliness and addiction are typically culture-linked phenomena; dementia, except to the extent that it is age-dependent, is not. The position regarding schizophrenia is different again: there is some consensus around the view that it occurs in all cultures to roughly the same extent (though this is disputed in various quarters, as the background analysis in the chapter on schizophrenia makes clear), suggesting that its aetiology is independent of socio-cultural influences. Whether and to what extent most mental problems are dependent on such influences is unfortunately either unknown or unclear, however, albeit it seems likely that the various types of problem vary in the extent of their culture-dependence.

Why does such a distinction between more and less culture-linked problems matter? The answer is essentially very brief: their meaning is different. Unlike diseases which can affect people everywhere and at all times, culture-linked problems -experienced, defined and treated as mental - must be seen as signals: not only are they important in themselves, they also confront society with the fact that some individuals and groups have to pay a price for it to function as it does. Culture-linked problems need not only to be controlled, treated or made manageable but also and above all interpreted.

Mental suffering in general faces society with three main questions:

- how can it be prevented?
- if prevention is impossible, how can it be minimized or eliminated?
- if elimination is impossible, how can it be made bearable?

(cf. NRV 1989).

These questions tend to be interpreted somewhat technocratically in terms such as:

- what measures are needed?
- what kind of research should be promoted?- what kinds of therapeutic technique should be developed?

Typical culture-linked problems prompt a further question, however: if the functioning of our society engenders, reinforces or aggravates mental problems, is that price worth paying? And that takes us into the area of social and political choice.

A parallel question may help clarify the point. (Geographic) mobility is important in our society and highly valued, so highly in fact that traffic continues to grow despite the high price paid in the form of around 2,000 road deaths every year and serious environmental damage. This situation does not of course reflect any deliberate, positive decision on the part of society - rather it is the aggregate end result of innumerable individual choices - but neither is it the outcome of some law of nature: it can be altered if we so choose. The same may well apply in some degree to culture-linked mental problems.

To avoid misunderstanding it is important to note, finally, that the strong/weak culture-dependence spectrum is quite distinct from, for example, the severe/mild and psychosocial/psychiatric spectrums: strongly culture-dependent problems can be very severe, suicide being a conspicuous example.

9.8 *Culture-dependence and the four themes*

This study has looked at four themes within the overall field of mental health whose classification according to the extent of their culture-dependence produces the following picture.

Mental health issues and the extent of their culture-dependence

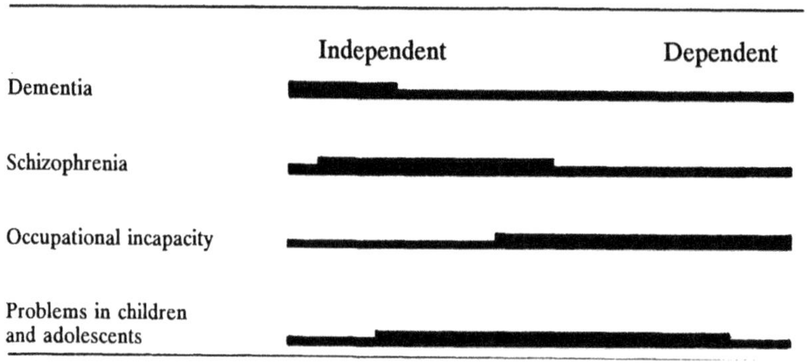

The lines in the diagram indicate the four problems' assumed position and spread across the culture-dependence spectrum.

Dementia is largely independent of social and cultural influences. Schizophrenia is, subject to many qualifications, somewhat more culture-dependent; its spread is also greater, indicating that some aspects of the condition are significantly affected by social and cultural circumstances and others little if at all (it is likely, for example, that the severity of the disorder and the forms in which it manifests itself depend partly on social and cultural circumstances, whereas the schizophrenic disposition appears to be unrelated to such factors). Emotional and behavioural problems in children and adolescents are widely spread across the culture-dependence spectrum, as is - albeit probably to a lesser extent - occupational incapacity due to mental problems. This of course reflects the fact that the latter two themes are concerned with population groups rather than diseases and their symptoms. Both youngsters' problems and occupational incapacity are markedly culture-dependent, the latter probably even more strongly than the former.

As section 9.2 indicated, a considerable increase in the prevalence of dementia can be expected to result from the aging of the population and, probably, from a gradual further increase in the life expectancy of demented patients, while the prevalence of schizophrenia is likely to change little if at all. Emotional and behavioural problems in children and adolescents and occupational incapacity due to mental problems are clearly growing and will continue to do so unless current trends are reversed.

The general picture that emerges is one of culture-independent problems whose prevalence is constant (while dementia is growing, the reasons are not culture-linked) and of culture-dependent problems whose prevalence is increasing. To what extent can this conclusion be extended to the whole field of mental health and its care?

This question can be tackled in two ways: the first is quantitative and involves considering how much of the mental health field is covered by the four themes of this study; the second, more qualitative, approach focuses on the extent to which the remainder of the field is comparable with the parts investigated. In quantitative terms the four themes probably account for more than half of all mental health problems, but no exact indication can be given since two of the themes concern mental conditions (dementia and schizophrenia), one focuses on a population group (problems in children and adolescents) and one (incapacity due to mental problems) is best defined as a social-insurance category, and of these the latter two in principle encompass all possible conditions.

Among the major problems not investigated in their own right are addiction, depression and anxiety disorders. Their positioning in the spectrum of culture-dependence does not differ in essential respects from that of the four themes considered; they tend to be more culture-dependent than dementia and schizophrenia but much less so than the great majority of mental health problems leading to occupational incapacity within the meaning of the disability-insurance legislation. The most extensive of the problem categories not considered in this study seem to locate somewhere in the middle of the spectrum (it is perhaps only addictions that should be located primarily at the culture-dependent end), while those on which we have focused are nearer its extremes.

Bearing all these considerations in mind we may conclude that, given the spread of the four themes across the spectrum of culture-dependence, general pronouncements relating to the whole field of mental health and its care are justified on the basis of what has been investigated here.

9.9 *The value of a socio-cultural approach*

If we are right in believing that mental problems and their growing prevalence must be seen and understood primarily in the light of processes of social and cultural change, then social and cultural conditions and their mutability are the obvious place to start looking for answers; and a prime need if we are to find answers is to extend the public debate on the links between social and cultural developments and the genesis, persistence and severity of mental problems. Once again a comparison with problems in another field may help clarify the point.

In the last two decades a great public and political debate on the implications of economic growth has got underway in the western world: are we paying too high a price for our material prosperity in the form of, first, the exhaustion of natural resources and, subsequently, the gradual destruction of the entire ecosystem? An in principle similar, if somewhat less dramatic, debate is possible in connection with mental problems: are we perhaps also paying a price for economic advancement in terms of mental ill-health? It is quite conceivable that rapid technological progress, with all that it implies by way of changing demands on individuals and changing interpersonal relations, is producing a situation in which growing numbers of people are mentally unable to fit into society and can no longer contribute to its further development, with the result that they are marginalized as mental patients.

In "Mental Health Policies and Programmes for the Twenty-first Century: A Personal View" Norman Sartorius, the head of the World Health Organization's Mental Health Division, writes that: "Unless mental health surges upward in the hierarchy of values, most of the efforts of mental health programs will be ephemeral. (...) Dehumanization of medicine and development has a pernicious counterpart in the medicalization of life problems. Issues that should be approached by broad social measures are declared medical and dumped onto the overstrained health-service system" (Sartorius 1987, 152-3). Sartorius believes that far too low a value is attached to mental health: mental health (or perhaps more realistically "the avoidance of mental ill-health") should but does not serve as a general reference point, a touchstone for appraising the development of our society; it is not one of our guiding principles.

Sartorius's alarm cry appears justified. Looking at the position in the Netherlands today, it is very striking that the concept of mental health has been narrowed right down to that of 'care'; the idea of a 'mentally healthy society' has never been fully developed. While the notion that mental health could be systematically promoted gained some support in the 1950s and 1960s, it was interpreted in a somewhat moralistic, elitist and patriarchal manner which would certainly not find favour today and has rightly fallen out of use. The sad thing is that little effort seems to have been made to give the notion a new focus with contemporary relevance. There are openings enough: the drive for equal opportunities, the fight against discrimination and the development of alternative forms of criminal justice, for example, could very well be seen as elements in a new movement for mental health. Unfortunately, mental health - or rather mental ill-health - seems currently to have been entirely reduced to the aggregate of all mental disorders requiring treatment, care, support and funding. Every article, every policy document, focuses on health care rather than health, and mental health problems are simply referred to an overburdened care system attacked by politicians for opening its doors too wide and by clients, actual or potential, for not opening them wide enough.

Such criticisms notwithstanding, the notion of mental health is a recurring element in successive government policy documents. A 1970 statement put the central focus on mental health (the term 'psycho-hygiene' was still used at that time), while one issued four years later ('Structuurnota Gezondheidszorg') was concerned very much with the organization of care; this was also the focus of a further statement in 1984 ('Nieuwe Nota Geestelijke Volksgezondheid'). Mental health as a more positive concept (under the heading of prevention and relevant policies in other fields) reappeared in 'Nota 2000' (1986), to be fleshed out in the section of the 1989 statement ('Ontwerp Kerndocument Gezondheidsbeleid') concerned with the prevention of mental illness.

Looking back it is striking that while the sections of these papers dealing with the care system's organization and funding and the distribution within it of powers and functions have repeatedly prompted to fierce debate, those concerned with mental health as such have tended to vanish from view quite rapidly. One reason for this is that the promotion of mental health is very a much more difficult area for policy-making than the care of the mentally ill; another, probably, is that well organized interests exist in the area of mental health care but not in that of mental health itself. This is of course no excuse for ignoring links between social and cultural developments and mental health; the issue needs to be raised and debated continually, and this should be seen as a task not just for the government but for a whole range of organizations and interests in society.

9.10 *Two core notions: normality and identity*

Since so little attention has been focused on mental health as an aspect of social and cultural reality (as distinct from the organization, substance and funding of mental health care), we also have little systematic understanding of the interactions that occur between processes of change in society and in the human mind. In what follows we therefore consider only two core notions in this field, namely normality and identity.

By 'normality' we mean all the (mainly implicit) requirements which people feel they should set for themselves and others under such headings as tolerance, sociability, the ability to process information, the capacity for acceptance and adjustment and the suppression of aggression. One effect of the highly complex and rapidly changing nature of modern society seems to be that, without our generally being aware of the process, the criteria which determine normality are being drawn ever more tightly. We need more and more knowledge and skills, psychologically as well as in other respects, if we are to function as full - i.e. normal - members of society. This narrowing of normality affects all major social institutions, including education, the organization of production, but also e.g. marriage and the family.

Education, for example, not only extends over an ever longer period, it also demands ever higher standards: this is reflected in the large numbers of children - maladjusted, mildly mentally handicapped, learning-disabled - referred to various types of special school. This new trend does not of course indicate the presence of new problems, since each generation of children has the same potentialities as earlier and later generations; it is our expectations regarding the minimum standards that children must achieve that are changing, along with the society in which they will have to function. More and more has to be invested in children if they are later to be able to function in society in a manner regarded as normal; it therefore takes longer and longer to prepare them to enter 'normal society', i.e. that section of society deemed normal: that of adults with jobs and families. Moreover even those who do eventually find themselves part of normal society must with increasing frequency undertake some form of retraining if they are not fall by the wayside.

Similar tendencies affect the world of work. People's chances of being unable to cope are increasing, as witness the large numbers of 'unemployables' and of workers shunted onto disability benefit for reasons which have little to do with what has traditionally been considered illness. Despite the fact that on average people not on disability benefit now remain healthy for longer the standard age of compulsory retirement has been lowered (though not far enough, apparently, since in some occupations - such as teaching - the modal age at which people cease to be able to cope has already fallen to between 50 and 55).

The boundaries of what is seen as normal have also narrowed in the area of marriage and the family. We have gradually reached a situation in which women are not regarded, and do not regard themselves, as being of the right age to have children until they are approaching thirty - between 1970 and 1987 the average age of mothers at the time of the birth of their first child rose from 24.4 to 27.0 years (CBS 1988) - while once they pass 35 they are deemed on medical grounds to be beyond safe child-bearing age. At the same time it is increasingly seen as tragic that women who want children should be unable to have them, necessitating complex medical interventions. Something similar has happened in marital relationships: as partners' expectations of one another have risen, particularly in psychological terms, so too has the number of insuperable disappointments, rendering relationships increasingly unstable. This would not in itself be a problem were it not that stable relationships are still considered highly desirable: they remain the normative model. This is also true of coping at a 'normal' school or of being employed.

The significance of this is that while fewer and fewer people now belong to the section of society which is felt to represent the norm, i.e. to which most people gear their behaviour, aspirations and expectations, it has not lost any of its normative power. Large groups of people do not really form part of this section of society and the many schemes designed to ensure a reasonable minimum standard of living have made it possible to leave them outside it, subsisting on their study grant, disability benefit or lone parent's allowance.

Interestingly, it is precisely such groups that make use of mental health facilities: the divorced and their children, the single, benefit claimants, children who cannot cope at school, and so on. It requires a high degree of 'mental fitness' to be able to function as a full member of our society, and those who do not possess it are seen, and see themselves, as mentally ill. In the modern welfare state a lack of social competence is manifested as a lack of mental competence.

The second core notion is that of *identity*. The anthropologist R. Linton (1936) was the first to distinguish between 'ascribed' and 'achieved' roles. In traditional communities most social positions and the roles which flow from them are set in advance and entered at birth; in modern society they have to be constructed. The positions that people occupy in society are of great importance to their sense of identity, and evidence has gradually accumulated that in our kind of society to a large extent it is not just our social but our personal identity that we have to build for ourselves. This is because almost nothing is given. We choose almost everything ourselves, or rather we must ourselves choose much of what shapes our personal identity: not just our jobs, partners, homes but also whether or not to have children, what language to speak, what religion to profess and so on.

This world of almost unlimited choice has the drawback of assuming that the individual is capable of determining, on the basis of his or her own self, the answer to the question "Who am I and who do I want to be?". A society marked by advanced technology, rapid change and above all a strong focus on the individual demands the type of personality that, having acquired a number of fundamental certainties early in life, has the basis on which to exercise the freedom to build an identity of his or her own. This condition cannot by any means always be met, nor ever could in the past; the problem we face today is that those with a weak or disturbed identity find it very much more difficult to cope in our self-centred society. Such people still have to make choices for themselves; there is no longer any system of pre-allocated positions and universal values and norms to tell the individual: "this is how the world is; this is your place in it; act accordingly". Identity has changed from a cultural datum into a cultural challenge, increasing the likelihood that those who enter the world with little sense of the route they should take will become psychologically disoriented and any lack of meaning, direction or sense in the individual's life will be experienced or defined as a mental shortcoming.

9.11 *Conclusions and policy options*

The starting point of this chapter was the distinction between those mental problems which are culture-dependent and those which are not, though it should be borne in mind that this is an oversimplification and that there is a continuum of conditions between the two extremes.

Expectations for the future vary markedly from one end of the continuum to the other.

As the population of old people grows, so too will the prevalence of mental problems and illnesses directly associated with the aging process. Aside from this important but entirely autonomous factor, we must assume that the prevalence of culture-independent conditions will not change significantly. At the other end of the continuum, however, we can expect an ongoingincrease, which will also increasingly manifest itself in a demand for professional treatment. This increase must in essence be understood as a consequence of two trends:

- our complex and rapidly changing society makes increasingly heavy demands on people in a variety of respects and increases the likelihood of their being unable to meet them. Those affected in this way are then regarded, or regard themselves, as inadequate or abnormal;

- there is a gradual tendency to designate and experience the discrepancy between individuals' capacities and society's norms as 'mental illness'.

With regard to the more *culture-independent* problems, such as schizophrenia, the core social and political question is this: what efforts are we prepared to make to enable those affected to lead as decent a life as possible? In concrete terms this means deciding how much investment should be devoted to improving the prevention and treatment of such conditions on the one hand and how much should to geared to other types of illness or indeed other social goals entirely on the other. There is evidence that, in proportion to the scale and severity of such conditions, relatively little investment of this sort (in education and research) is being made.

Where we still lack curative treatments, the political and social choice relates to the steps we are willing to take to create conditions which enable patients to enjoy as normal a life as possible despite their handicaps. Such steps involve not only financial but also organizational and interpersonal efforts: integrating people with mental problems into 'normal' society means a different, and in particular more flexible, approach to the organization of care (which then becomes mainly protection) and also confrontations which 'normal' society will in many cases see as a problem. This last point implies a need for a systematic programme of information and education aimed at increasing understanding and changing attitudes and for greater professional support for families and communities coping with people with mental problems. In general there seems still to be an overemphasis on curative care which, while understandable, gives rise to expectations which in many cases cannot (at least as yet) be fulfilled. In such cases it would be better to divert resources into limited social integration and crisis management. Were this the goal, large numbers of readmissions would no longer need to be seen as indicating deficient care, as now happens to a large extent.

The problems that we have designated *culture-dependent* (again it must be emphasized they are at one end of a continuum rather than forming a separate category) require a different approach, since they have a signalling function and must be recognized and treated accordingly. If we merely monitor developments without seeking to influence underlying causes, then there is no reason to suppose that the need for professional mental care will depart from the extrapolations detailed in chapter 4: in broad terms, the proportion of the Dutch population receiving care from the mental health services at any one time will rise from 1.5% in 1980 to 2% in 1990 and 2.5%

in 2000. This growing need for care cannot be dismissed on the grounds that it is in some sense wrongly expressed: needs that are in large measure socially and culturally generated are not for that reason any less genuine, and a 'cultural illness' is just as real in its impact and consequences as any other.

In the light of these observations and expectations there would appear to be three broad options for future policy.

First, developments could be left to run their course with the resulting growth in the need for care being met only to a very limited extent. If as seems likely the trends of the 1980s were to continue through the 1990s the need for mental health care would grow by around 2% a year. Holding the growth in provision to, say, 1% a year would produce a somewhat dismal picture, in that the result would be an increasing number of people who could no longer adequately fit in with what society regards as 'normal' and who would therefore be marginalized: chronic alcoholics, school dropouts, young vagrants, the lonely, the chronically anxious, the depressive and suicidal, and so on.

The second possibility is to expand care provision broadly in line with growing demand, with relatively heavy investment in methods and techniques for enhancing people's capacity for adjustment: people would be given a respite, as it were, so that they could then return (if only temporarily) to the fray.

The third option involves deliberate psychosocial reform. The key notion here is that high levels of certain mental problems are seen as indicating unhealthy tendencies in society, which are then systematically analysed with a view to formulating coordinated policies geared to prevention. This is easier said than done, of course, and then it is no part of our task to develop a policy programme as part of this study. One or two points can nevertheless be made.

Implementing such an approach depends importantly on the growth of a general recognition that mental health can be socially promoted, even if we cannot say precisely to what extent: the question has hardly been raised, with the result that little research has been done and little is known. Even so considerable experience has been built up over the last twenty years regarding the prevention and control of mental health problems, and that experience needs to be systematized, evaluated and above all passed on. On the physical side we have seen, in little more than a decade, a minor revolution in the area of health protection and promotion and disease prevention: people are now very much more aware that their physical health depends very much on healthy lifestyles and a healthy environment, and the implications of this fact are increasingly widely accepted. There has been no comparable process on the mental side, however, and indeed there has been very little pressure in this direction (other than in the area of sexual abuse). Public awareness of the links between lifestyles and mental health will not develop unless stimulated, particularly where - as at present - the significance of mental health problems as indicators of underlying social problems is fairly consistently ignored and depoliticized as 'deficiencies of provision'. This is of course not to imply that we should stop treating and caring for people with mental health problems, but we need to do something else as well: such problems must be related to the contexts in which they develop, worsen and become insoluble, and they must be publicly debated. One of the great difficulties facing us is that mental problems are so exclusively seen as belonging to the private sphere of life that it has hitherto been virtually impossible to conduct a public debate on the issue. Symptomatic of the position is the average Dutch person's ignorance of the fact that large numbers of people are classed as unfit for work on mental grounds: the public does not know who these people are or how and why they became and have remained incapacitated, for the simple reason that they are defined virtually exclusively as benefit claimants, whose mental difficulties are of a private nature.

We need to rediscover and redefine a notion of mental health which is more than just another bureaucratic label.

Bibliography

Aarts L. *et al.*

Beschrijving van WAO-toetreders; deelrapport Determinantenonderzoek WAO (*Description of new disability-benefit claimants*; report on the determinants of entitlement).

SVr (Social Insurance Council), Zoetermeer, 1982.

Aarts L., P.R. de Jong

Arbeidsverleden en uitkeringshoogte als determinanten van WAO-toetreding; deelrapport Determinantenonderzoek WAO (*Job record and benefit amount as determinants of disability-benefit entitlement*; report on the determinants of entitlement).

SVr (Social Insurance Council), Zoetermeer, 1987.

Abrams L., M.A. Taylor

The genetics of schizophrenia: a reassessment using modern criteria.

American Journal of Psychiatry, 140 (1983), 2, 171-175.

Afdeling Sociale Psychiatrie, R.U. Groningen (Groningen University Department of Social Psychiatry)

Epidemiologische beschouwingen over vraag en aanbod in de geestelijke gezondheidszorg (Epidemiological considerations concerning supply and demand in mental health care).

Groningen, 1983.

Albee, G.W.

The argument for primary prevention.

Journal of Primary Prevention, 5 (1985), 4, 213-219.

Algemeen Arbeidsongeschiktheidsfonds/Arbeidsongeschiktheidsfonds (Disability Funds)

Jaarverslagen 1986, 1987 (Annual Reports for 1986, 1987).

Zoetermeer, 1988, 1989.

American Psychiatric Association (APA)

Diagnostic and Statistical Manual of Mental Disorders (DSM-III R).

Washington DC, 1987.

Arie, T.

Questions in the psychiatry of old age.

In: Ciba Foundation Symposium 134, *Research and the aging population.*

Wiley, Chichester, 1988.

Asselbergs, L.

Ambulante behandeling van schizophrenia, een literatuurstudie (*The ambulatory treatment of schizophrenia*, a review of the literature).

Netherlands Institute of Mental Health (NcGv) series 91, NcVg, Utrecht, 1986.

Asselbergs, L.
Sociaal beperkt, een empirisch onderzoek naar het sociaal functioneren van schizophrenie-patiënten in het Psychose Preventie Project, Rotterdam (*Socially limited*, an empirical study of the social functioning of schizophrenia patients in the Psychosis Prevention Project, Rotterdam).
Thesis, Netherlands Institute of Mental Health (NcGv) series 89-7, NcGv, Utrecht, 1989.
Baars, H.M.J.
Sociale netwerkbenadering in de gezondheidszorg, geïllustreerd aan praktijkvoorbeelden (The social network approach in health care, illustrated with practical examples).
Metamedica, 63 (1984), 68-77.
Baartman, H.E.M.
Tussen te kort komen en te kort doen.
Free University, Amsterdam, 1988.
Babigian, H.M.
Schizophrenia: epidemiology.
In: Kaplan, Sadock (eds.), *op. cit.*, 1985.
Bannister, D.
The logical requirements of research into schizophrenia.
British Journal of Psychiatry, 114 (1968), 181-188.
Barnhoorn, J.A.J.
Sociale psychiatrie, geestelijke hygiëne, geestelijke gezondheidszorg en geestelijke volksgezondheid (Social psychiatry, psychohygiene, mental health care and mental health).
MGv, 10 (1955), special number.
Barrett, R.J.
Interpretations of schizophrenia.
Culture, medicine and psychiatry, 12 (1988), 3, 357-388.
Bateson, G., D.D. Jackson, J. Haley and J.H. Weakland
Toward a theory of schizophrenia.
Behavioral Science, 1 (1956), 251-264.
Bax, E.H.
Maatschappelijke verandering en arbeidsongeschiktheid, de macro-determinanten van WAO-toetreding en uittreding nader verkend (Social change and occupational incapacity, exploring the macro-determinants of benefit entitlement and its termination).
The Hague, Ministry of Employment and Social Security, Social Security Research Committee, 1984.
Beard, J.H., T.J. Malamud, E. Rossman
Psychiatric rehabilitation and long-term rehospitalization rates. The findings of two research studies.
Schizophrenia Bulletin, 4 (1978), 622-635.
Bell, R.A. *et al.*
Change and psychopathology: epidemiological considerations.
Community Mental Health Journal, 17 (1981), 3, 203-213.

Bentall, R.P., H.F. Jackson, D. Pilgrim
Abandoning the concept of 'schizophrenia': some implications of validity arguments for psychological research into psychotic phenomena.
British Journal of Clinical Psychology, 27 (1988), 303-324.
Bentall, R.P., P.D. Slade
Reality testing and auditory hallucinations: a signal detection analysis.
British Journal of Clinical Psychology, 24 (1985), 159-169.
Berben, E., H. de Kort, M. van Ooyen-Houben
Ontwikkelingen binnen de vrijwillige pleegzorg (Developments in voluntary fostering).
Ministry of Welfare, Health and Cultural Affairs, Rijswijk, 1986.
Besseling, J.J.M.
Diagnose en arbeidsongeschiktheid, 1977-1983 (Diagnosis and occupational incapacity, 1977-1983).
GMD (Joint Medical Service) Notes no. 6, Amsterdam, 1986.
Bijker, H., E. de Groot, M. Wöstmann *et al.*
Waarheen? Een onderzoek naar het kiezen van tehuizen, pleeggezinnen en andere woonsituaties door plaatsende instanties voor minderjarigen (*Where?* An investigation into the choice of children's homes, foster families and other forms of accommodation by agencies responsible for the placement of minors).
Leiden State University Department of Social and Organizational Psychology, Leiden, 1981.
Bijl, R.V., J.C.M. Masthoorn
Van behoefte naar vraag (From need to demand).
Netherlands Institute of Mental Health (NcGv) series 89, Utrecht, 1986.
Bijl, R.V., E.J.H. ter Heine, J.W. Furer
Op zoek naar risicogroepen. Onderzoek naar risicogroepen met psychosociale problemen in de bevolking van de gezondheidsregio Nijmegen (Seeking out at-risk groups. A study of at-risk groups with psychosocial problems in the population of the Nijmegen health region).
Tijdschrift Sociale Gezondheidszorg, 64 (1986), 297-304.
Bijl, R.V., E.J.H. ter Heine, J.W. Furer
Onderzoek naar risicogroepen: een risico voor de GGZ (Research into at-risk groups: a risk for the mental health services).
MGv, 41 (1986), 5, 493-507.
Bijl, R.V., E. Ketting
Rapport vooronderzoek Scenario-project Geestelijke Volksgezondheid en Geestelijke Gezondheidszorg (Report on the preliminary study for the scenario project on mental health and mental health care).
Netherlands Institute of Mental Health (NcGv), Utrecht, May 1987.
Bijlsma, T., F. Koopmans
Ongelijkheid in de WAO: verschillen tussen mannen en vrouwen per bedrijfssector (Inequalities in disability-benefit entitlement; sex differences by industrial sector).
Sociaal Maandblad Arbeid, June 1985, 430-455.

Birren, J.E., R.B. Sloane (eds.)
Handbook of mental health and aging.
Prentice Hall, Englewood Cliffs NJ, 1980.
Blazer, D. *et al.*
Psychiatric disorders; a rural/urban comparison.
Archives of General Psychiatry, 42 (1985), July, 651-656.
Bleeker, J.A.C., H.J. Meillo, E. Bongers, L.G.P.D. Koppers
Chronische inrichtingspatiënten in De Bijlmer (Chronic institutional patients in De Bijlmer).
MGv, 42 (1987), 12, 1331-1343.
Boelen, K.W.J., G.J. Zwanniken
Psychische stoornissen bij bejaarden (Mental disorders in the elderly).
Leiden, 1975.
Bol, M.W.
Uithuisplaatsing. Beslissingscriteria in de justitiële kinderbescherming (Taking children into care. Decision-making criteria in the justice system).
Justitiële Verkenningen, 4 (1978), 4.
Bosch, F.A.J. van den, C. Petersen (eds.)
Arbeidsongeschiktheid; een multidisciplinaire benadering (Occupational incapacity; a multidisciplinary approach).
Deventer, 1981.
Bosch, F.A.J. van den, C. Petersen
De omvang van de verborgen werkloosheid in de WAO (The extent of hidden unemployment among disability-benefit claimants).
In: Bosch, Petersen (eds.), *op. cit.*, 1981, 77-95.
Bosch, R.J. van den, C.R. van Meer, P.M.A.J. Dingemans, D.H. Linszen (eds.)
Schizophrenie. Recente ontwikkelingen in onderzoek en behandeling (*Schizophrenia*. Recent developments in research and treatment).
Van Loghum Slaterus, Deventer, 1988.
Bosch, J.S.G. van de
Behandelbare vormen van dementie (Treatable forms of dementia).
In: CBIT, *op. cit.*, 1988.
Brenner, H.D., B. Hodel
Treatment of cognitive disorders in schizophrenia. Approaches and results.
In: C.N. Stefanis *et al.* (eds.), Psychiatry Today, VIII World Congress of Psychiatry, Abstracts.
Excerpta Medica, International Congress Series 899, Amsterdam, 1989.
Brinkgreve, C., J.H. Onland, A. de Swaan
De opkomst van het psychotherapeutisch bedrijf. Sociologie van de psychotherapie. Deel I (*The rise of the psychotherapy business*. The sociology of psychotherapy. Part I).
Spectrum, Utrecht, 1979.
Brinkman, W., H. Kars
Aanpassing en predictie van aanpassing (Adjustment and prediction of adjustment).
Staatsdrukkerij, The Hague, 1974.

Broekhuis, H.
Beoordeling en begeleiding bij arbeidsongeschiktheid (Assessment and support in connection with occupational incapacity).
Lelystad, 1986 (dissertation, Groningen).
Brogren, P.O.
Promotion of Mental Health.
Nordic School of Public Health, Gothenburg, 1985.
Brown, G.W., J.L.T. Birley
Crises and life changes and the onset of schizophrenia.
Journal of Health and Social Behavior, 9 (1968), 203-214.
Brown, G.W., T. Harris
Social origins of depression.
Tavistock, London, 1978.
Burger, A.S., L. Kimelman, A. Lurie
Patients as tenants in a group residence program.
Psychiatry Journal of the University of Ottawa, 2 (1977), 2, 124-128.
Buurmeijer, F.A., P.C. Hermans
Gezinsfunctioneren en individuele stoornissen (Family functioning and individual disorders).
Swets & Zeitlinger, Amsterdam, 1988.
Buys, P.C.
Curatieve gezondheidszorg, ziekteverzuim en arbeidsongeschiktheid (Curative health care, sickness absence and occupational incapacity).
Amsterdam, Stichting CCOZ, 1985.
Cammen, T.J.M. van der
The memory clinic; a new approach to the detection of dementia.
British Journal of Psychiatry, 150 (1987), 359-364.
CBIT (Central Supervisory Body for Peer Review)
Diagnostiek bij het dementie syndrome (Diagnosis and the dementia syndrome).
Report on Consensus meeting of 4 November 1988.
Utrecht, CBIT, 1988.
CBS (Central Bureau of Statistics) (H. Swinkels)
Trendcijfers Gezondheidsenquête (Health survey trend figures).
Maandbericht Gezondheidsstatistiek, 7 (1988), 8-9, 14-28.
CBS (Central Bureau of Statistics)
Statistiek rechtsbescherming en veiligheid (Statistics on the protection of rights and security).
Staatsuitgeverij, The Hague, 1985.
CBS (Central Bureau of Statistics)
Bevolkingsprognose voor Nederland, 1988-2050 (Population forecasts for the Netherlands, 1988-2050).
Statistisch Bulletin, 44 (1988), 50.
CBS (Central Bureau of Statistics)
Statistisch zakboek 1988 (1988 Statistical Handbook).
Staatsuitgeverij, The Hague, 1988a.

CBS (Central Bureau of Statistics)
Zelfdoding (Suicide).
Kwartaalbericht rechtbescherming en veiligheid, 1988b, 73-75.

Centraal Planbureau (Central Planning Office) (J.M.J. op de Beke)
Herziening trendmatig arbeidsaanbod 1985-2010 (Revised figures for labour-supply trends 1985-2010) (note 8710.0).
The Hague, August 1987.

Centrum PS
Vrijwilligers in de psychiatrie: Gekkenwerk? (Volunteers in psychiatry: crazy work?).
Conference report, 6 October 1989, Centrum PS, Amsterdam.

Chien, C.P., J.O. Cole
Landlord-supervised cooperative apartments. A new modality for community-based treatment.
American Journal of Psychiatry, 130 (1973), 2, 156-159.

Colerick, E.J., L.K. George
Predictors of institutionalization among caregivers of patients with Alzheimer disease.
Journal of the American Geriatrics Society, 34 (1986), 493-498.

Cooper, D.
Psychiatry and anti-psychiatry.
Paladin, London 1967.

Cooper, B., H. Bickel.
Population and the early detection of dementing disorders in old age: a review.
Psychological Medicine, 14 (1984), 81-95.

Crevel, H. van
Hoeveel diagnostiek bij dementie? (How much diagnosis in connection with dementia?).
Graadmeter (Health Council publication), 5 (1989), 3, 17-18.

Crow, T.J.
The two-syndrome concept: origins and current status.
Schizophrenia Bulletin, 11 (1985), 3, 471-486.

Cutting, J.C.
The psychology of schizophrenia.
Churchill Livingstone, Edinburgh, 1985.

Davies, P.
The genetics of Alzheimer's disease: a review and a discussion of the implications.
Neurobiology of Aging, 7 (1986), 459-466.

Deboutte, D., A. van de Ven, H. van Engeland
Jeugd, hulpverlening, geestelijke gezondheidszorg: een psychiatrisch-epidemiologische verkenning (Young people, care, mental health care: an exercise in psychiatric epidemiology).
RIAGG (Regional Institute of Ambulatory Mental Health Care) Rotterdam South & GGD (Joint Medical Service) Rotterdam, Rotterdam, 1987.

Deboutte, D.
Jeugd en hulp, een psychiatrisch-epidemiologische verkenning (*Young people and* care, an exercise in psychiatric epidemiology).
Acco, Leuven, 1989.
Dell'Acqua, G., M.G. Cogliati Dezza
The end of the mental hospital. A review of the psychiatric experience in Trieste.
Acta Psychiatrica Scandinavica, 71 (1985), Suppl. 316.
De Schalm
Jaarverslag 1988 (1988 Annual Report).
De Schalm, Haarlem, 1989.
Deutsch, A., H. Fishman
Encyclopedia of mental health.
Watts, New York, 1963.
Diesfeldt, H.F.A., L.R. van Houte, R.M. Moerkens
Duration of survival in dementia.
Acta Psychiatrica Scandinavica, 1986, 73, 366-371.
Diesfeldt, H.F.A., J. Jolles
Psychologische diagnostiek en behandeling bij (vermoeden van) dementieel syndroom (Psychological diagnosis and treatment in (suspected) cases of dementia syndrome).
In: Gezondheidsraad (Health Council): *Psychogeriatrische ziektebeelden (Psychogeriatric syndromes).*
The Hague, 1988.
Dijk, W.K. van
Het medisch model in sociale context (The medical model in a social context).
In: C. Rümke, P.W. Boche, W.K. van Dijk (eds.), *Van kinderanalyse tot Y-chromosoom (From child analysis to the Y chromosome)*
Deventer, Van Loghum Slaterus, 1973.
Dijkstra, S., F.A. Swets-Gronert
Dilemma's rond signalering en melding van kindermishandeling (Dilemmas in the detection and notification of child abuse). Final report on the first stage.
Netherlands Institute of Mental Health (NcGv), Utrecht, 1989.
Dincin, J., T.F. Witheridge
Psychiatric rehabilitation as a deterrent to recidivism.
Hospital and Community Psychiatry, 33 (1982), 8, 645-650.
Dohrenwend, B.P., B.S. Dohrenwend
Social status and psychiatric disorder.
Wiley, New York, 1969.
Dohrenwend, B.P.
Socio-cultural and social psychological factors in the genesis of mental disorders.
Journal of Health and Social Behavior, 16 (1975), 365-392.
Doornbos, K., L.M. Stevens (eds.)
De groei van het speciaal onderwijs (The growth of special education).
Staatsuitgeverij, The Hague, 1987.

Douben, N.H., M. Herweyer
Arbeidsmarkt, werkloosheid en arbeidsongeschiktheid (Labour market, unemployment and incapacity).
Maandschrift Economie, 7/8 (1979), 309-320.
Draijer, N.
De omgekeerde wereld; seksueel misbruik van kinderen in het gezin (The world turned upside down; sexual abuse of children in the family).
Ministry of Employment and Social Security, The Hague, 1985.
Draijer, N.
Seksueel misbruik van meisjes door verwanten; een landelijk onderzoek naar de omvang, de aard, de gezinsachtergronden, de emotionele betekenis en de psychische en psychosomatische gevolgen (*Sexual abuse of girls by relatives*; a national investigation into the scale, nature, family background, emotional significance and mental and psychosomatic consequences).
Ministry of Employment and Social Security, The Hague, 1988.
Dunham, H.W.
Community and schizophrenia. An epidemiological analysis.
Wayne State University Press, Detroit, 1965.
Eagles, J.M. *et al.*
The psychological well-being of supporters of the demented elderly.
British Journal of Psychiatry, 150 (1987), 293-298.
Emanuel, H.
Achtergronden van het arbeidsongeschiktheidsverschijnsel in Nederland (Background to occupational incapacity in the Netherlands).
In: Bosch, Petersen (eds.), *op. cit.*, 1981, 25-62.
Endicott, J., M.J. Herz, M. Gibbon
Brief versus standard hospitalization: the differential costs.
American Journal of Psychiatry, 135 (1978), 707-712.
Engeland, H. van
De invloed van biologische factoren op de ontwikkeling van het kind (The influence of biological factors on child development).
In Goudena *et al., op. cit.* 1988.
Erlenmeyer-Kimling, L., B. Cornblatt
Implications for preventive intervention from prospective research on children at risk for schizophrenia.
In: J.A. Steinberg and M.M. Silverman (eds.), *Preventing mental disorders*, NIMH, Rockville, 1987.
Eyck, J.H.M., M.P.M. de Goede (eds.)
Hulverlening aan arbeidsongeschikten (Services for the occupationally incapacitated).
Alphen a/d Rijn, 1981.
Fadden, G., P. Bebbington, L. Kuipers
The burden of care: the impact of functional psychiatric illness on the patient's family.
British Journal of Psychiatry, 150 (1987), 285-292.

Falloon, I.R.H., J.L. Boyd, C.W. McGill *et al.*
Family management in the prevention of exacerbations of schizophrenia. A controlled study.
New England Journal of Medicine, 306 (1982), 1437-1440.
Faris, R.E.L., H.W. Dunham
Mental disorders in urban areas: an ecological study of schizophrenia and other psychoses.
Chicago, University of Chicago Press, 1939.
Fengler, A.P., N. Goodrich
Wives of elderly disabled men: the hidden patient.
Gerontologist, 18 (1979), 175-183.
Fenton, F.R., L. Tessier, E. Strüning
A comparative trial of home and hospital psychiatric care. One-year follow-up.
Archives of General Psychiatry, 36 (1979), 10, 1073-1079.
Foudraine, J.
Wie is van hout? (Who is made of wood?).
Ambo, Baarn, 1971.
Frances, A.J., R.E. Hales (eds.)
APA Annual Review, Volume 5.
American Psychiatric Press, Washington, 1986.
Frederiks, J.A.M.
Dementie (Dementia).
Nederlands Tijdschrift Geneeskunde, 129 (1985), 46, 2199-2205.
Frederiks, J.A.M.
Neurologisch onderzoek (Neurological testing).
In: CBIT, *op. cit.*, 1988.
Freeman, M.D.A.
The rights and wrongs of children.
Francis Pinter, London, 1983.
Fuhrmann, W., F. Vogel
Genetic counseling.
Springer Press, New York, 1983.
Furer, J.W., B. Tax (eds.)
Somatische klachten, psychiatrische symptomen en psychosociale problemen. Eindrapport van het Regioproject Nijmegen, deel I (*Somatic complaints, psychiatric symptoms and psychosocial problems.* Final report on the Nijmegen Regional Project, part I).
Institute of Social Medicine, Nijmegen Catholic University, Nijmegen, 1987.
Gaag, M. van der
Cognitieve functiestoornissen bij schizophrenie: consequenties voor revalidatie en therapie (Cognitive functional disorders in schizophrenia: implications for rehabilitation and therapy).
In: Bosch *et al.* (eds.), *op. cit.*, 1988.
Gardner, H.
Developmental psychology.
Little, Brown & Company, Boston, 1982.

Gardner, A.
The assessment of dementia.
In: R.N. Gaind *et al.*, *Current themes in psychiatry*, vol. 3.
Spectrum Publishers, 1984.
Garralda, M.E., D. Bailey
Psychological deviance in children attending general practice.
Psychological Medicine, 16 (1986), 2, 423-429.
Gemeenschappelijke Medische Dienst (GMD) (Joint Medical Service of the Industrial Insurance Boards)
Jaarverslagen (Annual Reports).
Amsterdam, various years.
Gezondheidsraad (Health Council)
Advies inzake intensive care neonatologie (Intensive care neonatology: report and recommendations).
Staatsuigeverij, The Hague, 1982.
Gezondheidsraad (Health Council)
Advies Geestelijke Gezondheidszorg (Mental Health Care: report and recommendations).
The Hague, 1986.
Gezondheidsraad (Health Council)
Psychogeriatrische ziektebeelden (Psychogeriatric syndromes).
The Hague, 1988.
GHIGV (Chief Medical Inspectorate of Health)
Bureaus Vertrouwensartsen inzake kindermishandeling (Centres for the Confidential Notification of Child Abuse).
Data from child-abuse records, 1983. Ministry of Welfare, Health and Cultural Affairs, Rijswijk, 1986.
Giel, R., H.C. Sauer, C.J. Slooff, D. Wiersma
Over de epidemiologie van functionele psychosen en invaliditeit (The epidemiology of functional psychoses and invalidity).
Tijdschrift voor Psychiatrie, 22 (1980), 11-12, 710-722.
Giel, R.
Onze moeite met moeilijke mensen (Taking trouble with troublesome people).
Tijdschrift voor Psychiatrie, 26 (1984), 4, 244-261.
Gilhooly, M.L.M.
The impact of caregiving on wellbeing: factors associated with the psychological wellbeing of people supporting a dementing relative in the community.
British Journal of Medical Psychology, 57 (1984), 35-44.
Gilleard, C.J.
Problems posed for supporting relatives of geriatric and psychogeriatric day patients.
Acta Psychiatrica Scandinavica, 70 (1984), 198-208.
Gilleard, C.J.
Living with dementia.
Croom Helm, London, 1984.

Gilleard, C.J. *et al.*
Emotional distress among the supporters of the elderly mentally infirm.
British Journal of Psychiatry, 146 (1984), 172-177.
Glick, I.D., W.A. Hargreaves, J. Drues *et al.*
Short versus long hospitalization: a prospective controlled study. IV. One-year follow-up results for schizophrenicpatients.
American Journal of Psychiatry, 133 (1976), 509-514.
Gmür, M.
Schizophrenieverlauf und Entinstitutionalisierung (The course of schizophrenia and deinstitutionalization).
(Forum der Psychiatrie; Neue Folge 24).
Ferdinand Enke Verlag, Stuttgart, 1986.
Goddijn, J., T. Sandfort
Sociale ondersteuning bij de verwerking van traumatische seksuele ervaring in de jeugdjaren (Social support in coming to terms with traumatic sexual experiences in childhood).
Gedrag & Gezondheid, 16 (1988), 60-67.
Goffman, E.
Stigma.
Prentice Hall, Englewood Cliffs, NJ, 1963.
Goldberg, D., P. Huxley
Mental illness in the community; the pathway to psychiatric care.
Tavistock, London, 1980.
Goldstein, M.J.
Family factors that antedate the onset of schizophrenia and related disorders.
Acta Psychiatrica Scandinavica, 71 (1985), supplement 319, 7-18.
Goldstein, M.J., D. Kreisman
Gender, family environment and schizophrenia.
Psychological Medicine, 18 (1988), 4, 861-972.
Gottesman, I.I., J. Shields
Schizophrenia and genetics: a twin-study vantage point.
Academic Press, New York, 1972.
Gottesman, I.I., P. McGuffin, A.E. Farmer
Clinical genetics as clues to the 'real' genetics of schizophrenia (A decade of modest gains while playing for time).
Schizophrenia Bulletin, 13 (1987), 1, 23-47.
Goudena, P.P., H.J. Groenendaal, F.A. Swets-Gronert
Kind in geding: bedreigende en beschermende factoren in de psychosociale ontwikkeling van kinderen (*Child at stake*: threatening and protecting factors in children's psychosocial development).
Acco, Leuven, 1988.
Gove, W.R.
Sex differences in mental illness among adult men and women: an evaluation of four questions raised regarding the evidence on the higher rates of women.
Social Science and Medicine, 12b (1978), 187-198.

Graaf, W.J. de, P.E.M. Hupkens
Dementie als huisartsgeneeskundige opgave (Dementia as a challenge for general practice).
Huisarts en Wetenschap, 28 (1985), 'Huisarts en Praktijk' supplement, October, 25-29.
Graham, P., M. Rutter
Psychiatric disorder in the young adolescent: a follow-up study.
Proceedings of the Royal Society of Medicine, 66 (1973), 1227-1229.
Graham, P., M. Rutter
Adolescent disorders.
In: Rutter & Hersov, *op. cit.*, 1985.
Grosfeld, J.A.M.
De voorspelbaarheid van individuele verzuimduur (Predicting the duration of individual sickness absence).
Lisse, 1988.
Gudeman, J.E., B. Dicckcy, L. Rood *et al.*
Alternative to the back ward. The Quarterway house.
Hospital and Community Psychiatry, 32 (1981), 5, 330-334.
Gurland, B.
The borderlands of dementia.
Ageing, 15 (1981), 61-80.
Gurland, B., J. Copeland *et al.*
The mind and mood of ageing; mental health problems of the community elderly in New York and London.
Haworth Press, New York, 1983.
Haen, F. de
Substitutie in de GGZ duurder dan verwacht (Substitution in mental health care dearer than expected).
Het Ziekenhuis, 19 (1989), 8, 352-353.
Häfner, H., W. an der Heiden
The Mannheim Case Register: the long-stay population.
In: Ten Horn *et al., op. cit.*, 1986.
Häfner, H., W. an der Heiden
The evaluation of mental health care systems.
British Journal of Psychiatry, 155 (1989), 12-17.
Hagen, B., J. van Weeghel
Subsidieaanvragen Ziekenfondsraad inzake dagbesteding: een eerste analyse (Applications to the Health Insurance Funds Council for grants in connection with day activities: a first analysis).
Internal publication, Netherlands Institute of Mental Health (NcGv), Utrecht, 1989.
Hagendoorn, A. *et al.*
Het ascetische arbeidethos: een exploratie (The ascetic work ethic: an exploration).
Gedrag, 9 (1981), 1, 2-19.

Hagnell, O., J. Lanke, B. Rorsman, L. Ojesjo.
Does the incidence of age psychosis decrease? A prospective longitudinal study of a complete population investigated during the 25-year period 1947-1972: the Lundby Study.
Neuropsychobiology, 1981, 7, 201-211.
Hagnell, O. *et al.*
Current trends in the incidence of senile and multi-infarct dementia; a prospective study of a total population followed over 25 years: the Lundby Study.
Archiv für Psychiatrie und Nervenkrankheiten (1983), 233, 423-438.
Hagnell, O.
Mental disorder in the welfare state - Sweden.
A prospective longitudinal study psychiatric-epidemiological study of a total population over 25 years, 1947-1972. The Lundby Study.
American Journal of Social Psychiatry, VI, 4, autumn 1986, 230-248.
Harding, C.M., G.W. Brooks, T. Ashikaga, J.S. Strauss, A. Breier
The Vermont longitudinal study of persons with severe mental illness I.
American Journal of Psychiatry, 144 (1987), 6, 718-726.
Harding, C.M., G.W. Brooks, T. Ashikaga, J.S. Strauss, A. Breier
The Vermont longitudinal study of persons with severe mental illness II.
American Journal of Psychiatry, 144 (1987a), 6, 727-735.
Harding, C.M., J.S. Strauss, H. Hafez, P.B. Lierberman
Work and mental illness. Toward an integration of the rehabilitation process.
Journal of Nervous and Mental Disorders, 175 (1987b), 317-326.
Harris, M., H.C. Bergman
Case management with the chronically mentally ill: A clinical perspective.
American Journal of Orthopsychiatry, 57 (1987), 296-302.
Heeten, W. den *et al.*
Preventie van ongeschikte arbeid (Prevention of incapacitating work).
RIAM, Hoofddorp, 1987.
Held, M. *et al.*
A comprehensive treatment program for severely impaired geriatric patients.
Hospital and Community Psychiatry, 35 (1984), 156-160.
Henderson, A.S.
Epidemiology of mental illness.
In: H. Hafner *et al.* (eds.), *Mental health in the elderly: a review of the present state of research.*
Springer Verlag, Berlin, 1986.
Henderson, A.S.
The epidemiology of Alzheimer's disease.
British Medical Bulletin, 42 (1986), 1, 3-10.
Herz, M.I., J. Endicott, R.L. Spitzer
Day versus inpatient hospitalization: A controlled study.
American Journal of Psychiatry, 127 (1971), 1371-1382.

Heston, L.L. *et al.*
Dementia of the Alzheimer type.
Archives of General Psychiatry, 38 (1981), 1085-1090.
Heydendael, P.H.J.M., M.H.R. Nuy
De thuisloze: een sociaal kwetsbare figuur (The homeless person: a socially vulnerable figure).
MGv, 38 (1983), 11, 1177-1188.
Hilverink, H.G.
Arbeidsongeschikt of arbeid ongeschikt? (Incapacitated for work or by work?)
In: Bosch, Petersen (eds.), *op. cit.*, 63-75.
Hirsch, S.R.
Reducing exposure and risk to neuroleptics when treating schizophrenics.
In: C.N. Stefanis *et al.* (eds.), *Psychiatry Today, VIII World Congress of Psychiatry, Abstracts.*
Excerpta Medica, International Congress Series 899, Amsterdam, 1989.
Hodiamont, P.P.G.
Het zoeken van zieke zielen (Seeking sick souls).
Thesis, Nijmegen Catholic University, Nijmegen, 1986.
Hoencamp, E. *et al.*
Rapportage en de sociale wetgeving. De niet-strafrechtelijke forensisch psychiatrische en psychologische beoordeling (Assessment reports and social-welfare legislation. Non-criminal forensic psychiatric and psychological assessment).
Gouda Quint (in collaboration with Willem Pompe Institute, Utrecht), Arnhem, 1988.
Hoencamp, E., J.A. Schipper
Psychiatrische expertises voor de Raad van Beroep. Ervaringen met 456 rapportages (Psychiatric reports to the Social Security Appeals Tribunal. Experience of 456 reports).
MGv, 40 (1985), 1, 3-18.
Hoencamp, E., K. Rijnhart
Psychiatrische criteria in relatie tot arbeidsongeschiktheid (Psychiatric criteria in relation to incapacity for work).
In: E. Hoencamp *et al.*, *op. cit.*, 1988.
Hoeven, E. van der
De politiereactie op delinquent gedrag van jeugdigen (Police response to juvenile delinquency).
Justitiële Verkenningen, 12 (1986), 569-588.
Hogarty, G.E., S.C. Goldberg, N.R. Scholler
Drug and sociotherapy in the aftercare of schizophrenic patients II. Two-year relapse rate.
Archives of General Psychiatry, 31 (1974), 603-608.
Hoksbergen, R., J. Spann, B. Waardenburg
Bittere ervaringen; uithuisplaatsing van buitenlandse adoptiekinderen (Bitter experiences; taking foreign adoptive children into care).
Swets & Zeitlinger, Amsterdam/Lisse, 1988.

Holman, B., J. Wennink
De hospitalisatiethesis, een dubieuze thesis (The hospitalization thesis, a dubious thesis).
Tijdschrift voor Psychiatrie, 27 (1985), 2, 83-93.
Holzer, C.E., B.M. Shea
The increased risk for specific psychiatric disorders among persons of low socio-economic status.
American Journal of Social Psychiatry, VI, 4, autumn 1986, 259-271.
Horn, G.H.M.M. ten, J.L. Wouters, A. Brug
De Geestelijke Gezondheidszorg voor kinderen tot en met 12 jaar (Mental health care for children up to the age of 12).
Tijdschrift voor Psychiatrie, 27 (1985), 2, 128-138.
Horn, G.H.M.M. ten, R. Giel, W.H. Gulbinat, J.H. Henderson (eds.)
Psychiatric case registers in public health.
Elsevier, Amsterdam, 1986.
Horn, G.H.M.M. ten
Epidemiologisch onderzoek naar dementie (Epidemiological studies of dementia).
In: Houweling *et al.* (eds.), *op. cit.*, 1987.
Houben, A.H.G.M.
De psychiatrische expertise in de procedure bij de Raad van Beroep (Psychiatric reports in the Social Security Appeals Tribunal procedure).
In: E. Hoencamp *et al., op. cit.*, 1988.
Houben, A.H.G.M.
De psychiatrische rapportering in beroepsprocedures over geschillen betreffende arbeidsongeschiktheid (Psychiatric reports in appeals procedures in disputes concerning occupational incapacity).
Tijdschrift Sociale Gezondheidszorg, 62 (1984), 17, 688-690.
Hoult, J., I. Reynolds
Schizophrenia. A comparative trial of community-oriented psychiatric care.
Acta Psychiatrica Scandinavica, 69 (1984), 359-372.
Hout, M.A. van den
Geestelijke gezondheidskunde (Mental health and hygiene).
Limburg State University, Maastricht, 1988 (Lecture).
Houweling, T.J., M.W. Ribbe, F. van 't Hooft *et al.* (eds.)
Symposium publication *"Oud(-er) worden nu" ("Getting old(er) today").*
Amsterdam Gerontological Institute (GIA), Amsterdam, 1987.
Hullenaar, R.H.J. van 't, D.B.J. van Koningsveld
Afgebrand of afgedankt, een onderzoek naar oorzaken van arbeidsongeschiktheid (Burned out or thrown out, an investigation into the causes of incapacity for work).
Swets & Zeitlinger, Lisse, 1986.
Iedema, P., P. Baart
Geestelijke Gezondheidszorg en arbeidsproblematiek (Mental health care and labour problems).
RIAGG (Regional Institute of Ambulatory Mental Health Care) Oost-Veluwe, Apeldoorn, 1986.

Ineichen, B.
Measuring the rising tide: how many dementia cases will there be by 2001?
British Journal of Psychiatry, 150 (1987), 193-200.
Innovatie Commissie Basisschool (Primary Education Reform Committee)
De zorg voor de leerlingen in het onderwijs. Zesde advies (*Caring for schoolchildren*. Sixth report and recommendations).
Staatsuitgeverij, The Hague, 1978.
IWRV (Interdepartmental working group on residential and semi-residential facilities for young people)
Interim Report II.
Ministry of Justice, The Hague, 1980.
Jacobs, C., E. Ketting
GGZ in getallen 1989 (Mental health care in figures, 1989).
Netherlands Institute of Mental Health (NcGv) series 89-4, NcGv, Utrecht, 1989.
Jacobs, C., E. Ketting
GGZ in getallen 1990 (Mental health care in figures, 1990).
Netherlands Institute of Mental Health (NcGv), Utrecht, 1990 .
Janssen, M.
Psychiatrische research steeds a-socialer (Psychiatric research is increasingly antisocial).
Gek'ooit, 1 (1982), 5, 13.
Jolles, J.
Vroege diagnostiek met behulp van neuropsychologisch onderzoek (Early diagnosis using neuropsychological tests).
In: CBIT *op. cit.*, 1988.
Jorm, A.F., A.E. Korten, A.S. Henderson
The prevalence of dementia: a quantitative integration of the literature.
Acta Psychiatrica Scandinavica, 76 (1987), 465-479.
Junger-Tas, J.
Uithuisplaatsing van kinderen (Taking children into care).
Coordinating committee for child-protection research and Working group on integration of youth protection (WIJN), The Hague, 1983.
Junger-Tas, J.
Taak en functie van de jeugdpolitie (Duties and responsibilities of the juvenile police).
Justitiële verkenningen, 12 (1986), 629-649.
Kabela, M.
Een psychiatrische visie op werkstoornissen (A psychiatric view of work disorders).
MGv, 40 (1985), 1, 19-39.
Kabela, M.
Psychiatrisch oordeel beoordeeld; de psychiatrische beoordeling van arbeidsongeschiktheid (Psychiatric assessment assessed; the psychiatric assessment of occupational incapacity).
Swets & Zeitlinger, Amsterdam/Lisse, 1988.

Kadushin, A., J.A. Martin
Child abuse; An interactional event.
Columbia University Press, New York, 1981.
Kalverboer
Longitudinaal onderzoek bij risikogroepen: problemen en perspectieven (Longitudinal studies of at-risk groups: problems and prospects).
In: P.P. Goudena *et al., op. cit.*, 1988.
Kane, J.M.
Somatic therapy.
In: Frances & Hales (eds.), *op. cit.*, 1986.
Kaplan, H.I., B.J. Sadock (eds.)
Comprehensive textbook of psychiatry.
Williams & Wilkins, Baltimore, 1985.
Katzman, R.
Alzheimer's disease.
New England Journal of Medicine, 314 (1986), 15, 964-973.
Kay, D.W.K. *et al.*
Old-age mental disorders in Newcastle on Tyne; Part I, a study of prevalence; Part II, a study of possible social and medical causes.
British Journal of Psychiatry, 110 (1964), 146-158, 668-682.
Kay, D.W.K. *et al.*
Mental illness and hospital usage in the elderly: a random sample followed up.
Comprehensive Psychiatry, 11 (1970), 26-35.
Kay, D.W.K., K. Bergmann
Epidemiology of mental disorders among the aged in the community.
In: Birren *et al.* (eds.), *op. cit.*, 1980.
Kay, D.W.K.
Genetics, Alzheimer's disease and senile dementia.
British Journal of Psychiatry, 154 (1989), 311-320.
Kendler, K.S.
Genetics of Schizophrenia.
In: Frances & Hales (eds.), *op. cit.*, 1986.
Kessler, R.C., J.A. McRae
Trends in the relationship between sex and psychological distress: 1957-1976.
Americal Sociological Review, 46 (1981), 443-452.
Kienhorst, C.W.M.
Suïcidaal gedrag bij jongeren; onderzoek naar omvang en kenmerken (*Suicidal behaviour in young people*; an investigation into its extent and characteristics).
Ambo, Baarn, 1988.
Kiesler, C.A.
Mental hospitals and alternative care. Noninstitutionalization as potential public policy for mental patients.
American Psychologist, 37 (1982), 8, 802-805.

Kind en Ziekenhuis (Children and Hospital)
Handvest Kind en Ziekenhuis (The "Children and Hospital" Charter).
Landelijke Vereniging Kind en Ziekenhuis (National "Children and Hospital" Association), Amsterdam, 1989.
Klerk, J.M. de, C.J. Ptersen, C.G. Diependaal
Diagnosecategorie V: psychische stoornissen en de WAO: een nadere beschrijving.
Tijdschrift Sociale Gezondheidszorg, 61 (1983), 434-440.
Klerk, J.M. de, C.J. Petersen, C.G. Diependaal
Diagnosecategorie V: Psychische stoornissen; Verslag 2, dossierstudie (Diagnostic category V: Mental disorders; Report 2, dossier study).
GMD Notes 4, Amsterdam, 1986.
Knepper, S.
De psychiatrische arbeids(on)geschiktheidsbeoordeling voor de administratieve rechter (Administrative tribunals and the psychiatric assessment of capacity and incapacity for work).
Tijdschrift Sociale Gezondheidszorg, 62 (1984), 17, 681-684.
Knepper, S.
Sociale verzekeringsgeneeskunde: crisis of ontwikkeling? (Social insurance medicine: crisis or development?).
Medisch Contact, 1, (3 jan. 1986), 17-21
Knepper, S.
Het deskundigenrapport in de verzekeringsgeneeskunde
Nederlands Tijdschrift voor Geneeskunde, 131 (1987), 22, 938-942.
Knorth, E.J.
Opname op maat; een verkennend onderzoek naar de intakeprocedure als begin van residentiële jeugdhulpverlening *(Admission tailor-made*; an exploratory study of the admission procedure as the start of residential youth welfare provision).
Acco, Leuven, 1987.
Knorth, E.J.
Iedere dag veertig. Opname van jeugdigen in tehuizen (Forty a day. Admission of young people to residential homes).
Tijdschrift Jeugdonderzoek, 2 (1989), 1, 13-19.
Knulst, M.
Thuisloos (Homeless).
Leeftijd, 1987, 7/8, 37-38.
Kobasa, S.C., S.R. Maddi, S. Kahn
Hardiness and health: A prospective study.
Journal of Personal and Social Psychology, 42 (1982), 168-177.
Koegel, P., M. Audrey Burnam, K. Rodger, K. Farr
The prevalence of specific psychiatric disorders among homeless individuals in the inner city of Los Angeles.
Archives of General Psychiatry, 45 (1988), 12, 1085-1092.
Koele, P., H. Beerends, S. van Goozen
De statistische analyse van het psychiatrisch oordeel (The statistical analysis of the psychiatric assessment).
De Psycholoog, January 1989, 8-11.

Koenders, R.F.
Overheidsbeleid en geestelijke volksgezondheid 1940-1988 (Public policy and mental health 1940-1988).
Arnhem, 1989 (Doctoral thesis in political studies, Nijmegen Catholic University).
Kompier, M.
Stadsbuschauffeur, een beroep met hoge risico's voor de gezondheid (Driving city buses, a health-threatening job).
KNVTO - Nederlands Transport, no. 2, 1984, 8-14.
Kooistra, M.
Uithuisplaatsing van jonge kinderen, hoe en waarom? Een oriënterend onderzoek naar procedures en beoordelingscriteria met betrekking tot uithuisplaatsing en plaatsing in tehuis of pleeggezin van jonge kinderen op grond van een justitieel maatregel in de regio Rotterdam (*Taking young children into care, how and why?* A fact-finding study of procedures and assessment criteria relating to the taking into care of young children and their placement in children's homes or foster families under child-care orders in the Rotterdam region).
Utrecht State University, Utrecht, 1982.
Korf, D., H. Hoogenhout
Thuis op straat (At home in the street).
Platform GGZ (Mental health care forum), Amsterdam, 1989.
Kubie, L.S.
Multiple fallacies in the concept of schizophrenia.
Journal of Mental Disorders, 152 (1971), 331-.
Kuiper, P.C.
Hoofdsom der psychiatrie (Adding up psychiatry).
Bijleveld, Utrecht, 1976.
Kuné, J.B.
Enige ontwikkelingen rond de AAW/WAO, IV (Developments in the area of disability benefit, IV).
Tijdschrift Sociale Geneeskunde, 60 (1982).
Laing, R., A. Esterson
Gezin en waanzin. Een onderzoek naar de gezinsachtergrond van een aantal schizofrenen (Family and madness. A study of the family background of a number of schizophrenics).
Boom, Meppel, 1974.
Lamb, H.R., J. Zusman
Primary prevention in perspective.
American Journal of Psychiatry, 136 (1979), 12-17.
Lamberts, H.
Incidentie en prevalentie van gezondheidsproblemen in de huisartspraktijk (Incidence and prevalence of health problems in general practice).
Huisarts en Wetenschap, 25 (1982), 401-414.
Langsley, D.G., D.M. Kaplan
The treatment of families in crisis.
Grune & Stratton, New York, 1968.

Leff, J.P., C. Vaughn
Expressed emotion in families. Its significance for mental illness.
The Guildford Press, London, 1985.
Leff, J.P., I.K. Wing
Trial of maintenance therapy in schizophrenia.
British Medical Journal, 3 (1971), 593-604.
Levenson, A.J.
Acute schizophrenia: an efficacious outpatient treatment approach as an alternative to full-time hospitalization.
Disorders of the Nervous System, 38 (1977), 242-245.
Liberman, R.P., K.T. Mueser, C.J. Wallace *et al.*
Training skills in the psychiatrically disabled. Learning coping and competence.
Schizophrenia Bulletin, 12 (1986), 631-647.
Liem, R., J. Liem
Social class and mental illness reconsidered: the role of economic stress and social support.
Journal of Health and Social Behavior, 19 (1978), 139-156.
Lieshout, P. van
Veertig jaar geestelijke volksgezondheid. Een analyse van het Maandblad Geestelijke Volksgezondheid (Forty years of mental health. An analysis of the journal "Maandblad Geestelijke Volksgezondheid").
MGv, 40 (1985), 12, 1243-1274.
Links, P.S.
Community surveys of the prevalence of childhood psychiatric disorders: a review.
Child Development, 54 (1983), 531-548.
Linn, M.W., E.M. Caffey, C.S. Klett
Hospital versus community care for psychiatric patients.
Archives of General Psychiatry, 34 (1977), 78-83.
Linton, R.
The study of man: an introduction.
Appleton-Century, 1936.
LMR (Landelijke Medische Registratie)
National Medical Records
Utrecht, SIG, various years.
Maas, P.J. van der
Arbeidsverzuim en arbeidsongeschiktheid in verband met psychische afwijkingen (Absence and incapacity in connection with mental disorders).
Arts en Sociale Verzekering, 13 (1975), 24-35.
Maas, P.J. van der
Lang zullen we leven. Over volksgezondheid, vergrijzing en vervuiling (Long may we live. Health, aging and pollution).
Erasmus University, Rotterdam, 1989.

Maccoby, E.E., J.A. Martin
Socialization in the context of the parent-child interaction.
In: P.H. Mussen (ed.), *Handbook of child psychology*, volume 4: Socialization, personality and social development.
Wiley & Sons, New York, 1983.
Marshall, J.R.
The genetics of schizophrenia revisited.
Bulletin of the British Psychological Society, 37 (1984), 177-181.
Matsuyama, S.S.
Genetic factors in dementia of the Alzheimer type.
In: Reisberg (ed.), *op. cit.*, 1983.
Matsuyama, S.S., L.F. Jarvik
Genetics and mental functioning in senescence.
In: Birren & Sloane (eds.), *op. cit.*, 134-148.
Mattes, J.A., B. Rosen, D.F. Klein *et al.*
Comparison of the clinical effectiveness of "short" versus "long" stay psychiatric hospitalization, II: results of a three-year post-hospitalization follow-up.
Journal of Nervous and Mental Disorders, 165 (1977), 187-394.
McFarlane, W.R. (ed.)
Family therapy in schizophrenia.
The Guildford Press, New York, 1983.
McGlashen, T.H.
The prediction of outcome in chronic schizophrenia IV. The Chestnut Lodge follow-up study.
Archives of General Psychiatry, 43 (1986), 167-176.
McGlashen, T.H.
Schizophrenia: psychosocial treatments and the role of psychosocial factors in its etiology and pathogenesis.
In: Frances & Hales (eds.), *op. cit.*, 1986.
McGuffin, P., I.I. Gottesman
Genetic influences on normal and abnormal development.
In: Rutter, Hersov, *op. cit.*, 1985.
Mednick, S.A., E. Mura, F. Schulsinger, B. Mednick
Perinatal conditions and infant development in children with schizophrenic mothers.
Social Biology, 18 (1971), 103-113.
Merens-Riedstra, H.S.
Leven zonder werk (Living without work).
Deventer, 1983.
Millcr, E.
Epidemiology.
In: J.M.S. Pearce (ed.), op. cit., *(1984).*
Ministry of Employment and Social Security
Rapportage Arbeidsmarkt 1987 (1987 Labour Market Report).
The Hague, September 1987.

Ministry of Health and Environmental Protection
Nota betreffende de GGZ (Statement on mental-health care).
Leidschendam, 1970.
Ministry of Health and Environmental Protection
Structuurnota Gezondheidszorg (Statement on the Structure of Health Care).
Leidschendam, 1974.
Ministry of Welfare, Health and Cultural Affairs
Nota Geestelijke Gezondheidszorg (Nieuwe Nota) (Statement on Mental-Health Care (New Statement)).
The Hague, 1984.
Ministry of Welfare, Health and Cultural Affairs
Preventie Geestelijke Volksgezondheid, Discussienota behorend bij het ontwerp-Kerndocument Gezondheidszorg (Preventive Mental-Health Care, discussion paper accompanying the draft Statement on the Core of Health Care).
Rijswijk, 1989.
Ministry of Welfare, Health and Cultural Affairs
Doelgericht veranderen; ontwerp-kerndocument gezondheidsbeleid voor de jaren 1990-1995 (Systematic change; draft statement on the core of health policy for the years 1990-1995).
Rijswijk, 1989.
Ministry of Welfare, Health and Cultural Affairs
Financieel Overzicht Zorg 1988 (Financial Overview of Care, 1988).
The Hague, 1988.
Ministry of Welfare, Health and Cultural Affairs
Onzichtbare banden met thuis (Invisible links with home).
The Hague, 1989.
Mirmiran, M., *et al.*
Environmental influences on brain and behaviour in aging and dementia.
In: D.F. Swaab *et al.* (eds.) - Aging of the brain and Alzheimer's disease.
Progress in Brain Research, vol. 70, 443-459.
Elsevier, Amsterdam, 1986.
Mirsky, A.F., C.C. Duncan
Etiology and expression of schizophrenia: neurobiological and psychosocial factors.
Annual Review of Psychology, 37 (1986), 291-319.
Mol, A., P. van Lieshout
Ziek is het woord niet; medicalisering, normalisering en de veranderende taal van huisartsgeneeskunde en geestelijke gezondheidszorg, 1945 - 1985 (*Sick isn't the word*; medicalization, normalization and the changing language of general practice and mental-health care, 1945-1985).
SUN, Nijmegen, 1989.
Mootz, M.
Samenhang in de geestelijke gezondheidszorg voor volwassenen (Coherence in adult mental-health care).
Social and Cultural Planning Office (SCP), Document 28, Rijswijk, 1985.

Mortimer, J.A. *et al.*
Epidemiology of dementing illness.
In: J.A. Mortimer & J.M. Schuman (eds.), *The epidemiology of dementia.*
New York, 1981.
Mosher, L.R., A.Z. Menn, S. Matthews
Soteria: Evaluation of a homebased treatment for schizophrenia.
American Journal of Orthopsychiatry, 45 (1975), 455-469.
Mowbray, C.T., P. Chamberlain, M. Jennings, C. Reed
Consumer-run mental health services: results from five demonstration projects.
Community Mental Health Journal, 24 (1988), 2, 151-156.
Muilwijk, G.
Wij die door zwarte gaten gevlogen zijn. Over psychoses. Pleidooi voor een positieve benadering (*We who have flown through black gates*. Concerning psychoses. A plea for a positive approach).
Utrecht, 1988.
Murphy, H.B.M., A.C. Raman
The chronicity of schizophrenia in indigenous tropical people.
British Journal of Psychiatry, 118 (1971), 489-497.
Myers, J.K., M.M. Weissman *et al.*
Six-month prevalence of psychiatric disorders in three communities.
Archives of General Psychiatry, 41 (1984), 10, 959-967.
NIDI (Netherlands Inter-University Demographic Institute)
Aspecten van het bevolkingsvraagstuk anno 1987 (Population issues in 1987).
Ministry of Education and Science, WPRB, Zoetermeer, 1988.
Nijhuis, F., J. Soeter
Werk en ziekte (Work and illness).
Limburg State University, Maastricht, 1982.
Nijnatten, C. van
Moeder Justitia en haar kinderen; de ontwikkeling van het psycho-juridisch complex in de kinderbescherming. Dissertatie (*Mother Justice and her children; the development of the psycho-judicial complex in child protection.* Dissertation).
Swets & Zeitlinger, Lisse, 1986.
Nijnatten, C.H.C.J van, A.J.M. van Bavel
Het grensgebied tussen kinderbescherming en jeugdpsychiatrie (The border area between child protection and child psychiatry).
MGv, 39 (1984), 1, 15-32.
NRV (National Health Council)
Advies functies GGZ (Deel 1, de inhoud; Deel 2, organisatie) (*Report and recommendations on functions in mental-health care* (Part 1, substance; Part 2, organization).
NRV, Zoetermeer, 1989.
NRV (National Health Council)
Advies dagbesteding en dagopvang in de geestelijke gezondheidszorg (Report and recommendations on day activities and care in mental-health care).
NRV, Zoetermeer, June 1987.

NRV (National Health Council)
Discussienota substitutie in de gezondheidszorg (Discussion paper on the substitution of outpatient for inpatient provision in health care).
NRV, Zoetermeer, January 1989.
Nuy, M.H.R., P.H.J.M. Heydendael
Het labyrint van zwervers (The labyrinth of vagrants).
Metamedica, 66 (1987), 2, 102-117.
NVAGG (Netherlands Association for Ambulatory Mental-Health Care)
Statistisch zakboekje 1987 (Statistical handbook for 1987).
NVAGG, Utrecht. 1988.
Offord, D.R., R.J. Alder, M.H. Boyle
Prevalence and sociodemographic correlates of conduct disorder.
American Journal of Social Psychiatry, 6 (1986), 272-278.
Offord, D.R., M.H. Boyle, P. Szatmari *et al.*
Ontario child health study; II Six-month prevalence of disorder and rates of service utilization.
Archives of General Psychiatry, 44 (1987), 832-836.
Oosterbaan, H., W. Zeldenrust
Gescheiden wegen. Sociale netwerken, protoprofessionalisering, psychische problemen en hulpzoekend gedrag bij gescheiden mensen (Separate ways. Social networks, protoprofessionalization, mental-health problems and help-seeking among the separated and divorced).
Netherlands Institute for Mental Health (NcGv) series 84, NcGv, Utrecht, 1985.
Overman, W., A. Soudemire
Guidelines for legal and financial counseling of Alzheimer's disease patients and their families.
American Journal of Psychiatry, 145 (1988), 1495-1500.
Owen, M.J., S.A. Whatley
Polymorphic DNA markers and mental disease.
Psychological Medicine, 1988, 18, 529-533.
Panhuis, P.J.A. van
Ziekte en/of gebrek in de psychiatrie (Sickness and/or shortcomings in psychiatry).
Tijdschrift Sociale Gezondheidszorg, 65 (1987), 14, 467-471.
Pasamanick, B., F. Scarpitti, S. Dinitz
Schizophrenics in the community: An experimental study in the prevention of hospitalization.
Appleton, New York, 1967.
Pearce, J.M.S. (ed.)
Dementia, a clinical approach.
Blackwell Scientific Publications, Oxford, 1984.
Pearce, J.M.S.
Dementing illness.
In: J.M.S. Pearce, *op. cit.*, 1984.
Perry, E.
Acetylcholine and Alzheimer's Disease.
British Journal of Psychiatry, 152 (1988), 737-740.

Petry, D.
Chroniciteit in Maastricht en Triëst (Chronicity in Maastricht and Trieste).
In: M. van der Kamp *et al.* (eds.), *De patiënt als burger*, een bezoek aan de democratische psychiatrie in Triëst (*The patient as citizen*, an experience of democratic psychiatry in Trieste).
SWP, Utrecht, 1989.

Peute, L.J.M.
Dementie als belasting voor de familie (Dementia as a burden on the family).
Tijdschrift voor Psychiatrie, 30 (1988), 2, 82-93.

Philipsen, H.
Afwezigheid wegens ziekte (Absent through illness).
Groningen, dissertation, 1969.

PIGG
Patient registers in intramural mental-health care, general psychiatric hospitals)
GHIGV (Chief Mental-Health Inspectorate), SIG (Health-Care Information Centre), NZR (National Hospitals Council), various years.

Pijl, Y.J.
Het toelatingsonderzoek in het LOM- en MLK-onderwijs (Special-education admissions tests).
Groningen State University (dissertation), Groningen, 1989.

Ploeg, J.D. van der
Elfhonderd jeugdigen in tehuizen (Eleven hundred youngsters in homes).
Working group on the integration of youth protection (WIJN), Utrecht, 1979.

Ploeg, J.D. van der
Diagnostiek in het (semi)residentieel hulpverleningsveld (Diagnostics in the practice of residential and semiresidential care).
In: J. Rispens *et al.* (eds.), *Diagnostiek in de hulpverlening (Diagnostics in medical and welfare services).*
Swets & Zeitlinger, Lisse, 1984.

Polak, P.R., M.W. Kirby
A model to replace psychiatric hospitals.
Journal of Nervous and Mental Disorders, 162 (1976), 13-22.

Preston, G.A.N.
Dementia in elderly adults: prevalence and institutionalization.
Journal of Gerontology, 41 (1986), 2, 261-167.

Pries, H., E. v.d. Poel, A. ter Laak, D. Kal
Het leven na de inrichting (Life after the institution).
Platform GGZ Amsterdam (Mental-Health Care Forum), Amsterdam, 1985.

Pugliesi, K.
Social support and self-esteem as intervening variables in the relationship between social roles and women's well-being.
Community Mental Health Journal, 25 (1989), 2, 87-100.

Putten, P. van der
Arbeidsongeschiktheidsverklaring bij overheidswerknemers (Determination of incapacity in state employees).
Tijdschrift Sociale Gezondheidszorg, 63 (1985), 7, 281-286.
Raad voor het Jeugdbeleid (Youth Policy Council)
Jeugd met en zonder toekomst (Youth with and without a future).
Studiegroep Toekomstverkenningen (Futures Study Group), Amsterdam, 1986a.
Raad voor het Jeugdbeleid (Youth Policy Council)
Spelregels bij weglopen (Running away, the rules of the game).
Studiegroep Toekomstverkenningen (Futures Study Group), Amsterdam, 1986b.
Raad voor het Jeugdbeleid (Youth Policy Council)
Toekomst gevraagd; commentaar op de notitie jeugdige minderheden (Future wanted; commentary on the statement on minority youngsters).
Ministry of Welfare, Health and Cultural Affairs, The Hague, 1989.
Reardon, G.T., A. Rifkin, A. Schwartz, A. Myerson, S.G. Siris
Changing patterns of neuroleptic dosage over a decade.
American Journal of Psychiatry, 146 (1989), 6, 726-729.
Regier, D.A., J.H. Boyd *et al.*
One-month prevalence of mental disorders in the United States.
Archives of General Psychiatry, 45 (1988), 11, 977-986.
Reisberg, B. (ed.)
Alzheimer's disease.
Free Press, New York, 1983.
Reisel, A.D.
Rehabilitatie van de chronisch psychiatrische patiënt. Behandelplanning en behandelmethodieken (*Rehabilitation of chronic psychiatric patients.* Treatment planning and methods).
Report of study day, 16 May 1986, Rotterdam.
RIAGG Zuid, Rotterdam, 1986.
Reveley, A.
Genetic counselling for schizophrenia.
British Journal of Psychiatry, 147 (1985), 107-112.
RIAGG (Regional Institute of Ambulatory Mental-Health Care), De Hagen, Preventive-Care Section.
Verslag van het onderzoek met betrekking tot RIAGG-cliënten in de ZW/WAO (Report on the study of Regional Institute clients receiving sickness or disability benefit).
Enschede, 1985.
Richman, A., A. Barry
More and more is less and less; the myth of massive psychiatric need.
British Journal of Psychiatry, 146 (1985), 164-168.
Richman, N., J. Stevenson, P.J. Graham
Preschool to school: a behavioural study.
Academic Press, London, 1982.

Richman, N.
Disorders in pre-school children.
In: Rutter & Hersov, *op. cit.*, 1985.
Ridder, D. de, J. Visser
Tussen de lijnen. De relatie tussen eerstelijn en geestelijke gezondheidszorg nader onderzocht (The relationship between the primary care sector and mental-health care).
NcGv/Nivel, Utrecht, 1988.
Riksen-Walraven, J.M.A., P. Geerts
Sociale ondersteuning en veerkracht: een vicieuze spiraal? (Social support and resilience: a vicious spiral?).
In: Goudena *et al., op. cit.*, 1988.
Romme, M.A.J., A.D.M.A.C. Escher
Leren omgaan met het horen van stemmen (Learning to cope with hearing voices).
MGv, 44 (1989), 7/8, 825-831.
Rose, S., R.C. Lewontin, L.J. Kamin
Not in our genes.
Penguin Books, Harmondsworth, 1984.
Roth, M.
Some strategies for tackling the problems of senile dementia and related disorders within the next decade.
Danish Medical Bulletin, 32 (1985), 1, 92-111.
Rubin, E.H., C.F. Zorumski, W.J. Burke
Overlapping symptoms of geriatric depression and Alzheimer-type dementia.
Hospital and Community Psychiatry, 39 (1988), 10, 1074-1079.
Ruijzendaal, H.
Vooroordelen in psychiatrische rapporten (Prejudices in psychiatric reports).
Social Maandblad Arbeid, May 1985, 383-397.
Russel, D.
Psychiatric diagnosis and the oppression of women.
International Journal of Social Psychiatry, vol. 31/4, winter 1985, 298-305.
Rutter, M., P. Graham, W. Yule
A neuropsychiatric study in childhood.
Heinemann, London, 1970.
Rutter, M., J. Tizard, K. Whitmore
Education, health and behaviour.
Longman, London, 1970.
Rutter, M.
Why are London children so disturbed?
Proceedings of the Royal Society of Medicine, 66 (1973).
Rutter, M.
Psychopathology and development: links between childhood and adult life.
In: Rutter & Hersov, *op. cit.*, 1985.
Rutter, M., M. Gould
Classification.
In: Rutter & Hersov, *op. cit.*, 1985.

Rutter, M., L. Hersov (eds.)
Child and adolescent psychiatry; modern approaches.
Blackwell, Oxford, 1985.
Sandfort, T.
Het belang van de ervaring; over seksuele contacten in de vroege jeugdjaren en seksueel gedrag en beleven op latere leeftijd (*The importance of experience*; sexual contacts in childhood and sexual behaviour and perceptions in later life).
Homostudies, Utrecht, 1988.
Sarbin, T.R., J.C. Mancuso
Schizophrenia: medical diagnosis or moral verdict?
Pergamon Press, New York, 1980.
Sartorius, N.
Mental Health Policies and Programs for the Twenty-first Century: A Personal View.
Integrated Psychiatry 1987, 5, 151-158.
Scheff, T.J.
Being mentally ill: a sociological theory.
Aldine, Chicago, 1966.
Schene, A.
Psychiatrische deeltijdbehandeling: een overzicht (*Psychiatric day treatment*: an overview).
Netherlands Institute of Mental Health (NcGv) Series 83, Utrecht, 1985.
Schipper, J.A., E. Hoencamp
Psychiaters en psychiatrise expertise (Psychiatrists en psychiatric reports).
Tijdschrift Sociale Gezondheidszorg, 62 (1984), 17, 684-688.
Schnitzler, J.G.
De psychiater in de niet-strafrechtelijke rechtspleging (Psychiatrists in non-criminal legal procedures).
In: W. Goudsmit *et al.* (eds.), *Psychiatrie en recht*: hoofdstukken uit de forensische psychiatrie (*Psychiatry and law*: chapters from forensic psychiatry).
Van Loghem Slaterus, Deventer, 1977.
Scholte, E.M.
Jeugd, politie en hulpverlening: preventieve hulp aan jongeren met psychosociale problemen (*Young people, the police and welfare*: preventive help for youngsters with psychosocial problems).
Acco, Leuven, 1988.
Schwab, J.J., M.W. Schwab
Sociocultural roots of mental illness, An epidemiological survey.
Plenum, New York, 1978.
Scott, J.P., K.A. Roberto, J.T. Hutton
Families of Alzheimer's victims, family support to the caregivers.
Journal of the American Geriatrics Society, 34 (1986), 348-354.
SCP (Social and Cultural Planning Office) (M. van Delft, M. Niphuis-Nell)
Eenoudergezinnen: ontstaan, leefsituatie en voorzieningengebruik (One-parent families: genesis, situation and use of services).
Sociale en Culturele Studies 9, Samson, Alphen a/d Rijn, 1988.

SCP (Social and Cultural Planning Office) (J. Timmermans)
Samenhang in de zorg voor jeugdigen (Coherence in youth care).
Document 43, SCP, Rijswijk, 1987.
SCP (Social and Cultural Planning Office)*Social and Cultural Report 1988.*
SCP, Rijswijk, 1988.
SCP (Social and Cultural Planning Office) (J.W. Becker *et al.*)
Enige aspecten van arbeid in de toekomst (Aspects of work in the future).
Sociale en Culturele Studies 7, The Hague, 1986.
Shaffer, D.
Brain damage.
In: Rutter & Hersov, *op. cit.*, 1985.
SIVIS
Nursing-home information service.
Utrecht, SIG (Health-Care Information Centre), various years.
Sloane, R.B.
Organic Brain Syndrome.
In: Birren & Sloane (eds.), *op. cit.*, 1980.
Slooff, C.J.A.J.
De klassifikatie en het beloop van schizophrene en reaktieve psychosen (Classification and course of schizophrenic and reactive psychoses).
Dissertation, Krips Repro, Meppel, 1984.
Slooff, C.J.
Het beloop en de afloop van schizophrene psychosen (Course and outcome of schizophrenic psychoses).
In: R.J. van den Bosch *et al.* (eds.), *op. cit.*, 1988.
Slooff, C.J.
Schizophrenie Stichting Nederland (Netherlands Schizophrenia Foundation).
Introduction given during press presentation on 1 November 1989, Schizophrenie Stichting Nederland, Soesterberg, 1989.
Slot, T., H. Steinbuch
Arbeidsongeschikt door een psychische ziekte (Incapacitated by mental illness).
GMD (Joint Medical Service) Notes 14, Amsterdam, 1988.
Sluss, T.K. *et al.*
The use of longitudinal studies in the investigation of risk factors for senile dementia - Alzheimer-type.
In: J.A. Mortimer, L.M. Schuman (eds.), *The epidemiology of dementia.*
Oxford University Press, New York, 1981.
Small, G.W., D.A. Greenberg
Biologic markers, genetics and Alzheimer's disease.
Archives of General Psychiatry, 45 (1988), 945-947.
Smit, R.
Thuislozen zullen er altijd blijven (There will always be homeless people).
Woningraad, 1986, 25/26, 5-9.
Social Insurance Council (SVr)
Samenvatting van het onderzoeksrapport "Determinanten van WAO-toetreding, een eerste totaalbeeld" (Determinants of eligibility to disability benefit, an initial overall picture; summary of the research report).
Zoetermeer, 1982.

Social Insurance Council (SVr), Disability Funds Aof and Aaf
Jaarverslagen 1986, 1987 (Annual Reports, 1986, 1987).
Zoetermeer, 1988, 1989.
Spruijt, P. (ed.)
Leven in een stiefgezin (Living in a stepfamily).
Giordano Bruno, Amersfoort, 1988.
Spruijt, A.P. (ed.)
Stiefgezinnen: gewoon of anders? (Stepfamilies: ordinary or different?).
Giordano Bruno, Amersfoort, 1988.
Stapert, W.H.G.M.
Systeemdenken in de kinderpsychiatrie (System-oriented thinking in child psychiatry).
In: Milders, C.F.A., W. van Tilburg (eds.), *Systeemdenken en psychiatrie; een kritische oriëntatie (System-oriented thinking and psychiatry; a critical examination).*
Van Gorcum, Assen, 1988.
Stein, L.I., M.A. Test
Alternatives to mental hospital treatment.
Archives of General Psychiatry, 37 (1980), 4, 392-397.
Stephens, J.H., C. Astrup, W.T. Carpenter *et al.*
A comparison of nine systems to diagnose schizophrenia.
Psychiatry Research, 6 (1982), 127-143.
Strauss, J.S., W.T. Carpenter
Schizophrenia.
Plenum, New York, 1981.
Strauss, J.S.
What does rehabilitation accomplish? Discussion.
Schizophrenia Bulletin, 12 (1986), 720-723.
Strauss, J.S., J. Rakfeldt, C.M. Harding, P. Lieberman
Psychological and social aspects of negative symptoms.
British Journal of Psychiatry, 155 (1989), Supplement 7, 128-132.
Strömgren, E.
Genetic factors in the origin of schizophrenia.
In: H.M. van Praag (ed.), *On the origin of schizophrenic psychoses.*
De Erven Bohn, Amsterdam, 1975.
STG (Steering Committee on Future Health Scenarios)
Ouder worden in de toekomst; Scenario's over gezondheid en vergrijzing 1984-2000 (Growing old in the future; health and aging scenarios 1984-2000).
STG, Utrecht, 1985.
STG (Steering Committee on Future Health Scenarios), Scenario Committee on Aging
Ontwikkelingen met betrekking tot het zelfstandig wonen van ouderen; ouder worden in de toekomst - tussenbalans 2 (Developments in independent living for old people; Growing old in the future - intermediate balance 2).
STG, Rijswijk, 1988.

Swaab, D.F., E. Fliers
Clinical strategies in the treatment of Alzheimer's disease.
In: D.F. Swaab *et al.* (eds.), *Progress in Brain Research,* vol. 70, 413-427.
Elsevier, Amsterdam, 1986.
Szasz, T.
Schizophrenia. The sacred symbol of psychiatry.
Basic Books, New York, 1976.
Tanja, T.A., A. Hofman
De epidemiologie van seniele dementie (The epidemiology of senile dementia).
Nederlands Tijdschrift Geneeskunde, 129 (1985), 46, 2206-2209.
Tantam, D. (ed.)
Social Psychiatry and rehabilitation.
Current Opinion in Psychiatry, 1 (1988), 2, 189-271.
Timmermans, J.
Jeugdhulpverlening en medische dienstverlening zijn slecht op elkaar gestemd (Youth welfare services and medical services are badly coordinated).
Tijdschrift voor Jeugdhulpverlening, 17 (1989), 77-86.
Torrey, E.F.
Surviving schizophrenia. A family manual.
Harper and Row, New York, 1983.
Torrey, E.F.
Prevalence studies in schizophrenia.
British Journal of Psychiatry, 150 (1987), 598-608.
Torrey, E.F.
Schizophrenia: fixed incidence or fixed thinking?
Psychological Medicine, 19 (1989), 2, 285-287.
Tranchina, P.
Norma e antinorma. Esperienze di psicanalisi e di lotte antistituzionali.
Feltrinelli, Milan, 1979.
Trimbos, C.J.B.J.
De geestelijke gezondheidszorg in Nederland (Mental-health care in the Netherlands).
Utrecht/Antwerp, 1959.
Turner, J.C., W.J. TenHoor
The NIMH community support program: pilot approach to a needed social reform.
Schizophrenia Bulletin, 4 (1978), 3, 319-344.
Tusenius, A.A.
De gevolgen van echtscheiding voor kinderen (The effects of divorce on children).
Tijdschrift voor Psychiatrie, 31 (1989), 1, 15-28.
Tweede Kamer der Staten Generaal (Lower House of Parliament)
Culturele minderheden in het beroepsonderwijs. Verslag van een mondeling overleg (*Cultural minorities in vocational education.* Report of oral consultation).
1988-89 session, 20643 no. 4, The Hague, 1989a.

Tweede Kamer der Staten Generaal (Lower House of Parliament)
Financieel Overzicht Jeugdhulpverlening 1989 (Financial Overview of Youth Welfare Services 1989).
1988-89 session, 20879 nos. 1-2, The Hague, 1988.
Tweede Kamer der Staten Generaal (Lower House of Parliament)
Groeibeheersing in het (voortgezet) speciaal onderwijs (Controlling the growth of special education).
1988-89 session, 20578 no. 26, The Hague, 1989b.
Tweede Kamer der Staten Generaal (Lower House of Parliament)
Jeugdige Minderheden (Minority Youngsters).
1988-89 session, 20941 nos. 1-5, The Hague, 1989c.
Tweede Kamer der Staten Generaal (Lower House of Parliament)
Nota 2000.
1985-86 session, 19500 nos. 1-2, The Hague, 1986.
Veen, H. van der
Een pleidooi voor actieve resocialisatie. Beschermende woonvormen en beleid (A plea for active resocialization. Sheltered living and public policy).
MGv, 38 (1983), 2, 125-134.
Veerman, J.W.
Bedreigende en beschermende factoren in de gezinsomgeving: gegevens uit onderzoek (Threatening and protecting factors in the family environment: research data).
In: Goudena *et al., op. cit.*, 1988.
Veldhuizen, J.R. van, D. Wiersma, L.M. Ram
Opnamevervangende dagbehandeling in ontwikkeling (Day treatment as an alternative to hospitalization).
MGv, 43 (1988), 1, 3-18.
Verbeek, J. *et al.*
Arbeidsongeschiktheid in het Amsterdamse onderwijs (Occupational incapacity among Amsterdam teachers).
Tijdschrift Sociale Gezondheidszorg, 67 (1989), 161-164.
Verhey, F.R.J. *et al.*
De geheugenkliniek: multi-disciplinaire benadering bij stoornissen van het geheugen en andere cognitieve functies (The memory clinic: a multidisciplinary approach to disorders of the member and other cognitive functions).
In: (T.J. Houweling *et al.*, (ed.), *op. cit.*, 1987.
Verhulst, F.C.
Mental health in Dutch children; an epidemiological study.
Krips Repro, Meppel, 1985.
Verhulst, F.C.
De ontwikkeling van het kind (Child development).
Van Gorcum, Assen, 1989.
Verhulst, F.C., M. Althaus
Persistence and change in behavioral/emotional problems reported by parents of children aged 4-14: an epidemiological study.
Acta Psychiatrica Scandinavica, 77 (1988), supplement 339.

Verhulst, F.C., J.H. van der Lee
Merendeel kinderen met gedrags-emotionele problemen krijgen geen hulp; bevolkingsonderzoek onder 4- tot 17-jarigen (Most children with behavioral/emotional problems get no help; a survey of 4-17-year-olds).
Tijdschrift voor Jeugdhulpverlening, 16 (1988), 618-627.
Vikan, A.
Psychiatric epidemiology in a sample of 1510 ten-year-old children; I Prevalence.
Journal of Child Psychology and Psychiatry, 26 (1985), 55-75.
Vink, M.T., P. van der Kam, H.F.A. Diesfeldt
Gedragsproblemen in verzorgingstehuizen (Behavioural problems in old-people's homes).
Tijdschrift Gerontologie en Geriatrie, 20 (1989), 1, (Feb.), 3-11.
Vlaminck, P.
Psychose Preventie Project. Eindverslag (*Psychosis Prevention Project*. Final Report).
Eburon, Delft, May 1989.
VNG/SGBO
Dak- en thuislozen. Aantallen, opvang en gemeentelijk beleid - een inventariserend onderzoek (Homeless people. Numbers, facilities and municipal policy - a survey).
VNG/SGBO (Association of Dutch Municipalities, Research in Social Geography and Administration), January 1990.
Vrooland, V.C. (ed.)
Werk en gezondheid: over ziekteverzuim en humanisering van de arbeid (Work and health: sickness absence and the humanization of work).
Samson, Alphen a/d Rijn, 1982.
WAGG (Federation of Employers in Ambulatory Mental-Health Care)
Personeel in de AGGZ 1987 (Ambulatory mental-health care staff 1987).
WAGG, Utrecht, 1988.
Warner, R.
Recovery from schizophrenia: Psychiatry and political economy.
Routledge and Kegan Paul, London, 1985.
Washburn, S., M. Vannicelli, R. Longabush, B.J. Schoff
A controlled comparison of psychiatric day treatment and inpatient hospitalization.
Journal of Consultative and Clinical Psychology, 44 (1976), 665-675.
Watt, N.F., E.J. Anthony, L. Wynne, J. Rolf (eds.)
Children at risk for schizophrenia. A longitudinal perspective.
Cambridge University Press, New York, 1984.
Weelden, J. van
Uw kind hoort niet op onze school (Your child shouldn't be at this school).
Working group on the integration of youth protection (WIJN)/Child Foundation, Utrecht/Amsterdam, 1981.
Weiner, H.
Schizophrenia: etiology.
In: Kaplan & Sadock (eds.), *op. cit.*, 1985.

Weissman, M.M., J.K. Myers *et al.*
Psychiatric disorders (DSM-III) and cognitive impairment among the elderly in a US urban community.
Acta Psychiatrica Scandinavica, 71 (1985), 366-379.
Werkgroep Etnopsychiatrie (Ethnopsychiatry Working Group)
Etnische groeperingen in het PZ Santpoort: cijfers, meningen, inzichten, beleidskonklusies (Ethnic groups in Santpoort Psychiatric Hospital: figures, opinions, ideas, policy conclusions).
Santpoort Psychiatric Hospital, Santpoort, 1986.
Wiersma, D., R. Giel, A. de Jong, C.J. Slooff
Social class and schizophrenia in a Dutch cohort.
Psychological Medicine, 13 (1983), 141-150.
Wiersma, D., R. Giel, H.W. Hoek, A. de Jong, F. Nienhuis, M. Ruphan, A.J. Tholen.
Chronische patiënten in de geestelijke gezondheidszorg: een epidemiologische verkenning van hun behoefte aan zorg (Chronic mental patients: an epidemiological exploration of their care needs).
Tijdschrift voor Psychiatrie, 30 (1988), 6, 388-400.
Wiersma, D.
Psychosociale stress en langdurige arbeidsongeschiktheid (Psychosocial stress and long-term incapacity).
Groningen State University, Groningen, 1980.
Wijnstra, J.
Verwijzing van leerlingen uit etnische en culturele minderheden naar het speciaal onderwijs (Referral of pupils from ethnic and cultural minorities to special schools).
CITO (Central Institute for the Development of Testing), Arnhem, 1986.
Wilmink, F.W.
Patient, physician, psychiatrist. Assessment of mental health problems in primary care.
Dissertation, Groningen, 1989.
Wing, J.K., G.W. Brown
Institutionalism and schizophrenia. A comparative study of three mental hospitals, 1960-1968.
Cambridge University Press, Cambridge, 1970.
WODC (Research and Documentation Division, Ministry of Justice)
Deviant gedrag en slachtofferschap onder jongens van etnische minderheden (Deviant behaviour and victimization among boys from ethnic minorities).
Ministry of Justice, The Hague, 1989.
Wolkind, S., M. Rutter
Sociocultural factors.
In: Rutter & Hersov, *op. cit.*, 1985.
World Health Organization
Dementia in later life: research and action.
WHO Technical Report 730, Geneva, 1986.

World Health Organization - Europe
Prevention of mental, psychosocial and neurological disorders in the European region (EUR/PSF/88.1).
Copenhagen, 1988.
World Health Organization
Primary prevention of schizophrenia in high-risk groups.
Copenhagen, 1975.
World Health Organization
Report of the International Pilot Study of Schizophrenia, vol. 1.
WHO, Geneva, 1973.
World Health Organization
Schizophrenia: an international follow-up study.
Wiley, Chichester, 1979.
WRR (Scientific Advisory Council on Government Policy)
Allochtonenbeleid (Policy on ethnic minorities).
Reports to the Government, no. 36.
Staatsuitgeverij, The Hague, 1989.
Wynne, L., M.T. Singer, J.J Bartko, M.L. Toohey
Schizophrenics and their families: recent research on parental communication.
In: J.M. Tanner (ed.), *Developments in psychiatric research.*
Hodder & Stoughton, London, 1977.
Zarit, S.H. *et al.*
Subjective burden of husbands and wives as caregivers: a longitudinal study.
Gerontologist, 26 (1986), 260-266.
Zubin, J., J. Magaziner, S.R. Steinhauer
The metamorphosis of schizophrenia: from chronicity to vulnerability.
Psychological Medicine, 13 (1983), 551-571.

Appendix 1

Basic assumptions of the exploratory and target-setting scenarios

All the exploratory scenarios make a number of identical assumptions. In relation to *economic* trends they arebased on the intermediate (low-growth) variant from the Central Planning Office forecasting exercise for 1985-2010. In broad terms this involves:

- average annual growth in real national income of 2.75%, equal to the long-term average since the beginning of the century;
- some fall in unemployment, though with the level remaining high;
- average annual growth of 3% in private consumption and industrial investment;
- a sharp rise in the proportion of women in the workforce.

Available resources (in real terms) for 'formal' mental health care are assumed to rise in line with national income, i.e. at 2.75% annually, implying an increase over twenty years from five to 8.6 billion guilders.

Demographic trends are assumed to follow the intermediate variant in the 1988 population forecasts of the Central Bureau of Statistics. In broad terms this involves:

- a rise in the population of the Netherlands from 14.9 million in 1990 to 16.1 million in 2010;
- a rise in the proportion of over-65s from 12.8% of the population in 1990 to 15.2% in 2010. The number of very elderly persons is assumed to increase more sharply still andthe proportion of young people to continue falling.

With regard to *policy and legislation* in the field of health care in general and mental health care in particular, the trends and developments currently visible are assumed to continue over the next twenty years without any radical change of direction or intensity. In concrete terms this means the following: some stress on *health education and preventive care*, albeit not more than at present; continued *substitution of extramural for intramural care*, with facilities for the former being stimulated as the latter is cut back; increasing *public funding* for care; maintenance of current levels of *quality* of care; the *research* budget keeps pace with the growth in GNP; *relevant policies in other areas* are further coordinated.

The target-setting scenarios serve primarily to indicate the measures needed to achieve goals set for the year 2010. Where the exploratory scenarios focus on the consequences of various autonomous developments in society with no radical changes in public policy, the target-setting scenarios focus on alternatives in the area of necessary and concrete measures and assume a number of (autonomous) environmental factors to remain constant.

The target-setting scenarios assume those trends which can be regarded as largely autonomous (specifically those concerned with demographic and economic trends and developments in medical technology over the next twenty years) to parallel those described in the reference scenarios. Other developments mentioned in the context of the exploratory scenarios can be influenced to a greater or lesser extent.

The objectives formulated are regarded as attainable by the majority of the experts making up the Delphi panels.